Bayesian Adaptive Methods for Clinical Trials

Chapman & Hall/CRC Biostatistics Series

Chapman & Hall/CRC Biostatistics Series

Published Titles

1. *Design and Analysis of Animal Studies in Pharmaceutical Development*, Shein-Chung Chow and Jen-pei Liu
2. *Basic Statistics and Pharmaceutical Statistical Applications*, James E. De Muth
3. *Design and Analysis of Bioavailability and Bioequivalence Studies, Second Edition, Revised and Expanded*, Shein-Chung Chow and Jen-pei Liu
4. *Meta-Analysis in Medicine and Health Policy*, Dalene K. Stangl and Donald A. Berry
5. *Generalized Linear Models: A Bayesian Perspective*, Dipak K. Dey, Sujit K. Ghosh, and Bani K. Mallick
6. *Difference Equations with Public Health Applications*, Lemuel A. Moyé and Asha Seth Kapadia
7. *Medical Biostatistics*, Abhaya Indrayan and Sanjeev B. Sarmukaddam
8. *Statistical Methods for Clinical Trials*, Mark X. Norleans
9. *Causal Analysis in Biomedicine and Epidemiology: Based on Minimal Sufficient Causation*, Mikel Aickin
10. *Statistics in Drug Research: Methodologies and Recent Developments*, Shein-Chung Chow and Jun Shao
11. *Sample Size Calculations in Clinical Research*, Shein-Chung Chow, Jun Shao, and Hansheng Wang
12. *Applied Statistical Design for the Researcher*, Daryl S. Paulson
13. *Advances in Clinical Trial Biostatistics*, Nancy L. Geller
14. *Statistics in the Pharmaceutical Industry, Third Edition*, Ralph Buncher and Jia-Yeong Tsay
15. *DNA Microarrays and Related Genomics Techniques: Design, Analysis, and Interpretation of Experiments*, David B. Allsion, Grier P. Page, T. Mark Beasley, and Jode W. Edwards
16. *Basic Statistics and Pharmaceutical Statistical Applications, Second Edition*, James E. De Muth
17. *Adaptive Design Methods in Clinical Trials*, Shein-Chung Chow and Mark Chang
18. *Handbook of Regression and Modeling: Applications for the Clinical and Pharmaceutical Industries*, Daryl S. Paulson
19. *Statistical Design and Analysis of Stability Studies*, Shein-Chung Chow
20. *Sample Size Calculations in Clinical Research, Second Edition*, Shein-Chung Chow, Jun Shao, and Hansheng Wang
21. *Elementary Bayesian Biostatistics*, Lemuel A. Moyé
22. *Adaptive Design Theory and Implementation Using SAS and R*, Mark Chang
23. *Computational Pharmacokinetics*, Anders Källén
24. *Computational Methods in Biomedical Research*, Ravindra Khattree and Dayanand N. Naik
25. *Medical Biostatistics, Second Edition*, A. Indrayan
26. *DNA Methylation Microarrays: Experimental Design and Statistical Analysis*, Sun-Chong Wang and Arturas Petronis
27. *Design and Analysis of Bioavailability and Bioequivalence Studies, Third Edition*, Shein-Chung Chow and Jen-pei Liu
28. *Translational Medicine: Strategies and Statistical Methods*, Dennis Cosmatos and Shein-Chung Chow
29. *Bayesian Methods for Measures of Agreement*, Lyle D. Broemeling
30. *Data and Safety Monitoring Committees in Clinical Trials*, Jay Herson
31. *Design and Analysis of Clinical Trials with Time-to-Event Endpoints*, Karl E. Peace
32. *Bayesian Missing Data Problems: EM, Data Augmentation and Noniterative Computation*, Ming T. Tan, Guo-Liang Tian, and Kai Wang Ng
33. *Multiple Testing Problems in Pharmaceutical Statistics*, Alex Dmitrienko, Ajit C. Tamhane, and Frank Bretz
34. *Bayesian Modeling in Bioinformatics*, Dipak K. Dey, Samiran Ghosh, and Bani K. Mallick
35. *Clinical Trial Methodology*, Karl E. Peace and Ding-Geng (Din) Chen
36. *Monte Carlo Simulation for the Pharmaceutical Industry: Concepts, Algorithms, and Case Studies*, Mark Chang
37. *Frailty Models in Survival Analysis*, Andreas Wienke
38. *Bayesian Adaptive Methods for Clinical Trials*, Scott M. Berry, Bradley P. Carlin, J. Jack Lee, and Peter Muller

Chapman & Hall/CRC Biostatistics Series

Bayesian Adaptive Methods for Clinical Trials

Scott M. Berry
Berry Consultants
College Station, Texas

Bradley P. Carlin
University of Minnesota
Minneapolis, Minnesota

J. Jack Lee
The University of Texas
MD Anderson Cancer Center
Houston, Texas

Peter Müller
The University of Texas
MD Anderson Cancer Center
Houston, Texas

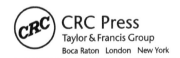

CRC Press
Taylor & Francis Group
Boca Raton   London   New York

CRC Press is an imprint of the
Taylor & Francis Group, an **informa** business

A CHAPMAN & HALL BOOK

CRC Press
Taylor & Francis Group
6000 Broken Sound Parkway NW, Suite 300
Boca Raton, FL 33487-2742

International Standard Book Number: 978-1-4398-2548-8 (Hardback)

Library of Congress Cataloging-in-Publication Data

Bayesian adaptive methods for clinical trials / Scott M. Berry ... [et al.].
    p. ; cm. -- (Chapman & Hall/CRC biostatistics series ; 38)
    Includes bibliographical references and indexes.
    Summary: "As has been well-discussed, the explosion of interest in Bayesian methods over the last 10 to 20 years has been the result of the convergence of modern computing power and elcient Markov chain Monte Carlo (MCMC) algorithms for sampling from and summarizing posterior distributions. Practitioners trained in traditional, frequentist statistical methods appear to have been drawn to Bayesian approaches for three reasons. One is that Bayesian approaches implemented with the majority of their informative content coming from the current data, and not any external prior information, typically have good frequentist properties (e.g., low mean squared error in repeated use). Second, these methods as now readily implemented in WinBUGS and other MCMC-driven software packages now offer the simplest approach to hierarchical (random effects) modeling, as routinely needed in longitudinal, frailty, spatial, time series, and a wide variety of other settings featuring interdependent data. Third, practitioners are attracted by the greater flexibility and adaptivity of the Bayesian approach, which permits stopping for elcacy, toxicity, and futility, as well as facilitates a straightforward solution to a great many other specialized problems such as dosing, adaptive randomization, equivalence testing, and others we shall describe. This book presents the Bayesian adaptive approach to the design and analysis of clinical trials"--Provided by publisher.
    ISBN 978-1-4398-2548-8 (hardcover : alk. paper)
    1. Clinical trials--Statistical methods. 2. Bayesian statistical decision theory. I. Berry, Scott M. II. Series: Chapman & Hall/CRC biostatistics series ; 38.
    [DNLM: 1. Clinical Trials as Topic. 2. Bayes Theorem. QV 771 B357 2011]

R853.C55B385 2011
615.5072'4--dc22

2010022618

To

OUR FAMILIES

Contents

Foreword

It's traditional to get a foreword written by an *éminence grise*, generally an aging researcher who has seen better days. I can provide plenty of *grise* although I am possibly a bit short on *éminence*. Perhaps I best qualify through sheer long-service in trying to promote Bayesian clinical trials, having started my small contribution to this epic effort nearly 30 years ago with Laurence Freedman, eliciting prior opinions from oncologists about the plausible benefits of new cancer therapies.

This fine book represents the most recent and exciting developments in this area, and gives ample justification for the power and elegance of Bayesian trial design and analysis. But it is still a struggle to get these ideas accepted. Why is this? I can think of four main reasons: ideological, bureaucratic, practical and pragmatic.

By *ideological*, I mean the challenge facing the "new" idea of using probability theory to express our uncertainty about a parameter or existing state of the world – our epistemic uncertainty. Of course "new" is ironic, given it is nearly 250 years since Bayes formalized the idea, but the idea is still unfamiliar and disturbing to those brought up on classical ideas of probability as long-run frequency. One can only sympathize with all that effort to master the correct definition of a p-value and a confidence interval, only to be told that the intuitive meanings can be right after all.

I really enjoy introducing students to this beautiful idea, but tend to leave Bayes' theorem to subsequent lectures. In fact I sometimes feel the role of Bayes' theorem in Bayesian analysis is overemphasized: the crucial element is being willing to put a distribution over a parameter, and it is not always necessary even to mention the "B-word." Natural examples include models for informative dropout in clinical trials, and the size of possible biases in historical studies: in these situations there may be no information in the data about the parameter, and so Bayes' theorem is not used.

But of course there are *bureaucratic* obstacles: as the authors of this book make clear, regulatory agencies perform a gate-keeping role where the Neyman-Pearson framework of decision-making without a loss function still has merits. Although the posterior distribution tells us what it is reasonable to believe given the evidence in a specific study, the regulators do need to consider a continuous sequence of drug approval decisions. So quantifying Type I and Type II error can still be a valuable element of trial design, and one that is excellently covered in this book.

Then there are *practical* problems: can we actually do the analysis, or is the mathematics too tricky and there's no software to help us along? The authors have done a great job in discussing computation and providing software, but I am sure would still admit that there's some way to go before all these wonderful techniques are easily available to the average trial designer. But it will happen.

Finally, the crucial *pragmatic* test. Do these techniques help us do things we could not do before? This has been the factor that has led to increasingly widespread penetration of Bayesian methods into subject domains over the last 20 years or so: people can fit models and make inferences that were previously impossible or very cumbersome. And this is where this book wins hands down, since adaptive trials are so natural, ethical and efficient, that everyone wants to do them.

This book, based on the many years of cumulative experience of the authors, manages to deal with all these difficulties. Adaptive studies are a perfect application for a Bayesian approach, and I am confident that this book will be a major contribution to the science and practice of clinical trials.

DAVID J. SPIEGELHALTER
MRC Biostatistics Unit and University of Cambridge
April 2010

Preface

As has been well discussed, the explosion of interest in Bayesian methods over the last 10 to 20 years has been the result of the convergence of modern computing power and efficient Markov chain Monte Carlo (MCMC) algorithms for sampling from and summarizing posterior distributions. Practitioners trained in traditional, frequentist statistical methods appear to have been drawn to Bayesian approaches for three reasons. One is that Bayesian approaches implemented with the majority of their informative content coming from the current data, and not any external prior information, typically have good frequentist properties (e.g., low mean squared error in repeated use). Second, these methods as now readily implemented in WinBUGS and other MCMC-driven software packages now offer the simplest approach to hierarchical (random effects) modeling, as routinely needed in longitudinal, frailty, spatial, time series, and a wide variety of other settings featuring interdependent data. Third, practitioners are attracted by the greater flexibility and adaptivity of the Bayesian approach, which permits stopping for efficacy, toxicity, and futility, as well as facilitates a straightforward solution to a great many other specialized problems such as dose-finding, adaptive randomization, equivalence testing, and others we shall describe.

This book presents the Bayesian adaptive approach to the design and analysis of clinical trials. The ethics and efficiency of such trials can benefit from Bayesian thinking; indeed the Food and Drug Administration (FDA) Center for Devices and Radiological Health (CDRH) has been encouraging this through its document *Guidance for the Use of Bayesian Statistics*; see www.fda.gov/MedicalDevices/DeviceRegulationandGuidance/GuidanceDocuments/ucm071072.htm. The FDA Center for Drug Evaluation and Research (CDER) and Center for Biologics Evaluation and Research (CBER) has issued its own *Guidance for Industry: Adaptive Design Clinical Trials for Drugs and Biologics*: www.fda.gov/downloads/Drugs/GuidanceComplianceRegulatoryInformation/Guidances/UCM201790.pdf. This document also mentions Bayes, albeit far less prominently. The recent series of winter Bayesian biostatistics conferences at the University

of Texas M.D. Anderson Cancer Center in Houston are also testament to
the growing role Bayesian thinking plays in this field.

The outline of the book is as follows. In Chapter 1 we summarize the
current state of clinical trial design and analysis, present the main ideas behind the Bayesian alternative, and describe the potential benefits of such an
alternative. We also describe what we mean by the word "adaptive" in the
book's title. Chapter 2 then gives an overview of the basic Bayesian methodological and computational tools one needs to get started as a Bayesian
clinical trialist. While this whirlwind tour is not a substitute for a full
course in Bayesian methods (as from Gelman et al., 2004, or Carlin and
Louis, 2009), it should enable those with a basic understanding of classical
statistics to get "up and running" on the material. This chapter also includes overviews of hierarchical modeling (with special emphasis on its role
in Bayesian metaanalysis) and the basics of Bayesian clinical trial design
and analysis. The idea here is to establish the basic principles that will be
expanded and made phase- and endpoint-specific in subsequent chapters.

The next two chapters of the book (Chapters 3–4) follow standard clinical
trials practice by giving Bayesian tools useful in "early" and "middle" phase
clinical trials, roughly corresponding to phases I and II of the U.S. drug
regulatory process, respectively. While our own professional affiliations have
led us to focus primarily on oncology trials, the techniques we describe are
readily adapted to other disease areas. We also place primary emphasis on
"partially Bayesian" designs that concentrate on probability calculations
utilizing prior information and Bayesian updating while still maintaining
good frequentist properties (power and Type I error). An exception to this
general rule is Section 4.6, where we discuss "fully Bayesian" designs that
incorporate a utility function (and often more informative priors) within
a more formal decision-theoretic framework. Chapter 4 also contains brief
reviews of two recent trials utilizing Bayesian adaptive designs, BATTLE
and I-SPY 2.

Chapter 5 deals with late (phase III) studies, an important area and
the one of potentially greatest interest to statisticians seeking final regulatory approval for their compounds. Here we emphasize modern adaptive
methods, seamless phase II–III trials for maximizing information usage and
minimizing trial duration, and describe in detail a case study of a recently
approved medical device. Finally, Chapter 6 deals with several important
special topics that fit into various phases of the process, including the use of
historical data, equivalence studies, multiplicity and multiple comparisons,
and the related problem of subgroup analysis. The historical data material
is particularly relevant for trials of medical devices, where large historical
databases often exist, and where the product being evaluated (say, a cardiac pacemaker) is evolving slowly enough over time that worries about the
exchangeability of the historical and current data are relatively low.

Since this is not a "textbook" per se, we do not include homework problems at the end of every chapter. Rather, we view this book as a handbook enabling those engaged in clinical trials research to update and expand their toolkit of available techniques, so that Bayesian methods may be used when appropriate. See `http://www.biostat.umn.edu/~brad/data3.html` and `http://biostatistics.mdanderson.org/SoftwareDownload/` on the web for many of our datasets, software programs, and other supporting information. The final sections of Chapters 2–6 link to these software sites and provide programming notes on the `R` and `WinBUGS` code we recommend.

We owe a debt of gratitude to those who helped in our writing process. In particular, the second author is very grateful to Prof. Donald Berry and the Division of Quantitative Sciences at the University of Texas M.D. Anderson Cancer Center for allowing him to spend his fall 2008 sabbatic time in the same U.S. state as the other three authors. Key staff members worthy of special mention are Martha Belmares and the incomparable Lydia Davis. Sections 1.1, 1.2, 1.4, and 2.4 are based on Prof. Berry's previous work in their respective areas. Indeed, many sections of the book owe much to the hard work of our research colleagues, including Lee Ann Chastain, Nan Chen, Jason Connor, Laura Hatfield, Brian Hobbs, Haijun Ma, Ashish Sanil, and Amy Xia. We also thank the 2010 spring semester "Topics in Clinical Trials" class at Rice University and the University of Texas Graduate School of Biomedical Sciences," taught by the third author, for commenting on the text and testing the supporting software. Rob Calver and David Grubbs at Chapman and Hall/CRC/Taylor & Francis Group were pillars of strength and patience, as usual. Finally, we thank our families, whose ongoing love and support made all of this possible.

SCOTT M. BERRY	College Station, Texas
BRADLEY P. CARLIN	Minneapolis, Minnesota
J. JACK LEE	Houston, Texas
PETER MÜLLER	Houston, Texas

March 2010

CHAPTER 1

Statistical approaches for clinical trials

1.1 Introduction

Clinical trials are prospective studies to evaluate the effect of interventions in humans under prespecified conditions. They have become a standard and an integral part of modern medicine. A properly planned and executed clinical trial is the most definitive tool for evaluating the effect and applicability of new treatment modalities (Pocock, 1983; Piantadosi, 2005; Cook and Demets, 2008).

The standard statistical approach to designing and analyzing clinical trials and other medical experiments is *frequentist*. A primary purpose of this book is to describe an alternative approach called the *Bayesian* approach. The eponym originates from a mathematical theorem derived by Thomas Bayes (1763), an English clergyman who lived from 1702 to 1761. Bayes' theorem plays a fundamental role in the inferential and calculational aspects of the Bayesian approach. The Bayesian approach can be applied separately from frequentist methodology, as a supplement to it, or as a tool for designing efficient clinical trials that have good frequentist properties. The two approaches have rather different philosophies, although both deal with empirical evidence and both use probability. Because of the similarities, the distinction between them is often poorly understood by nonstatisticians.

A major difference is flexibility, in both design and analysis. In the Bayesian approach, experiments can be altered in midcourse, disparate sources of information can be combined, and expert opinion can play a role in inferences. This is not to say that "anything goes." For example, even though nonrandomized trials can be used in a Bayesian analysis, biases that can creep into some such trials can, in effect, make legitimate conclusions impossible. Another major difference is that the Bayesian approach can be decision-oriented, with experimental designs tailored to maximize objective functions, such as company profits or overall public health benefit.

Much of the material in this book is accessible to nonstatisticians. However, to ensure that statisticians can follow the arguments and reproduce the results, we also include technical details. Not all of this technical development will be accessible to all readers. Readers who are not interested in technicalities may skim or skip the mathematics and still profitably focus on the ideas.

Certain subjects presented in this book are treated in a rather cursory fashion. References written from the same perspective as the current report but that are somewhat more comprehensive in certain regards include (Berry, 1991; 1993). The text by Berry (1996) and its companion computing supplement by Albert (1996) explain and illustrate Bayesian statistics in very elementary terms and may be helpful to readers who are not statisticians. Other readers may find more advanced Bayesian texts accessible. These texts include Box and Tiao (1973), Berger (1985), DeGroot (1970), Bernardo and Smith (1994), Lee (1997), Robert (2001), Gelman, Carlin, Stern, and Rubin (2004), and Carlin and Louis (2009). Berry and Stangl (1996) is a collection of case studies in Bayesian biostatistics; it gives applications of modern Bayesian methodology. Finally, the lovely text by Spiegelhalter et al. (2004) is an outstanding introduction to Bayesian thinking in many problems important to biostatisticians and medical professionals generally, one of which is clinical trials.

Turning to the area of computing, Gilks, Richardson, and Spiegelhalter (1996) is a collection of papers dealing with modern Bayesian computer simulation methodology that remains relevant since it was so many years ahead of its time at publication. Two other recent Bayesian computing books by Albert (2007) and Marin and Robert (2007) are also important. Both books adopt the R language as their sole computing platform; indeed, both include R tutorials in their first chapters. Albert (2007) aims at North American first-year graduate or perhaps advanced undergraduate students, building carefully from first principles and including an R package, LearnBayes, for implementing many standard methods. By contrast, the level of formality and mathematical rigor in Marin and Robert (2007) is at least that of its fairly mature stated audience of second-year master's students. In the present book, we also use R as our "base" computing platform, consistent with its high and accelerating popularity among statisticians. However, we also take advantage of other, mostly freely available packages when they offer the most sensible solutions. In particular, we rely on WinBUGS, both by itself and as called from R by the BRugs library. This popular software has emerged as the closest thing to an "industry standard" that exists in the applied Bayesian statistical community.

We now offer a simple example to help show some of the primary features of the frequentist perspective. We will return to this setting in Example 2.2 to show the corresponding Bayesian solution and its features.

Example 1.1 Suppose an experiment is conducted in which a device is used to treat $n = 100$ patients, and a particular outcome measurement is made on each. The design value for the device is a measurement of 0, but as is usual, there is variability from the design value even under ideal

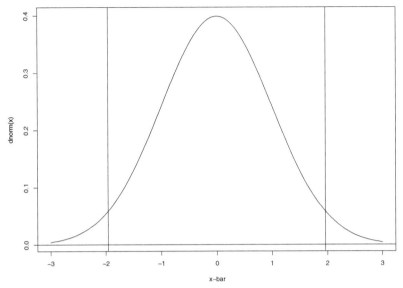

Figure 1.1 *Frequentist sampling distribution of the test statistic, $\bar{x}$, when $\mu = 0$. Each of the tails (left of –1.96 and right of 1.96) has area under the curve equal to 0.025, so that the two-sided p-value is 0.05.*

conditions. The goal of the experiment is to assess whether the mean μ of the measurements in some population of devices is in fact 0: The null hypothesis is that $\mu = \mu_0 = 0$. Suppose that the average $\bar{x}$ of the 100 measurements is 1.96 and the standard deviation σ is 10. In a frequentist analysis, one calculates a z-score,

$$z = \frac{\bar{x} - \mu_0}{\sigma/\sqrt{n}} = \frac{\bar{x} - 0}{10/\sqrt{100}} = \bar{x} = 1.96 \ .$$

Since 1.96 is the 97.5 percentile of the standard normal distribution, the null hypothesis is rejected at the (two-sided) 5% level of significance. Put another way, the results are statistically significant with a p-value of 0.05.

This p-value statement is poorly understood by most nonstatisticians. Its interpretation is as follows. If the population mean μ is indeed 0, observing a value of $\bar{x}$ as extreme as that observed or more so (that is, either larger than or equal to 1.96, or smaller than or equal to –1.96) has probability 0.05 when the null hypothesis is true. The p-value of 0.05 is the sum of the areas of the two tail regions indicated in Figure 1.1. The density shown in this figure is for $\bar{x}$, conditioning on the null hypothesis being true. Because p-values are tail areas, they include probabilities of observations that are possible, but that were not actually observed. ■

1.2 Comparisons between Bayesian and frequentist approaches

This section addresses some of the differences between the Bayesian and frequentist approaches. Later sections will discuss other differences and give details of the comparisons made here. Listing differences gives a one-sided view; there are many similarities between the two approaches. For example, both recognize the need for controls when evaluating an experimental therapy. Still, with this caveat, here are some of the key differences between the two approaches:

1. *Probabilities of parameters:* All unknowns have probability distributions in the Bayesian approach. In the frequentist approach, probabilities are defined only on the data space. In particular, Bayesians associate probabilities distributions with parameters while frequentists do not. These distributions are called the *prior* and *posterior* distributions. The former summarizes information on the parameters *before* the data are collected, while the latter conditions on the data once observed.

2. *Using all available evidence:* The fundamental inferential quantity in the Bayesian approach is the posterior distribution of the various unknown parameters. This distribution depends on all information currently available about these parameters. In contrast, frequentist measures are specific to a particular experiment. This difference makes the Bayesian approach more appealing in a sense, but assembling, assessing, and quantifying information from outside the trial makes for more work. One approach to combining data is *hierarchical modeling*. This is especially easy to implement from a Bayesian point of view, and leads to borrowing of estimative strength across similar but independent experiments. The use of hierarchical models for combining information across studies is a Bayesian approach to *metaanalysis*; see Example 2.7.

3. *Conditioning on results actually observed:* Bayesian inferences depend on the current study only through the data actually observed, while frequentist measures involve probabilities of data (calculated by conditioning on particular values of unknown parameters) that were possible given the design of the trial, but were not actually observed. For example, in Example 1.1, the value of $\bar{x}$ that was observed was precisely 1.96, yet the p-value included the probability of $\bar{x} > 1.96$ and also of $\bar{x} \leq -1.96$ (assuming the null hypothesis). On the other hand, in the Bayesian approach all probabilities condition only on $\bar{x} = 1.96$, the actual observed data value. See discussions of the *Likelihood Principle* in Berger and Wolpert (1984), Berger and Berry (1988), Carlin and Louis (2009, pp. 8, 51), as well as Subsection 2.2.3.

4. *Flexibility:* Bayesian inferences are flexible in that they can be updated continually as data accumulate. For example, the reason for stopping a trial affects frequentist measures but not Bayesian inferences. (See dis-

cussions of the likelihood principle referred to in item 3 above.) Frequentist measures require a complete experiment, one carried out according to the prespecified design. Some frequentists are not hampered by such restrictions, and reasonably so, but the resulting conclusions do not have clear inferential interpretations. In a Bayesian approach, a sample size need not be chosen in advance; before a trial, the only decision required is whether or not to start it. This decision depends on the associated costs and benefits, recognizing when information will become available should the trial start. Once a trial or development program has begun, decisions can be made (at any time) as to whether to continue. Certain types of deviations from the original plan are possible: the sample size projection can be changed, the drugs or devices involved can be modified, the definition of the patient population can change, etc. Such changes can weaken some conclusions (unless they are prespecified, which we advocate), but Bayesian analyses may still be possible in situations where frequentist analyses are not.

5. *Role of randomization:* Randomized controlled trials are the gold standard of medical research. This is true irrespective of statistical approach. Randomization minimizes the possibility of selection bias, and it tends to balance the treatment groups over covariates, both known and unknown. There are differences, however, in the Bayesian and frequentist views of randomization. In the latter, randomization serves as the basis for inference, whereas the basis for inference in the Bayesian approach is subjective probability, which does not require randomization.

6. *Predictive probabilities:* A Bayesian approach allows for calculating predictive probabilities, such as the probability that Ms. Smith will respond to a new therapy. Probabilities of future observations are possible in a formal frequentist approach only by conditioning on particular values of the parameters. Bayesians average these conditional probabilities over unknown parameters, using the fact that an unconditional probability is the expected value of conditional probabilities.

7. *Decision making:* The Bayesian approach is ideal for and indeed is tailored to decision making. Designing a clinical trial is a decision problem. Drawing a conclusion from a trial, such as recommending a therapy for Ms. Smith, is a decision problem. Allocating resources among R&D projects is a decision problem. When to stop device development is a decision problem. There are costs and benefits involved in every such problem. In the Bayesian approach these costs and benefits can be assessed for each possible sequence of future observations. Consider a particular decision. It will give rise to one among a set of possible future observations, each having costs and benefits. These can be weighed by their corresponding predictive probabilities. The inability of the frequen-

tist approach to find predictive probabilities makes it poorly suited to decision making; see Section 4.6.

All of this is *not* to say that the frequentist approach to clinical trials is totally without merit. Frequentism fits naturally with the regulatory "gate-keeping" role, through its insistence on procedures that perform well *in the long run* regardless of the true state of nature. And indeed frequentist operating characteristics (Type I and II error, power) are still very important to the FDA and other regulators; see Subsections 1.4.2 and 2.5.4.

1.3 Adaptivity in clinical trials

The bulk of this chapter (and indeed the entire book) is devoted to describing the intricacies of the Bayesian approach, and its distinction from corresponding frequentist approaches. However, we pause briefly here to describe what we mean by the word "adaptive" in the book's title. Certainly there are a large number of recent clinical trial innovations that go under this name, both frequentist and Bayesian. But perhaps it won't come as a surprise at this point that the two camps view the term rather differently. Concerned as they must be with overall Type I error, frequentists have sometimes referred to any procedure that changes its stopping boundaries over time while still protecting overall Type I error rate as "adaptive." More recently, both frequentists and Bayesians mean a procedure that alters something *based on the results of the trial so far*. But of course this is a serious shift in the experimental design, and thus one that must be reflected in the Type I error calculation. By contrast, freedom from design-based inference means Bayesians are free to enter a trial with nothing more than a stopping rule and a (possibly minimally informative) prior distribution. In particular, note we need not select the trial's sample size in advance (although a maximum sample size is often given). Any procedure we develop can be simulated and checked for frequentist soundness, but this is not required for the Bayesian procedure to be sensibly implemented.

But all this raises the questions of what sorts of adaptation do we envision in our trials, and in what sorts of settings (e.g., early versus late phase). Of course, these two questions are related, since the task at hand depends on the phase. But certainly it is true that as of the current writing, a great many non-fixed-sample-size trials are running across a variety of phases of the regulatory process. In early phase studies it seems ethically most important to be adaptive, since the patients are often quite ill, making sudden treatment changes both more needed and possibly more frequent. Phase I drug studies are typically about safety and dose-finding, meaning in the latter case that the dose a patient receives is not fixed in advance, but rather determined by the outcomes seen in the patients treated to date. The traditional approach for doing this, the so-called "3 + 3" design (see Subsection 3.1.1) is constructed from sensible rules, but turns out to be a bit simpleminded with respect to its learning; model-based procedures (described in Subsection 3.2) use the information in the data to better advantage. We might also be interested in trading off efficacy and toxicity where both are explicitly observed; here the *EffTox* approach and software of Thall and Cook (2004) offers an excellent example of an adaptive dose-finding trial (see Subsection 3.3). The problems created by *combination therapies*, where we seek to estimate the joint effect of two concurrently given treatments (which may well interact in the body) is another setting in which adaptivity is paramount; see Subsection 3.4.

In phase II, we typically seek to establish efficacy while still possibly guarding against excess toxicity, and also against *futility*, i.e., continuing a trial that is unlikely to *ever* produce a significant result even if all available patients are enrolled. In such settings, we again wish to be adaptive, stopping the trial early if any of the three conclusions (efficacy, toxicity, or futility) can be reached early; see Section 4.3. We may also wish to drop unproductive or unpromising study arms, again a significant alteration of the design space but one that in principle creates no difficulties within the Bayesian model-based paradigm.

Another form of adaptivity often encountered in phase II is that of *adaptive randomization*. For example, our trial's goal may be to maintain the advantages of randomizing patients to treatment assignment while allowing the assignment of more patients to the treatments that do better in the trial. Note that this sort of adaptive dose allocation is distinct from *deterministic* adaptive treatment assignment, such as so-called "play-the-winner" rules (see e.g. Ware, 1989). In Section 4.4 we focus on *outcome-adaptive* (or *response-adaptive*) designs, as opposed to covariate-adaptive designs that seek to balance covariates across treatments. In particular, Subsection 4.4.4 offers a challenging example where we wish to adapt in this way while also facing the issue of delayed response (where some patients' observations are either totally or partially unknown at the time of analysis).

In phase III and beyond, the need for adaptivity may be reduced but ethical treatment of the patients and efficient use of their data requires as much flexibility as possible. For an adaptive trial featuring all of the aforementioned complications including delayed response, see Subsection 5.2.3. Indeed, a particular trial might start with multiple doses of a particular drug, and with the intention that it consist of two consecutive phases: the first to determine the appropriate dose, and the second to compare its efficacy to a reference standard. Such *seamless* phase II-III trials are adaptive in a variety of ways. For one thing, a decision may be made to abandon the drug at any time, possibly eliminating phase III entirely. This type of confirmatory trial is sometimes referred to as a "learn and confirm trial"; see Section 5.7.

Finally, in some settings the need for adaptivity outstrips even the above designs' abilities to adapt the dose, randomization fraction, total sample size, number of arms, and so on. Here we are imagining settings where a specific *decision* must be made upon the trial's conclusion. Of course, every clinical trial is run so that a decision (say, the choice of best treatment) may be made, and so in this sense the field of *statistical decision theory* would appear to have much to offer. But to do this, we must agree on the unit of analysis (say, research dollars, or patient quality-adjusted life years (QALYs)), as well as the cost-benefit function we wish to consider. For instance, we may wish to choose the treatment that maximizes the QALYs saved subject to some fixed cost per patient, where this can be agreed upon via a combination of economic and moral grounds. An immediate complication here is the question of *whose* lives we are valuing: just those enrolled in the trial, or those of every potential recipient of the study treatment. Still, in settings where these ground rules can be established, Bayesian decision theoretic approaches seem very natural. Inference for sequentially arriving data can be complex, since at every stage a decision must be made whether to enroll more patients (thus incurring their financial and ethical costs), or to stop the trial and make a decision. Sadly, the *backward induction* method needed to solve such a problem in full generality is complex, but feasible given appropriate computing methods and equipment (see e.g. Carlin et al., 1998; Brockwell and Kadane, 2003). In some settings, relatively straightforward algorithms and code are possible; the case of constructing screening designs for drug development (see Subsection 4.6.2) offers an example.

Throughout the book we will attempt to be clear on just what aspect(s) of the trial are being adapted, and how they differ from each other. This task is larger than it might have initially seemed, since virtually *every* trial we advocate is adaptive in some way.

1.4 Features and use of the Bayesian adaptive approach

Researchers at the University of Texas M.D. Anderson Cancer Center are increasingly applying Bayesian statistical methods in laboratory experiments and clinical trials. More than 200 trials at M.D. Anderson have been designed from the Bayesian perspective (Biswas et al., 2009). In addition, the pharmaceutical and medical device industries are increasingly using the Bayesian approach. Many applications in all these settings use adaptive methods, which will be a primary focus of this text. The remainder of this section outlines several features that make the Bayesian approach attractive for clinical trial design and analysis.

1.4.1 The fully Bayesian approach

There are two overarching strategies for implementing Bayesian statistics in drug and medical device development: a fully Bayesian approach, and a hybrid approach that uses Bayes' rule as a tool to expand the frequentist envelope. Choosing the appropriate approach depends on the context in which it will be used. Is the context that of company decision making, or does it involve only the design and analysis of registration studies? Pharmaceutical company decisions involve questions such as whether to move on to phase III (full-scale evaluation of efficacy), and if so, how many doses and which doses to include, whether to incorporate a pilot aspect of phase III, how many phase III trials should be conducted, and how many centers should be involved. Other decision-oriented examples are easy to imagine. An investment capitalist might wonder whether or not to fund a particular trial. A small biotechnology company might need to decide whether to sell itself to a larger firm that has the resources to run a bigger trial.

These questions suggest a decision analysis using what we call a fully Bayesian approach, using the likelihood function, the *prior* distribution, and a *utility* structure to arrive at a decision. The prior distribution summarizes available information on the model parameters before the data are observed; it is combined with the likelihood using *Bayes' Theorem* (2.1) to obtain the posterior distribution. A utility function assigns numerical values to the various gains and losses that would obtain for various true states of nature (i.e., the unknown parameters). It is equivalent to a *loss function*, and essentially determines how to weigh outcomes and procedures. Bayesian statistical decision theory suggests choosing procedures that have high utility (low loss) when averaged with respect to the posterior.

Fully Bayesian analysis is the kind envisioned by the great masters De-Finetti (reprinted 1992), Savage (1972), and Lindley (1972), and continues to be popular in business contexts, where there is often a lone decisionmaker whose prior opinions and utility function can be reliably assessed. In a drug or device evaluation, a decisionmaker may initially prefer a certain action a. After assessing the decisionmaker's prior distribution and utilities, we may discover that the optimal action is in fact b, perhaps by quite a margin. This can then lead to an exploration of what changes to the prior and utility structure are required in order for a to actually emerge as optimal. Such a process can be quite revealing to the decisionmaker!

Still, in the everyday practice of clinical trials, the fully Bayesian approach can be awkward. First, except in the case of internal, company-sponsored trials, there are often multiple decisionmakers, all of whom arrive at the trial with their own prior opinions and tolerances for risk. Second, when data arrive sequentially over time (as they typically do in clinical trials), calculations in the fully Bayesian vein require a complex bookkeeping system known as *backward induction*, in which the decision as to whether to stop or continue the trial at each monitoring point must account for both the informational value of the next observations, and the cost of obtaining them (though again, see Carlin et al., 1998, and Brockwell and Kadane, 2003 for approaches that avoid backward induction in a class of clinical trials). Third, the process of eliciting costs and benefits can be a difficult process, even for seasoned experts trained in probabilistic thinking. Moreover, the appropriate scales for the losses (monetary units, patient lives, etc.) are often difficult to work with and lead to decision rules that seem somewhat arbitrary.

For these and other reasons, fully Bayesian approaches have largely failed to gain a foothold in regulatory and other later-phase clinical trial settings. As such, with the notable exception of Sections 4.6 and 6.4.2, we will mostly focus on the less controversial and easier-to-implement "probability only" approach, where we use Bayesian techniques to summarize all available information, but do not take the further step of specifying utility functions.

1.4.2 Bayes as a frequentist tool

In the context of designing and analyzing registration studies, the Bayesian approach can be a tool to build good frequentist designs. For example, we can use the Bayesian paradigm to build a clinical trial that requires a smaller expected sample size regardless of the actual parameter values. The design may be complicated, but we can always find its frequentist operating characteristics using simulation. In particular, we can ensure that the false-positive rate is within the range acceptable to regulatory agencies.

Bayesian methods support sequential learning, allowing updating one's posterior probability as the data accrue. They also allow for finding predictive distributions of future results, and enable borrowing of strength across studies. Regarding the first of these, we make an observation, update the probability distributions of the various parameters, make another observation, update the distributions again, and so on. At any point we can ask which observation we want to make next; e.g., which dose we want to use for the next patient. Finding predictive distributions (the probabilities that the next set of observations will be of a specific type) is uniquely Bayesian. Frequentist methods allow for calculations that are conditional on particular values of parameters, so they are able to address the question of prediction only in a limited sense. In particular, frequentist predictive probabilities that change as the available data change are not possible.

The Bayesian paradigm allows for using historical information and results of other trials, whether they involve the same drug, similar drugs, or possibly the same drug but with different patient populations. The Bayesian approach is ideal for borrowing strength across patient and disease groups within the same trial and across trials. Still, we caution that historical information typically cannot simply be regarded as exchangeable with current information; see Section 6.1.

Some trials that are proposed by pharmaceutical and device companies are deficient in ways that can be improved by taking a Bayesian approach. For example, a company may regard its drug to be most appropriate for a particular disease, but be unsure just which subtypes of the disease will be most responsive. So they propose separate trials for the different subtypes. To be specific, consider advanced ovarian cancer, a particularly difficult disease to achieve tumor responses. In exploring the possible effects of its drug, suppose a company was trying to detect a tumor response rate of 10%. It proposed to treat 30 patients in one group and 30 patients in the complementary group, but to run two separate trials. All 60 patients would be accrued with the goal of achieving at least one tumor response. Suppose there were 0 responses out of the 30 patients accrued in Trial 1 and 0 responses out of 25 patients accrued so far in Trial 2. By design, they would still add 5 more patients in Trial 2. But this would be folly, since so far, we would have learned two things: first, the drug is not very active, and second, the two patient subgroups respond similarly. It makes sense to incorporate what has been learned from Trial 1 into Trial 2. A Bayesian hierarchical modeling analysis (see Section 2.4) would enable this, and a reasonable such analysis would show that with high probability it is futile (and ethically questionable) to add the remaining 5 patients in Trial 2.

Bayesian designs incorporate sequential learning whenever logistically possible, use predictive probabilities of future results, and borrow strength across studies and patient subgroups. These three Bayesian characteristics have implications for analysis as well as for design. All three involve modeling in building likelihood functions.

Bayesian goals include faster learning via more efficient designs of trials and more efficient drug and medical device development, while at the same time providing better treatment of patients who participate in clinical trials. In our experience, physician researchers and patients are particularly attracted by Bayesian trial designs' potential to provide effective care while not sacrificing scientific integrity.

Traditional drug development is slow, in part because of several characteristics of conventional clinical trials. Such trials usually have inflexible designs, focus on single therapeutic strategies, are partitioned into discrete phases, restrict to early endpoints in early phases but employ different long-term endpoints in later phases, and restrict statistical inferences to information in the current trial. The rigidity of the traditional approach inhibits progress, and can often lead to clinical trials that are too large or too small. The adaptivity of the Bayesian approach allows for determining a trial's sample size while it is in progress. For example, suppose a pharmaceutical company runs a trial with a predetermined sample size and balanced randomization to several doses to learn the appropriate dose for its drug. That is like saying to a student, "Study statistics for N hours and you will be a statistician." Perhaps the student will become a statistician long before N. Or there may be no N for which this particular student could become a statistician. The traditional approach is to pretend that the right dose for an experimental drug is known after completing the canonical clinical trial(s) designed to answer that question. More realistically, we never "know" the right dose.

A clinical trial should be like life: experiment until you achieve your objective, or until you learn that your objective is not worth pursuing. Better methods for drug and device development are based on decision analyses, flexible designs, assessing multiple experimental therapies, using seamless trial phases, modeling the relationships among early and late endpoints, and synthesizing the available information. Flexible designs allow the data that are accruing to guide the trial, including determining when to stop or extend accrual.

We advocate broadening the range of possibilities for learning in the early phases of drug and device development. For example, we might use multiple experimental oncology drugs in a single trial. If we are going to defeat cancer with drugs, it is likely to be with selections from lists of many drugs and their combinations, not with any single drug. We will also have to learn in clinical trials which patients (based on clinical and biological characteristics) benefit from which combinations of drugs. So we need to be able to study many drugs in clinical trials. We might use, say, 100 drugs in a partial factorial fashion, while running longitudinal genomic and proteomic experiments. The goal would be to determine the characteristics of the patients who respond to the various combinations of drugs – perhaps an average of 10 drugs per patient – and then to validate these observations in the same trial. We cannot learn about the potential benefits of combinations of therapies unless we use them in clinical trials. Considering only one experimental drug at a time in clinical trials is an inefficient way to make therapeutic advances.

Regarding the process of learning, in the Bayesian paradigm it is natural to move beyond the notion of discrete phases of drug development. An approach that is consistent with the Bayesian paradigm is to view drug development as a continuous process. For example, *seamless* trials allow for moving from one phase of development to the next without stopping patient accrual. Another possibility is allowing for the possibility of ramping up accrual if the accumulating data warrant it. Modeling relationships among clinical and early endpoints will enable early decisionmaking in trials, increasing their efficiency. Synthesizing the available information involves using data from related trials, from historical databases, and from other, related diseases, such as other types of cancer.

1.4.3 Examples of the Bayesian approach to drug and medical device development

Here we offer some case studies to illustrate the Bayesian design characteristics of predictive probabilities, adaptive randomization, and seamless phase II/III trials.

Predictive probability

Predictive probability plays a critical role in the design of a trial and also in monitoring trials. For example, conditioning on what is known about patient covariates and outcomes at any time during a trial allows for finding the probability of achieving statistical significance at the end of the trial. If that probability is sufficiently small, the researchers may deem that continuing is futile and decide to end the trial. Assessing such predictive probabilities is especially appropriate for data safety monitoring boards (DSMBs) quite apart from the protocol, but it is something that can and should be explicitly incorporated into the design of a trial.

A drug trial at M.D. Anderson for patients with HER2-positive neoadjuvant breast cancer serves as an example of using predictive probability while monitoring a trial (Buzdar et al., 2005). The original design called for balanced randomization of 164 patients to receive standard chemotherapy either in combination with the drug trastuzumab or not (controls). The endpoint was pathologic complete tumor response (pCR). The protocol specified no interim analyses. At one of its regular meetings, the institution's DSMB considered the results after the outcomes of 34 patients were available. Among 16 control patients there were 4 (25%) pCRs. Of 18 patients receiving trastuzumab, there were 12 (67%) pCRs. The DSMB calculated the predictive probability of statistical significance if the trial were to continue to randomize and treat the targeted sample size of 164 patients, which turned out to be 95%. They also considered that the trial's accrual rate had dropped to less than 2 patients per month. They stopped the trial and made the results available to the research and clinical communities. This was many years sooner than if the trial had continued to the targeted sample size of 164. The researchers presented the trial results at the next annual meeting of the American Society of Clinical Oncology. That presentation and the related publication had an important impact on clinical practice, as well as on subsequent research. See Sections 2.5.1, 4.2, and 5.2 for much more detail on predictive probability methods.

Adaptive randomization and early stopping for futility

An M.D. Anderson trial in the treatment of acute myelogenous leukemia (AML) serves as an example of adaptive randomization (Giles et al., 2003). That trial compared the experimental drug troxacitabine to the institution's standard therapy for AML, which was idarubicin in combination with cytarabine, also known as ara-C. It compared three treatment strategies: idarubicin plus ara-C (IA), troxacitabine plus ara-C (TA), and troxacitabine plus idarubicin (TI). The maximum trial size was set in advance at 75. The endpoint was complete remission (CR); early CR is important in AML. The trialists modeled time to CR within the first 50 days. The study design called for randomizing based on the currently available trial results.

In particular, when a patient entered the trial they calculated the probabilities that TI and TA were better than IA, and the probability that TA was better than TI, and used those current probabilities to assign the patient's therapy. If one of the treatment arms performed sufficiently poorly, its assignment probability would decrease, with better performing therapies getting higher probabilities. An arm doing sufficiently poorly would be dropped.

In the actual trial, the TI arm was dropped after 24 patients. Arm TA was dropped (and the trial ended) after 34 patients, with these final results for CR within 50 days: 10 of 18 patients receiving IA (56%, a rate consistent with historical results); 3 of 11 patients on TA (27%) and 0 of 5 patients on TI (0%).

These results and the design used have been controversial. Some cancer researchers feel that having 0 successes out of only 5 patients is not reason enough to abandon a treatment. For some settings we would agree, but not when there is an alternative that produces on the order of 56% complete remissions. In view of the trial results, the Bayesian probability that either TA or TI is better than IA is small. Moreover, if either has a CR rate that is greater than that of IA, it is not much greater.

The principal investigator of this trial, Dr. Francis Giles, MD, was quoted in *Cure* magazine (McCarthy, 2009) as follows:

> "I see no rationale to further delay moving to these designs," says Dr. Giles, who is currently involved in eight Bayesian-based leukemia studies. "They are more ethical, more patient-friendly, more conserving of resources, more statistically desirable. I think the next big issue is to get the FDA to accept them as the basis for new drug approvals."

Adaptive randomization: screening phase II cancer agents

The traditional approach in drug development is to study one drug at a time. Direct comparisons of experimental drugs with either standard therapies or other experimental drugs are unusual in early phases; combinations of experimental drugs are often frowned upon. Focusing on one drug means that hundreds of others are waiting their turns in the research queue. Simply because of its size, the queue is likely to contain better drugs than the one now being studied. A better approach is to investigate many drugs and their combinations at the same time. One might screen drugs in phase II in a fashion similar to screening in a preclinical setting. The goal is to learn about safety and efficacy of the candidate drugs as rapidly as possible. Another goal is to treat patients effectively, promising them in the informed consent process that if a therapy is performing better, then they are more likely to receive it.

Consider a one-drug-at-a-time example in phase II cancer trials. Suppose the historical tumor response rate is 20%. A standard design for a clinical trial has two stages. The first stage consists of 20 patients. The trial ends after the first stage if 4 or fewer tumor responses are observed, and also if 9 or more tumor responses are observed. Otherwise, we proceed to the second stage of another 20 patients. A positive result moves the drug into phase III, or to some intermediate phase of further investigation. Progress is slow.

Now consider an alternative adaptive design with many drugs and drug combinations. We assign patients to a treatment in proportion to the probability that its response rate is greater than 20%:

$$r = P(\text{rate} > 20\% \mid \text{current data}) \,.$$

We add drugs as they become available, and drop them if their probability of having a response rate greater than 20% is not very high. Drugs that have sufficiently large r move on to phase III.

As an illustration, consider 10 experimental drugs with a total sample size of 200 patients: 9 of the drugs have a mix of response rates 20% and 40%, and one is a "nugget," a drug with a 60% response rate. The standard trial design finds the nugget with probability less than 0.70. This is because the nugget may not be among the first seven or so drugs in the queue, and that is all that can be investigated in 200 patients. On the other hand, the adaptive design has better than a 0.99 probability of finding the nugget. That is because all drugs have some chance of being used early in the trial. Randomizing according to the results means that the high probability of observing a response when using the nugget boosts its probability of being assigned to later patients. So we identify the nugget with very high probability and we find the nugget much sooner: after 50 of 200 patients for an adaptive design, as opposed to 110 of the 200 in the standard design (conditioning on finding it at all). Adaptive randomization is also a better method for finding the drugs that have response rates of 40%.

If we have many more drugs (say, 100) and proportionally more patients (say, 2000), then the relative comparisons are unchanged from the earlier case. We find the 1-in-100 nugget drug essentially with certainty, and we find it much more quickly using adaptive randomization. The consequences of using adaptive randomization are that we treat patients in the trial more effectively, we learn more quickly, and we are also able to identify the better drug sooner, which allows it to move through the process more rapidly. Benefits accrue to both the patient and the drug developer.

These comparisons apply qualitatively for other endpoints, such as progression-free survival, and when randomization includes a control therapy. See Sections 4.4 and 5.2 for full details on adaptive randomization in phase II and III trials.

Seamless phase II and III trial designs

Consider a trial for which there is pharmacologic or pathophysiologic information about a patient's outcomes. In such a trial, clinicians may require biologic justification of an early endpoint. If the early endpoint is to serve as a surrogate for the clinical endpoint in the sense that it replaces the clinical endpoint, then we agree. But early endpoints can be used whether or not the biology is understood: all that is required is some evidence that it may be correlated with the clinical endpoint. The possibility of such correlation can be modeled statistically. If the data in the trial point to the existence of correlation (depending on treatment), then the early endpoint is implicitly exploited through the modeling process. If the data suggest a lack of correlation, then the early endpoint plays no role, and little is lost by having considered the possibility.

In one study, we modeled the possible correlation between the success of a spinal implant at 12 months and at 24 months. We didn't assume that those endpoints were correlated, but instead let the data dictate the extent to which the 12-month result was predictive of the 24-month endpoint. The primary endpoint was success at 24 months. The earlier endpoint at 12 months was not a "surrogate endpoint," but rather an auxiliary endpoint.

In another study, we modeled the possible relationship among scores on a stroke scale at early time points, weeks 1 through 12, but the primary endpoint was the week-13 score on the stroke scale. We did not employ anything so crude as "last observation carried forward," but instead built a longitudinal model and updated the model as evidence about relationships between endpoints accumulated in the trial.

An early endpoint in cancer trials is tumor response. Early information from tumor response can be used to construct a seamless phase II/III trial. In conventional cancer drug development, phase II addresses tumor response. Sufficient activity in phase II leads to phase III, which is designed to determine if the drug provides a survival advantage. A conventional phase II process generally requires more than 18 months, after which phase III generally requires at least another 2 years. In contrast, a comparably powered seamless phase II/III trial with modeling the relationship between tumor response and survival can take less than two years in total.

In a seamless trial, we start out with a small number of centers. We accrue a modest number of patients per month, randomizing to experimental and control arms. If the predictive probability of eventual success is sufficiently promising, we expand into phase III, and all the while, the initial centers continue to accrue patients. It is especially important to use the "phase II" data because the patients enrolled in the trial early have longer follow-up time and thus provide the best information about survival.

Our seamless design involves frequent analyses and uses early stopping determinations based on predictive probabilities of eventually achieving statistical significance. Specifically, we look at the data every month (or even every week), and use predictive probabilities to determine when to switch to phase III, to stop accrual for futility if the drug's performance is sufficiently bad, or to stop for efficacy if the drug is performing sufficiently well.

Inoue et al. (2002) compared the seamless design with more conventional designs having the same operating characteristics (Type I error rate and power) and found reductions in average sample size ranging from 30% to 50%, in both the null and alternative hypothesis cases. In addition, the total time of the trial was similarly reduced. We return to this subject in detail in Section 5.7.

Summary

The Bayesian method is by its nature more flexible and adaptive, even when the conduct of a study deviates from the original design. It is possible to incorporate all available information into the prior distribution for designing a trial, while recognizing that regulators and other reviewers may well have a different prior. Indeed, they may not have a prior at all, but will want to use statistical significance in the final analysis. The Bayesian approach addresses this with aplomb, since predictive probabilities can look forward to a frequentist analysis when all the data become available.

We note that a deviation in the conduct of a study from the original design causes the frequentist properties to change, whereas Bayesian properties (which always condition on whatever data emerge) remain unchanged. Bayesian methods are better able to handle complex hierarchical model structures, such as random effects models used in metaanalysis to borrow strength across different disease subgroups or similar treatments (see Example 2.7). Bayesian methods also facilitate the development of innovative trials such as seamless phase II/III trials and outcome-based adaptive randomization designs (Inoue et al., 2002; Thall et al., 2003; Berry, 2005; Berry, 2006; Zhou et al., 2008). In the next chapter we develop and illustrate the requisite Bayesian machinery, before proceeding on to its use in specific phase I-III trials in Chapters 3–5, respectively.

## CHAPTER 2

Basics of Bayesian inference

In this chapter we provide a brief overview of hierarchical Bayesian modeling and computing for readers not already familiar with these topics. Of course, in one chapter we can only scratch the surface of this rapidly expanding field, and readers may well wish to consult one of the many recent textbooks on the subject, either as preliminary work or on an as-needed basis. By contrast, readers already familiar with the basics of Bayesian methods and computing may wish to skip ahead to Section 2.5, where we outline the principles of Bayesian clinical trial design and analysis.

It should come as little surprise that the Bayesian book we most highly recommend is the one by Carlin and Louis (2009); the Bayesian methodology and computing material below roughly follows Chapters 2 and 3, respectively, in that text. However, a great many other good Bayesian books are available, and we list a few of them and their characteristics. First we must mention texts stressing Bayesian theory, including DeGroot (1970), Berger (1985), Bernardo and Smith (1994), and Robert (2001). These books tend to focus on foundations and decision theory, rather than computation or data analysis. On the more methodological side, a nice introductory book is that of Lee (1997), with O'Hagan and Forster (2004) and Gelman, Carlin, Stern, and Rubin (2004) offering more general Bayesian modeling treatments.

2.1 Introduction to Bayes' Theorem

As discussed in Chapter 1, by modeling both the observed data and any unknowns as random variables, the Bayesian approach to statistical analysis provides a cohesive framework for combining complex data models with external knowledge, expert opinion, or both. We now introduce the technical details of the Bayesian approach.

In addition to specifying the distributional model $f(\mathbf{y}|\boldsymbol{\theta})$ for the observed data $\mathbf{y} = (y_1, \ldots, y_n)$ given a vector of unknown parameters $\boldsymbol{\theta} = (\theta_1, \ldots, \theta_k)$, suppose that $\boldsymbol{\theta}$ is a random quantity sampled from a *prior* distribution $\pi(\boldsymbol{\theta}|\boldsymbol{\lambda})$, where $\boldsymbol{\lambda}$ is a vector of hyperparameters. For instance, y_i might be the empirical drug response rate in a sample of women aged 40 and over from clinical center i, θ_i the underlying true response rate for all such women in this center, and λ a parameter controlling how these true rates vary across centers. If λ is known, inference concerning θ is based on its *posterior* distribution,

$$p(\theta|\mathbf{y}, \lambda) = \frac{p(\mathbf{y}, \theta|\lambda)}{p(\mathbf{y}|\lambda)} = \frac{p(\mathbf{y}, \theta|\lambda)}{\int p(\mathbf{y}, \theta|\lambda)\, d\theta} = \frac{f(\mathbf{y}|\theta)\pi(\theta|\lambda)}{\int f(\mathbf{y}|\theta)\pi(\theta|\lambda)\, d\theta}. \qquad (2.1)$$

Notice the contribution of both the data (in the form of the likelihood f) and the previous knowledge or expert opinion (in the form of the prior π) to the posterior. Since, in practice, λ will not be known, a second stage (or *hyperprior*) distribution $h(\lambda)$ will often be required, and (2.1) will be replaced with

$$p(\theta|\mathbf{y}) = \frac{p(\mathbf{y}, \theta)}{p(\mathbf{y})} = \frac{\int f(\mathbf{y}|\theta)\pi(\theta|\lambda)h(\lambda)\, d\lambda}{\int \int f(\mathbf{y}|\theta)\pi(\theta|\lambda)h(\lambda)\, d\theta d\lambda}.$$

This multi-stage approach is often called *hierarchical modeling*, a subject to which we return in Section 2.4. Alternatively, we might replace λ by an estimate $\hat{\lambda}$ obtained as the maximizer of the marginal distribution $p(\mathbf{y}|\lambda) = \int f(\mathbf{y}|\theta)\pi(\theta|\lambda)d\theta$, viewed as a function of λ. Inference could then proceed based on the *estimated* posterior distribution $p(\theta|\mathbf{y}, \hat{\lambda})$, obtained by plugging $\hat{\lambda}$ into equation (2.1). This approach is referred to as *empirical Bayes* analysis; see Carlin and Louis (2009, Chapter 5) for details regarding empirical Bayes methodology and applications.

The Bayesian inferential paradigm offers attractive advantages over the classical, frequentist statistical approach through its more philosophically sound foundation, its unified approach to data analysis, and its ability to formally incorporate prior opinion or external empirical evidence into the results via the prior distribution π. Modeling the θ_i as random (instead of fixed) effects allows us to induce specific correlation structures among them, hence among the observations y_i as well.

A computational challenge in applying Bayesian methods is that for most realistic problems, the integrations required to do inference under (2.1) are often not tractable in closed form, and thus must be approximated numerically. Forms for π and h (called *conjugate* priors) that enable at least partial analytic evaluation of these integrals may often be found, but in the presense of nuisance parameters (typically unknown variances), some intractable integrations remain. Here the emergence of inexpensive, high-speed computing equipment and software comes to the rescue, enabling the application of recently developed Markov chain Monte Carlo (MCMC) integration methods, such as the Metropolis-Hastings algorithm (Metropolis et al., 1953; Hastings, 1970) and the Gibbs sampler (Geman and Geman, 1984; Gelfand and Smith, 1990). Details of these algorithms will be presented in Section 2.3.

Illustrations of Bayes' Theorem

Equation (2.1) is a generic version of what is referred to as *Bayes' Theorem* or *Bayes' Rule*. It is attributed to Reverend Thomas Bayes, an 18th-century nonconformist minister and part-time mathematician; a version of the result was published (posthumously) in Bayes (1763). In this subsection we consider a few basic examples of its use.

Example 2.1 *(basic normal/normal model).* Suppose we have observed a single normal (Gaussian) observation $Y \sim N\left(\theta, \sigma^2\right)$ with σ^2 known, so that the likelihood $f\left(y|\theta\right) = N\left(y|\theta, \sigma^2\right) \equiv \frac{1}{\sigma\sqrt{2\pi}}\exp\left(-\frac{(y-\theta)^2}{2\sigma^2}\right)$, $y \in \Re$, $\theta \in \Re$, and $\sigma > 0$. If we specify the prior distribution as $\pi\left(\theta\right) = N\left(\theta \,\middle|\, \mu, \tau^2\right)$ with $\boldsymbol{\lambda} = (\mu, \tau^2)'$ fixed, then from (2.1) we can compute the posterior as

$$
\begin{aligned}
p\left(\theta|y\right) &= \frac{N\left(\theta|\mu, \tau^2\right) N\left(y|\theta, \sigma^2\right)}{p\left(y\right)} \\
&\propto N\left(\theta|\mu, \tau^2\right) N\left(y|\theta, \sigma^2\right) \\
&= N\left(\theta \,\middle|\, \frac{\sigma^2}{\sigma^2 + \tau^2}\mu + \frac{\tau^2}{\sigma^2 + \tau^2}y, \, \frac{\sigma^2\tau^2}{\sigma^2 + \tau^2}\right).
\end{aligned} \tag{2.2}
$$

That is, the posterior distribution of θ given y is also normal with mean and variance as given. The proportionality in the second row arises since the marginal distribution $p(y)$ does not depend on θ, and is thus constant with respect to the Bayes' Theorem calculation. The final equality in the third row results from collecting like (θ^2 and θ) terms in the two exponential components of the previous line, and then completing the square.

Note that the posterior mean $E(\theta|y)$ is a weighted average of the prior mean μ and the data value y, with the weights depending on our relative uncertainty with respect to the prior and the likelihood. Also, the posterior *precision* (reciprocal of the variance) is equal to $1/\sigma^2 + 1/\tau^2$, which is the sum of the likelihood and prior precisions. Thus, thinking of precision as "information," we see that in the normal/normal model, the information in the posterior is the total of the information in the prior and the likelihood.

Suppose next that instead of a single datum we have a set of n observations $\mathbf{y} = (y_1, y_2, \ldots, y_n)'$. From basic normal theory we know that $f(\bar{y}|\theta) = N(\theta, \sigma^2/n)$. Since $\bar{y}$ is sufficient for θ, from (2.2) we have

$$
\begin{aligned}
p(\theta|\mathbf{y}) = p\left(\theta|\bar{y}\right) &= N\left(\theta \,\middle|\, \frac{(\sigma^2/n)}{(\sigma^2/n) + \tau^2}\mu + \frac{\tau^2}{(\sigma^2/n) + \tau^2}\bar{y}, \, \frac{(\sigma^2/n)\tau^2}{(\sigma^2/n) + \tau^2}\right) \\
&= N\left(\theta \,\middle|\, \frac{\sigma^2}{\sigma^2 + n\tau^2}\mu + \frac{n\tau^2}{\sigma^2 + n\tau^2}\bar{y}, \, \frac{\sigma^2\tau^2}{\sigma^2 + n\tau^2}\right).
\end{aligned}
$$

Again we obtain a posterior mean that is a weighted average of the prior (μ) and data-supported ($\bar{y}$) values. ∎

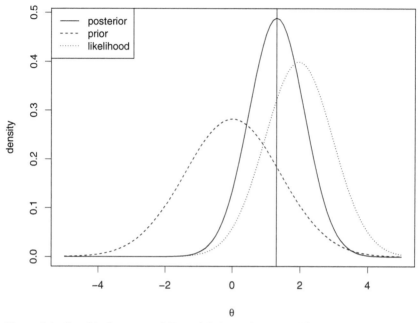

Figure 2.1 *Graphical version of Bayes' Rule in the normal/normal example. The vertical line marks the posterior mean, 1.31.*

Example 2.2 *(normal/normal model applied to a simple efficacy trial).*
Recall that in Example 1.1, a device is used to treat 100 patients and a particular outcome measurement is made on each. The average $\bar{y}$ of the 100 measurements is 1.96 and the standard deviation σ is 10. Suppose the prior distribution is normal with mean 0 and variance 2 (standard deviation $\sqrt{2}$). This prior density and the likelihood function of θ (taken from above) are shown in Figure 2.1 as dashed and dotted lines, respectively. As seen in Example 2.1, the posterior density by Bayes' Theorem is the product of the prior and likelihood, restandardized to integrate to 1. This (also normal) posterior density is shown in Figure 2.1 as a solid line. For ease of comparison, the three curves are shown as having the same area, although the area under the likelihood function is irrelevant since it is not a probability density in θ. Note the location of the posterior is a compromise between that of the prior and the likelihood, and it is also more concentrated than either of these two building blocks, since it reflects more information, i.e., the total information in both the prior and the data.

As seen in the previous example, there is a general formula for the posterior distribution of θ when both the sampling distribution and the prior distribution are normal. Figure 2.1 is representative of the typical case in that the posterior distribution is more concentrated than both the prior distribution and the likelihood. Also, the posterior mean is always between the prior mean and the maximum likelihood estimate. Suppose again the mean of the prior distribution for θ is μ and its variance is $\tau^2 = 1/h_0$; h_0 is the precision. If the sample size and population standard deviation are again n and σ, then the sample precision $h_s = n/\sigma^2$. Since precisions add in this normal model, the posterior precision is $h_{post} = h_0 + h_s$. The posterior mean, $E(\theta|\bar{y})$, is a weighted average of the prior mean and sample mean (called shrinkage), with the weights proportional to the precisions:

$$E(\theta|\bar{y}) = \frac{h_0}{h_0 + h_s}\mu + \frac{h_s}{h_0 + h_s}\bar{y} = \frac{h_0\mu + h_s\bar{y}}{h_0 + h_s} \ .$$

In our case, we have $\mu = 0$, $h_0 = 1/2$, $\bar{y} = 1.96$, $\sigma = 10$, $n = 100$, $h_s = 100/(10^2) = 1$, $h_{post} = h_0 + h_s = 3/2$ (so the posterior standard deviation is $\sqrt{2/3} = 0.816$), and $E(\theta|\bar{y}) = 1.96/(3/2) = 1.31$, as indicated in Figure 2.1.

The sample is twice as informative as the prior in this example, in the sense that $h_s = 2h_0$. Relative to the experiment in question, the prior information is worth the same as 50 observations (with the mean of these hypothetical observations being 0). In general, h_s/h_0 is proportional to n, and so for sufficiently large sample size, the sample information overwhelms the prior information. While this fact is comforting, the limiting case, $n \to \infty$, is not very interesting. Usually, unknown parameters become known in the limit and there is no need for statistics when there is no uncertainty. In practice, sampling has costs and there is a trade-off between increasing n and making an unwise decision based on insufficient information about a parameter. When the sample size is small or moderate, the ability to exploit prior information in a formal way is an important advantage of the Bayesian approach.

The posterior distribution of the parameters of interest is the culmination of the Bayesian approach. With the posterior distribution in hand, probabilities of hypotheses can be calculated, decisions can be evaluated, and predictive probabilities can be derived. As an example of the first of these, consider the hypothesis $\theta > 0$. Because our posterior distribution is normal with mean 1.31 and standard deviation 0.816, the probability of this hypothesis is 0.945, which is the area of the shaded region under the curve shown in Figure 2.2. ■

In these two examples, the prior chosen leads to a posterior distribution for θ that is available in closed form, and is a member of the same distributional family as the prior. Such a prior is referred to as a *conjugate* prior. We will often use such priors in our work, since, when they are available, conjugate families are convenient and still allow a variety of shapes wide enough to capture our prior beliefs.

Note that setting $\tau^2 = \infty$ in the previous examples corresponds to a prior that is arbitrarily vague, or *noninformative*. This then leads to a posterior of $p(\theta|y) = N(\theta|\bar{y}, \sigma^2/n)$, exactly the same as the likelihood for

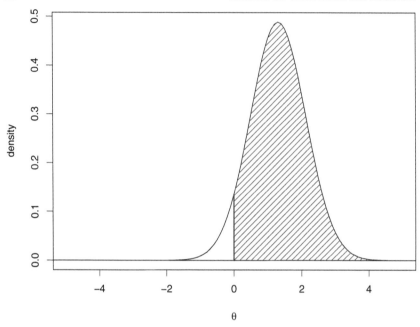

Figure 2.2 *Shaded area is the posterior probability that θ is positive.*

this problem. This arises since the limit of the conjugate (normal) prior here is actually a uniform, or "flat" prior, and thus the posterior is nothing but the likelihood, possibly renormalized so it integrates to 1 as a function of θ. Of course, the flat prior is *improper* here, since the uniform does not integrate to anything finite over the entire real line. However, the posterior is still well defined since the likelihood can be integrated with respect to θ. Bayesians use flat or otherwise improper noninformative priors in situations where prior knowledge is vague relative to the information in the likelihood, or in settings where we want the data (and not the prior) to dominate the determination of the posterior.

Example 2.3 *(normal/normal model with unknown sampling variance).* Consider the extension of the normal/normal model in Examples 2.1 and 2.2 to the more realistic case where the sample variance σ^2 is unknown. Transforming again to the precision $h = 1/\sigma^2$, it turns out the *gamma* distribution offers a conjugate prior. To see this, let h have a *Gamma*(α, β) prior with pdf

$$p(h) = \frac{\beta^\alpha}{\Gamma(\alpha)} h^{\alpha-1} e^{-h\beta}, \; h > 0 \; . \tag{2.3}$$

Since the likelihood for any one observation y_i is still

$$f(y_i|\theta, h) = \frac{h^{1/2}}{\sqrt{2\pi}} e^{-\frac{h}{2}(y_i-\theta)^2} \ ,$$

the posterior of h is proportional to the product of the full likelihood and the prior,

$$
\begin{aligned}
p(h|\mathbf{y}, \theta) \quad &\propto \quad \left[\prod_{i=1}^{n} f(y_i|\theta, h)\right] \times p(h) \\
&\propto \quad h^{n/2} e^{-\frac{h}{2}\sum_{i=1}^{n}(y_i-\theta)^2} \times h^{\alpha-1} e^{-h\beta} \\
&\propto \quad h^{n/2+\alpha-1} e^{-h[\beta+\frac{1}{2}\sum_{i=1}^{n}(y_i-\theta)^2]} \ ,
\end{aligned}
$$

where in all three steps we have absorbed any multiplicative terms that do not involve h into the unknown normalizing constant. Looking again at the form of the gamma prior in (2.3), we recognize this form as proportional to another gamma distribution, namely a

$$Gamma\left(n/2 + \alpha \ , \ \beta + \frac{1}{2}\sum_{i=1}^{n}(y_i - \theta)^2\right) \ . \qquad (2.4)$$

Thus the posterior for h is available via conjugacy.

Note that (2.4) is only a *conditional* posterior distribution, since it depends on the mean parameter θ, which is itself unknown. However, the conditional posterior for θ, $p(\theta|\mathbf{y}, h)$, is exactly the same as that previously found in Example 2.2, since the steps we went through then to get $p(\theta|\mathbf{y})$ are exactly those we would go through now; in both calculations, h is assumed fixed and known. Armed with these two *full conditional* distributions, it turns out to be easy to obtain Monte Carlo samples from the *joint* posterior $p(\theta, h|\mathbf{y})$, and hence the two *marginal* posteriors $p(\theta|\mathbf{y})$ and $p(h|\mathbf{y})$, using the Gibbs sampler; we return to this subject in Subsection 2.3.1.

Finally, regarding the precise choice of α and β, many authors (and even the WinBUGS software manual) use $\alpha = \beta = \epsilon$ for some small positive constant ϵ as a sort of "default" setting. This prior has mean $\alpha/\beta = 1$ but variance $\alpha/\beta^2 = 1/\epsilon$, making it progressively more diffuse as $\epsilon \to 0$. It is also a "minimally informative" prior in the sense that choosing a very small ϵ will have minimal impact on the full conditional in (2.4), forcing the data and θ to provide virtually all the input to this distribution. However, this prior becomes improper as $\epsilon \to 0$, and its shape also becomes more and more spiked, with an infinite peak at 0 and a very heavy right tail (to create the larger and larger variance). Gelman (2006) suggests placing a *uniform* prior on σ, simply bounding the prior away from 0 and ∞ in some sensible way – say, via a $Uniform(\epsilon, 1/\epsilon)$. We will experiment with both of these priors in subsequent examples.

As a side comment, Spiegelhalter et al. (2004) recommend a Jeffreys noninformative prior (see e.g. Carlin and Louis, 2009, Sec. 2.2.3) for the sampling standard deviation σ, i.e., $\pi(\sigma) = 1/\sigma$. This is in some sense a limiting version of the conjugate gamma prior above. However, Spiegelhalter et al. (2004) express a preference for the Gelman prior for standard deviations arising in random effects distributions. ∎

2.2 Bayesian inference

While the computing associated with Bayesian methods can be daunting, the subsequent inference is relatively straightforward, especially in the case of estimation. This is because once we have computed (or obtained an estimate of) the posterior, inference comes down merely to summarizing this distribution, since by Bayes' Rule the posterior summarizes everything we know about the model parameters in light of the data. In the remainder of this section, we shall assume for simplicity that the posterior $p(\boldsymbol{\theta}|\mathbf{y})$ itself (and not merely an estimate of it) is available for summarization.

Bayesian methods for estimation are also reminiscent of corresponding maximum likelihood methods. This should not be surprising, since likelihoods form an important part of the Bayesian calculation; we have even seen that a normalized (i.e., standardized) likelihood can be thought of a posterior when this is possible. However, when we turn to hypothesis testing, the approaches have little in common. Bayesians have a profound dislike for p-values, for a long list of reasons we shall not go into here; the interested reader may consult Berger (1985, Sec. 4.3.3), Kass and Raftery (1995, Sec. 8.2), or Carlin and Louis (2009, Sec. 2.3.3).

2.2.1 Point estimation

To keep things simple, suppose for the moment that θ is univariate. Given the posterior $p(\theta|\mathbf{y})$, a sensible Bayesian point estimate of θ would be some measure of centrality. Three familiar choices are the posterior mean,

$$\hat{\theta} = E(\theta|\mathbf{y}) \, ,$$

the posterior median,

$$\hat{\theta} \, : \, \int_{-\infty}^{\hat{\theta}} p(\theta|\mathbf{y})d\theta = 0.5 \, ,$$

and the posterior mode,

$$\hat{\theta} \, : \, p(\hat{\theta}|\mathbf{y}) = \sup_{\theta} p(\theta|\mathbf{y}) \, .$$

The lattermost estimate has historically been thought of as easiest to compute, since it does not require any integration: we can replace $p(\theta|\mathbf{y})$ by its unstandardized form, $f(\mathbf{y}|\theta)p(\theta)$, and get the same answer (since these two differ only by a multiplicative factor of the marginal distribution $p(\mathbf{y})$, which does not depend on θ). Existing code to find maximum likelihood estimates (MLEs) can be readily used with the product of the likelihood and the prior (instead of the likelihood alone) to produce posterior modes. Indeed, if the posterior exists under a flat prior $p(\theta) = 1$, then the posterior mode is nothing but the MLE itself.

Note that for symmetric unimodal posteriors (e.g., a normal distribution), the posterior mean, median, and mode will all be equal. However, for multimodal or otherwise nonnormal posteriors, the mode will often be the poorest choice of centrality measure. Consider for example the case of a steadily decreasing, one-tailed posterior: the mode will be the very first value in the support of the distribution — hardly central! By contrast, the posterior mean will sometimes be overly influenced by heavy tails (just as the sample mean $\bar{y}$ is often nonrobust against outlying observations). As a result, the posterior median will often be the best and safest point estimate. In the days prior to MCMC integration, it was also the most difficult to compute, but this difficulty has now been mitigated; see Section 2.3.

2.2.2 Interval estimation

The posterior allows us to make direct probability statements about not just its median, but any quantile. For example, suppose we can find the $\alpha/2$- and $(1 - \alpha/2)$-quantiles of $p(\theta|\mathbf{y})$, that is, the points q_L and q_U such that

$$\int_{-\infty}^{q_L} p(\theta|\mathbf{y})d\theta = \alpha/2 \ \text{ and } \ \int_{q_U}^{\infty} p(\theta|\mathbf{y})d\theta = \alpha/2 \ .$$

Then clearly $P(q_L < \theta < q_U|\mathbf{y}) = 1 - \alpha$; our confidence that θ lies in (q_L, q_U) is $100 \times (1 - \alpha)\%$. Thus this interval is a $100 \times (1 - \alpha)\%$ *credible set* (or simply *Bayesian confidence interval*) for θ. This interval is relatively easy to compute, and enjoys a direct interpretation ("the probability that θ lies in (q_L, q_U) is $(1 - \alpha)$") that the usual frequentist interval does not.

The interval just described is often called the *equal tail* credible set, for the obvious reason that it is obtained by chopping an equal amount of support $(\alpha/2)$ off the top and bottom of $p(\theta|\mathbf{y})$. Note that for symmetric unimodal posteriors, this equal tail interval will be symmetric about this mode (which we recall equals the mean and median in this case). It will also be optimal in the sense that it will have shortest length among sets C satisfying

$$1 - \alpha \leq P(C|\mathbf{y}) = \int_C p(\theta|\mathbf{y})d\theta \ . \tag{2.5}$$

Note that any such set C could be thought of as a $100 \times (1 - \alpha)\%$ credible set for θ. For posteriors that are not symmetric and unimodal, a better (shorter) credible set can be obtained by taking only those values of θ having posterior density greater than some cutoff $k(\alpha)$, where this cutoff is chosen to be as large as possible while C still satisfies equation (2.5). This *highest posterior density* (HPD) confidence set will always be of optimal length, but will typically be significantly more difficult to compute. The equal tail interval emerges as HPD in the symmetric unimodal case since there too it captures the "most likely" values of θ. Fortunately, many of the posteriors we will be interested in will be (at least approximately) symmetric unimodal, so the much simpler equal tail interval will often suffice. This is due to the following theorem:

Theorem 2.1 *(the "Bayesian Central Limit Theorem")*. Suppose that the data $X_1, \ldots, X_n \overset{\text{iid}}{\sim} f_i(x_i|\boldsymbol{\theta})$, and thus $f(\mathbf{x}|\boldsymbol{\theta}) = \prod_{i=1}^{n} f_i(x_i|\boldsymbol{\theta})$. Suppose the prior $\pi(\boldsymbol{\theta})$ and $f(\mathbf{x}|\boldsymbol{\theta})$ are positive and twice differentiable near $\hat{\boldsymbol{\theta}}^{\pi}$, the posterior mode (or "generalized MLE") of $\boldsymbol{\theta}$, assumed to exist. Then under suitable regularity conditions, the posterior distribution $p(\boldsymbol{\theta}|\mathbf{x})$ for large n can be approximated by a normal distribution having mean equal to the posterior mode, and covariance matrix equal to minus the inverse Hessian (second derivative matrix) of the log posterior evaluated at the mode. This matrix is sometimes notated as $[I^{\pi}(\mathbf{x})]^{-1}$, since it is the "generalized" observed Fisher information matrix for $\boldsymbol{\theta}$. More specifically,

$$I_{ij}^{\pi}(\mathbf{x}) = -\left[\frac{\partial^2}{\partial \theta_i \partial \theta_j} \log\left(f(\mathbf{x}|\boldsymbol{\theta})\pi(\boldsymbol{\theta}) \right) \right]_{\boldsymbol{\theta}=\hat{\boldsymbol{\theta}}^{\pi}}.$$

Other forms of the normal approximation are occasionally used. For instance, if the prior is reasonably flat, we might ignore it in the above calculations. This in effect replaces the posterior mode $\hat{\theta}^{\pi}$ by the MLE $\hat{\theta}$, and the generalized observed Fisher information matrix by the usual observed Fisher information matrix, $\hat{I}(\mathbf{x})$, where

$$
\begin{aligned}
\hat{I}_{ij}(x) &= -\left[\frac{\partial^2}{\partial \theta_i \partial \theta_j} \log f(\mathbf{x}|\boldsymbol{\theta}) \right]_{\boldsymbol{\theta}=\hat{\boldsymbol{\theta}}} \\
&= -\sum_{l=1}^{n} \left[\frac{\partial^2}{\partial \theta_i \partial \theta_j} \log f(x_l|\boldsymbol{\theta}) \right]_{\boldsymbol{\theta}=\hat{\boldsymbol{\theta}}}.
\end{aligned}
$$

■

The moniker "Bayesian Central Limit Theorem" appears to come from the fact that the theorem shows the posterior to be approximately normal for large sample sizes, just as the "regular" Central Limit Theorem provides approximate normality for frequentist test statistics in large samples. A general proof of the theorem requires only multivariate Taylor expansions; an outline in the unidimensional case is provided by Carlin and Louis (2009, p.109). The use of this theorem in Bayesian practice has diminished in the past few years, due to concerns about the quality of the approximation combined with the increasing ease of exact solutions implemented via MCMC. Still, the theorem provides a justification for the use of equal-tail credible intervals in most standard problems, and may also provide good starting values for MCMC algorithms in challenging settings.

2.2.3 Hypothesis testing and model choice

Hypothesis testing is perhaps the bedrock statistical technique in the analysis of clinical trials, and dates back to the celebrated foundational 1930s work of Jerzy Neyman and Egon Pearson (son of Karl, the founder of the journal *Biometrika* and developer of the chi-squared test and other fundamental methods for the analysis of 2×2 tables). As everyone reading this far into this text is no doubt aware, the basic setup compares two hypotheses,

$$H_0 : \theta = \theta_0 \text{ versus } H_A : \theta \neq \theta_0 .$$

Here, note that H_0 is the *null* hypothesis, and is the one our trial typically hopes to reject (since θ_0 is usually taken as 0, the case of no treatment efficacy). As already illustrated in Example 1.1, the frequentist approach is to compute a test statistic, and check to see if it is "extreme" enough relative to a reference distribution determined by the statistical model under the null hypothesis. Despite his famous and lifelong disagreement with Neyman, Fisher himself contributed to the effort by developing the *p-value*,

$$p = P\{T(\mathbf{Y}) \text{ more "extreme" than } T(\mathbf{y}_{obs}) \mid \boldsymbol{\theta}, H_0\} , \qquad (2.6)$$

where "extremeness" is in the direction of the alternative hypothesis. If the p-value is less than some prespecified Type I error rate α, H_0 is rejected; otherwise, it is not.

While Bayesians generally embrace Fisher's concept of likelihood, they also abhor p-values for a variety of reasons. Some of these are purely practical. For one thing, note the setup is asymmetric in the sense that H_0 can never be *accepted*, only rejected. While this is the usual goal, in the case of *equivalence testing* it is the alternative we actually hope to reject. This forces the frequentist into an awkward restructuring of the entire decision problem; see Section 6.2. Another practical problem with frequentist hypothesis testing is that the null hypothesis must be a "reduction" (special case) of the alternative; the hypotheses must be *nested*. But it is easy to imagine our interest lying in a comparison of nonnested hypotheses like

$$H_0 : \theta < \theta_0 \text{ versus } H_A : \theta \geq \theta_0 ,$$

or perhaps even nonnested models (quadratic versus exponential) or distributional (normal versus logistic) alternatives. Yet another practical difficulty (and one already mentioned in Example 1.1) is the common misinterpretation of the p-value by nonstatisticians (and even by many statisticians!) as the "probability that the null hypothesis is true," a misinterpretation reinforced by the fact that null hypotheses are rejected when p-values are small. But in fact only Bayesians can make claims about the probability that *any* hypothesis is true (or false), since only Bayesians admit that unknown model characteristics have distributions!

While these practical difficulties are enough to make one rethink the use of p-values in science, a much more fundamental difficulty is their violation of something called the *Likelihood Principle*. Originally postulated by Birnbaum (1962), its brief statement is as follows:

> **The Likelihood Principle:** In making inferences or decisions about θ after **y** is observed, all relevant experimental information is contained in the likelihood function for the observed **y**.

By taking into account not only the observed data **y**, but also the *unobserved* (but more extreme) values of **Y**, classical hypothesis testing violates the Likelihood Principle. This has great relevance for the practice of clinical trials since it effectively precludes the frequentist from "peeking" at the data as it accumulates. This is because additional looks at the data change the definition of "as extreme as the observed value or more so" in (2.6), and thus the p-value. But altering our decision regarding the efficacy of a drug or device simply because we decided to peek at the data an extra time is a clear violation of the Likelihood Principle; surely only the accumulating data itself should drive our decision here, not how many times we look at it or what might have happened had we stopped the experiment in a different way. The debate over the proper handling of this *multiplicity* problem is ongoing; c.f. Example 2.6 in Subsection 2.2.7, as well as the much fuller discussion and possible Bayesian remedies in Section 6.3.

We have seen that Bayesian inference (point or interval) is quite straightforward given the posterior distribution, or an estimate thereof. By contrast, hypothesis testing is less straightforward, for two reasons. First, there is less agreement among Bayesians as to the proper approach to the problem. For years, posterior probabilities and Bayes factors were considered the only appropriate method. But these methods are only suitable with fully proper priors, and for relatively low-dimensional models. With the recent proliferation of very complex models with at least partly improper priors, other methods have come to the fore. Second, solutions to hypothesis testing questions often involve not just the posterior $p(\theta|\mathbf{y})$, but also the *marginal* distribution, $p(\mathbf{y})$. Unlike the case of posterior and the predictive distributions, samples from the marginal distribution do not naturally emerge from most MCMC algorithms. Thus, the sampler must often be "tricked" into producing the necessary samples.

Recently, an approximate yet very easy-to-use model choice tool known as the Deviance Information Criterion (DIC) has gained popularity, as well as implementation in the `WinBUGS` software package. We will limit our attention in this subsection to Bayes factors and the DIC. The reader is referred to Carlin and Louis (2009, Sections 2.3.3 and 4.4–4.6) for further techniques and information, as well as a related posterior predictive criterion proposed by Gelfand and Ghosh (1998).

Bayes factors

We begin by setting up the hypothesis testing problem as a model choice problem, replacing the customary two hypotheses H_0 and H_A by two candidate parametric models M_1 and M_2 having respective parameter vectors $\boldsymbol{\theta}_1$ and $\boldsymbol{\theta}_2$. Under prior densities $\pi_i(\boldsymbol{\theta}_i)$, $i = 1, 2$, the marginal distributions of $\mathbf{Y}$ are found by integrating out the parameters,

$$p(\mathbf{y}|M_i) = \int f(\mathbf{y}|\boldsymbol{\theta}_i, M_i)\pi_i(\boldsymbol{\theta}_i)d\boldsymbol{\theta}_i \ , \ i = 1, 2 \ . \tag{2.7}$$

Bayes' Theorem (2.1) may then be applied to obtain the posterior probabilities $P(M_1|\mathbf{y})$ and $P(M_2|\mathbf{y}) = 1 - P(M_1|\mathbf{y})$ for the two models. The quantity commonly used to summarize these results is the *Bayes factor*, BF, which is the ratio of the posterior odds of M_1 to the prior odds of M_1, given by Bayes' Theorem as

$$BF \ = \ \frac{P(M_1|\mathbf{y})/P(M_2|\mathbf{y})}{P(M_1)/P(M_2)} \tag{2.8}$$

$$= \ \frac{\left[\frac{p(\mathbf{y}|M_1)P(M_1)}{p(\mathbf{y})}\right] / \left[\frac{p(\mathbf{y}|M_2)P(M_2)}{p(\mathbf{y})}\right]}{P(M_1)/P(M_2)}$$

$$= \ \frac{p(\mathbf{y} \mid M_1)}{p(\mathbf{y} \mid M_2)} \ , \tag{2.9}$$

the ratio of the observed marginal densities for the two models. Assuming the two models are *a priori* equally probable (i.e., $P(M_1) = P(M_2) = 0.5$), we have that $BF = P(M_1|\mathbf{y})/P(M_2|\mathbf{y})$, the posterior odds of M_1.

Consider the case where both models share the same parametrization (i.e., $\boldsymbol{\theta}_1 = \boldsymbol{\theta}_2 = \boldsymbol{\theta}$), and both hypotheses are simple (i.e., $M_1 : \boldsymbol{\theta} = \boldsymbol{\theta}^{(1)}$ and $M_2 : \boldsymbol{\theta} = \boldsymbol{\theta}^{(2)}$). Then $\pi_i(\boldsymbol{\theta})$ consists of a point mass at $\boldsymbol{\theta}^{(i)}$ for $i = 1, 2$, and so from (2.7) and (2.9) we have

$$BF = \frac{f(\mathbf{y}|\boldsymbol{\theta}^{(1)})}{f(\mathbf{y}|\boldsymbol{\theta}^{(2)})} \ ,$$

which is nothing but the likelihood ratio between the two models. Hence, in the simple-versus-simple setting, the Bayes factor is precisely the odds in favor of M_1 over M_2 *given solely by the data.*

A popular "shortcut" method is the *Bayesian Information Criterion* (BIC), also known as the *Schwarz criterion*, the change in which across the two models is given by

$$\Delta BIC = W - (p_2 - p_1) \log n \ , \tag{2.10}$$

where p_i is the number of parameters in model $M_i, i = 1, 2$, and

$$W = -2 \log \left[\frac{\sup_{M_1} f(\mathbf{y}|\boldsymbol{\theta})}{\sup_{M_2} f(\mathbf{y}|\boldsymbol{\theta})} \right] ,$$

the usual likelihood ratio test statistic. Schwarz (1978) showed that for nonhierarchical (two-stage) models and large sample sizes n, BIC approximates $-2 \log BF$. An alternative to BIC is the *Akaike Information Criterion* (AIC), which alters (2.10) slightly to

$$\Delta AIC = W - 2(p_2 - p_1) . \tag{2.11}$$

Both AIC and BIC are *penalized likelihood ratio* model choice criteria, since both have second terms that act as a penalty, correcting for differences in size between the models (to see this, think of M_2 as the "full" model and M_1 as the "reduced" model).

   The more serious (and aforementioned) limitation in using Bayes factors or their approximations is that they are not appropriate under noninformative priors. To see this, note that if $\pi_i(\boldsymbol{\theta}_i)$ is improper, then $p(\mathbf{y}|M_i) = \int f(\mathbf{y}|\boldsymbol{\theta}_i, M_i)\pi_i(\boldsymbol{\theta}_i)d\boldsymbol{\theta}_i$ necessarily is as well, and so BF as given in (2.9) is not well defined. While several authors (see, e.g., Berger and Pericchi, 1996; O'Hagan, 1995) have attempted to modify the definition of BF to repair this deficiency, we prefer the more informal yet still general approach we now describe.

The DIC criterion

Spiegelhalter et al. (2002) propose a generalization of the AIC, whose asymptotic justification is not appropriate for hierarchical (3 or more level) models. The generalization is based on the posterior distribution of the *deviance* statistic,

$$D(\boldsymbol{\theta}) = -2 \log f(\mathbf{y}|\boldsymbol{\theta}) + 2 \log h(\mathbf{y}) , \tag{2.12}$$

where $f(\mathbf{y}|\boldsymbol{\theta})$ is the likelihood function and $h(\mathbf{y})$ is some standardizing function of the data alone. These authors suggest summarizing the *fit* of a model by the posterior expectation of the deviance, $\overline{D} = E_{\theta|y}[D]$, and the *complexity* of a model by the effective number of parameters p_D (which may well be less than the total number of model parameters, due to the borrowing of strength across random effects). In the case of Gaussian models, one can show that a reasonable definition of p_D is the expected deviance minus the deviance evaluated at the posterior expectations,

$$p_D = E_{\theta|y}[D] - D(E_{\theta|y}[\boldsymbol{\theta}]) = \overline{D} - D(\bar{\boldsymbol{\theta}}) . \tag{2.13}$$

The *Deviance Information Criterion* (DIC) is then defined as

$$DIC = \overline{D} + p_D = 2\overline{D} - D(\bar{\boldsymbol{\theta}}) , \tag{2.14}$$

with smaller values of DIC indicating a better-fitting model. Both building blocks of DIC and p_D, $E_{\theta|y}[D]$ and $D(E_{\theta|y}[\theta])$, are easily estimated via MCMC methods (see below), enhancing the approach's appeal. Indeed, DIC may be computed automatically for any model in WinBUGS.

Although the p_D portion of this expression has meaning in its own right as an effective model size, DIC itself does not, since it has no absolute scale (due to the arbitrariness of the scaling constant $h(\mathbf{y})$, which is often simply set equal to zero). Thus only *differences* in DIC across models are meaningful. Relatedly, when DIC is used to compare nested models in standard exponential family settings, the unnormalized likelihood $L(\boldsymbol{\theta}; \mathbf{y})$ is often used in place of the normalized form $f(\mathbf{y}|\boldsymbol{\theta})$ in (2.12), since in this case the normalizing function $m(\boldsymbol{\theta}) = \int L(\boldsymbol{\theta}; \mathbf{y})d\mathbf{y}$ will be free of $\boldsymbol{\theta}$ and constant across models, hence contribute equally to the DIC scores of each (and thus have no impact on model selection). However, in settings where we require comparisons across different likelihood distributional forms, generally we must be careful to use the properly scaled joint density $f(\mathbf{y}|\boldsymbol{\theta})$ for each model.

Identification of what constitutes a *significant* difference is also somewhat subjective. Spiegelhalter et al. (2002) state that a DIC difference of 5 or 10 is typically thought of as "the smallest worth mentioning." Regarding the Monte Carlo variance of DIC, an informal approach is simply to recompute DIC a few times using different random number seeds, to get a rough idea of the variability in the estimates. With a large number of independent DIC replicates $\{DIC_l, \, l = 1, \ldots, N\}$, one could of course estimate $Var(DIC)$ by its sample variance,

$$\widehat{Var}(DIC) = \frac{1}{N-1} \sum_{l=1}^{N} (DIC_l - \overline{DIC})^2 \, .$$

But in any case, DIC is not intended for formal identification of the "correct" model, but rather merely as a method of comparing a collection of alternative formulations (all of which may be incorrect). This informal outlook (and DIC's approximate nature in markedly nonnormal models) suggests informal measures of its variability will often be sufficient. The p_D statistic is also helpful in its own right, since how close it is to the actual parameter count provides information about how many parameters are actually "needed" to adequately explain the data. For instance, a relatively low p_D in a random effects model indicates the random effects are greatly "shrunk" back toward their grand mean, possibly so much so that they are not really needed in the model.

DIC is remarkably general, and trivially computed as part of an MCMC run without any need for extra sampling, reprogramming, or complicated loss function determination. Moreover, experience with DIC to date suggests it works remarkably well, despite the fact that no formal justification for it is yet available outside of posteriors that can be well approximated by a Gaussian distribution (a condition that typically occurs asymptotically, but perhaps not without a moderate to large sample size for many models). Still, DIC is by no means universally accepted by Bayesians as a suitable all-purpose model choice tool, as the discussion to Spiegelhalter et al. (2002) almost immediately indicates. Model comparison using DIC is not invariant to parametrization, so (as with prior elicitation) the most sensible parametrization must be carefully chosen beforehand. Unknown scale parameters and other innocuous restructuring of the model can also lead to subtle changes in the computed DIC value.

Finally, DIC will obviously depend on what part of the model specification is considered to be part of the likelihood, and what is not. Spiegelhalter et al. (2002) refer to this as the *focus* issue, i.e., determining which parameters are of primary interest, and which should "count" in p_D. For instance, in a hierarchical model with data distribution $f(\mathbf{y}|\boldsymbol{\theta})$, prior $p(\boldsymbol{\theta}|\eta)$ and hyperprior $p(\eta)$, one might choose as the likelihood either the obvious conditional expression $f(\mathbf{y}|\boldsymbol{\theta})$, or the *marginal* expression,

$$p(\mathbf{y}|\eta) = \int f(\mathbf{y}|\boldsymbol{\theta})p(\boldsymbol{\theta}|\eta)d\boldsymbol{\theta} \ . \tag{2.15}$$

We refer to the former case as "focused on $\boldsymbol{\theta}$," and the latter case as "focused on η." Spiegelhalter et al. (2002) defend the dependence of p_D and DIC on the choice of focus as perfectly natural, since while the two foci give rise to the same marginal density $p(\mathbf{y})$, the integration in (2.15) clearly suggests a different model complexity than the unintegrated version (having been integrated out, the θ parameters no longer "count" in the total). They thus argue that it is up to the user to think carefully about which parameters ought to be in focus before using DIC. Perhaps the one difficulty with this advice is that in cases where the integration in (2.15) is not possible in closed form, the unintegrated version is really the only feasible choice. Indeed, the DIC tool in WinBUGS *always* focuses on the lowest level parameters in a model (in order to sidestep the integration issue), even when the user intends otherwise. Our view is that this is really "not a bug but a feature" of WinBUGS, since we would nearly always want the effective parameter count to be relative to the total parameter burden, as this provides an idea of how much the random effects have shrunk back toward their (posterior) grand means.

2.2.4 Prediction

An advantage of the Bayesian approach is the ability to find probability distributions of as yet unobserved results. Consider the following example:

Example 2.4 A study reported by Freireich et al. (1963) was designed to evaluate the effectiveness of chemotherapeutic agent 6-mercaptopurine

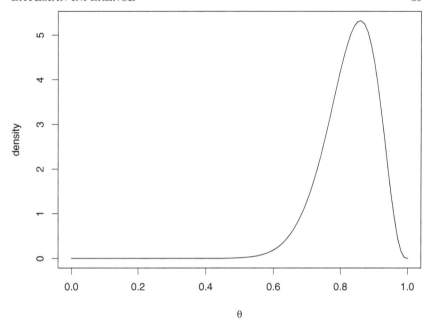

Figure 2.3 *Posterior density of θ, a Beta(19, 4).*

(6-MP) for the treatment of acute leukemia. Patients were randomized to therapy in pairs. Let θ be the population proportion of pairs in which the 6-MP patient stays in remission longer than the placebo patient. (To distinguish a probability θ from a probability *distribution* concerning θ, we will call it a population *proportion* or a *propensity*.) The null hypothesis is $H_0 : \theta = 1/2$, i.e., no effect of 6-MP. Let H_1 stand for the alternative, $H_1 : \theta \neq 1/2$. There were 21 pairs of patients in the study, and 18 of them favored 6-MP.

Suppose that the prior distribution is uniform on the interval $(0,1)$. The $Uniform(0, 1)$ distribution is also the $Beta(1, 1)$ distribution. Updating the $Beta(a, b)$ distribution after y successes and $n - y$ failures is easy because the beta prior is conjugate with the likelihood. As mentioned above, this means that the posterior distribution emerges as a member of the same distributional family as the prior. To see this in the beta-binomial case, from Bayes' Rule (2.1) we have

$$
\begin{aligned}
p(\theta|y) &\propto f(y|\theta)\pi(\theta) \\
&= \binom{n}{y}\theta^y(1-\theta)^{n-y} \times \frac{\Gamma(a+b)}{\Gamma(a)\Gamma(b)}\theta^{a-1}(1-\theta)^{b-1} \\
&\propto \theta^{y+a-1}(1-\theta)^{n-y+b-1} .
\end{aligned}
$$

Note in this last expression we have absorbed all multiplicative terms that do not involve θ into the unknown constant of proportionality. But now, we recognize this form as being proportional to a $Beta(y + a, n - y + b)$ density. Since this is the *only* density proportional to our form that still integrates to 1, this must be the posterior we are looking for. Thus, in our case ($y = 18$ and $n - y = 3$), the posterior distribution under H_1 is $Beta(19, 4)$, as plotted in Figure 2.3. Note this distribution is unimodal with mean $19/(19 + 4) = .8261$.

In the predictive context, suppose it is possible to take 5 additional observations. How useful would this be? A way to answer is to assess the consequences of getting k successes in the next 5 pairs of patients (for a total of 26 pairs in all) for $k = 0, 1, \ldots, 5$, and then to weigh these consequences by the predictive probabilities of the possible values of k.

To calculate the probabilities of future observations, we first find these probabilities assuming that the parameters are known, and also find the posterior (or current) distribution of the parameters. We then average the conditional distribution with respect to the posterior distribution of the parameters. This gives the unconditional predictive distribution of interest.

To illustrate, first consider a single additional, 22nd pair of patients, having binary outcome variable x_{22}. Assume that this pair is exchangeable with the first 21 pairs, $\mathbf{x} = (x_1, \ldots, x_{21})'$, for which $y = \sum_{i=1}^{21} x_i = 18$. One member of the new pair is assigned to 6-MP, and the other is assigned to placebo. The predictive probability that the 6-MP patient will stay in remission longer is the mean of the posterior distribution of θ. For the $Beta(19, 4)$ distribution considered separately, the predictive probability of success is given by *Laplace's Rule of Succession*: $19/(19+4) = 0.8261$ (Berry, 1996, Sec. 7.2). To prove this, note that the predictive distribution of x_{22} is

$$
f(x_{22}|\mathbf{x}) = \int f(x_{22}|\theta)p(\theta|\mathbf{x})d\theta
$$

$$
= \int \theta^{x_{22}}(1 - \theta)^{1-x_{22}} \frac{\Gamma(23)}{\Gamma(19)\Gamma(4)}\theta^{18}(1 - \theta)^3 d\theta .
$$

So the chance that the 22nd observation is a success ($x_{22} = 1$) is just

$$
P(x_{22} = 1|\mathbf{x}) = \int \frac{\Gamma(23)}{\Gamma(19)\Gamma(4)}\theta^{19}(1 - \theta)^3 d\theta
$$

$$
= \frac{\Gamma(23)}{\Gamma(19)\Gamma(4)} \frac{\Gamma(4)\Gamma(20)}{\Gamma(24)} \int \frac{\Gamma(24)}{\Gamma(20)\Gamma(4)}\theta^{19}(1 - \theta)^3 d\theta
$$

$$
= \frac{\Gamma(23)\Gamma(20)}{\Gamma(19)\Gamma(24)}
$$

$$
= \frac{19}{23} = .8261 ,
$$

the third equality arising since the "fixed up" integral equals 1, and the fourth arising since $\Gamma(z) = (z-1)\Gamma(z-1)$ for any z.

Now suppose that *two* more pairs of patients (both exchangeable with the first 21) are treated, one member of each pair with 6-MP and the other with placebo. The predictive probability of both being successes for 6-MP is not the square of 0.8261, but rather the probability of the first pair being a success times the probability of the second being a success *given* the result of the first. Using Laplace's Rule of Succession twice, we have

$$P(x_{22} = 1 \text{ and } x_{23} = 1 | \mathbf{x}) = P(x_{22} = 1 | \mathbf{x}) P(x_{23} = 1 | x_{22} = 1, \mathbf{x})$$
$$= \left(\frac{19}{23}\right)\left(\frac{20}{24}\right) = 0.6884 .$$

For 5 additional pairs, the predictive probability of 4 successes for 6-MP is

$$5 \left(\frac{22 \cdot 21 \cdot 20 \cdot 19 \cdot 4}{27 \cdot 26 \cdot 25 \cdot 24 \cdot 23}\right) = 0.3624 ,$$

the leading "5" arising since there are 5 possible orders in which the 4 successes could have arrived (SSSSF, SSSFS, ..., FSSSS), all of which lead to the same overall probability. Note that we could easily repeat this calculation for any number of successes and use the resulting table of probabilities in our decision regarding whether to stop the trial; see Chapters 3 and 4. ∎

2.2.5 Effect of the prior: sensitivity analysis

Bayes' Theorem makes it clear that the prior distribution influences the posterior distribution, and therefore it influences conclusions. This aspect of Bayesian analysis is regarded as negative by some. But the effect is positive in that it allows researchers and others to formally account for information that is available separate from the current experiment. Consider two people who come to markedly different conclusions from an experiment. Either they have been exposed to different additional information or they have processed the available evidence differently. In any case, we can infer that the experiment is not very informative. Edwards, Lindman, and Savage (1963) show that two reasonably open-minded people will eventually come to agree if both are exposed to the same data and both use Bayes' Theorem. The condition "reasonably open-minded" is meant to exclude people who "know" the answer in advance; if the two observers assign probability 1 to different values of a parameter, no amount of information will dissuade them from their original (and discordant) "knowledge."

Example 2.5 As an example showing that opinions tend to converge, consider control data presented by Smith, Spiegelhalter, and Parmar (1996): of 1934 patients in an intensive care unit, 566 developed respiratory tract infections. As seen in Example 2.4, for a $Beta(a, b)$ prior distribution, the

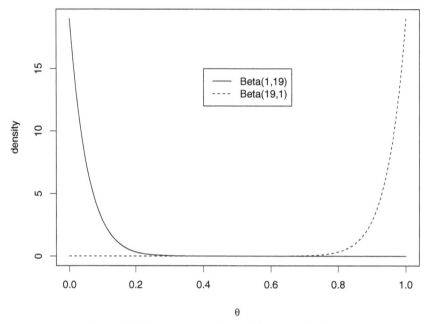

Figure 2.4 *Two rather different beta prior densities.*

posterior distribution for the probability θ of developing an infection is $Beta(a + 566, b + 1368)$. With such a large sample size, two people with prior opinions that are rather disparate would come to agree reasonably well. For example, suppose one person's (a, b) is (1,19) while the other's is (19,1) (as shown in Figure 2.4). Then the first's prior probability of infection is just 0.05, while the second's is a whopping 0.95. The first's posterior is $Beta(567, 1387)$ and the second's is $Beta(585, 1369)$, both of which are plotted in Figure 2.5. The corresponding predictive mean probabilities of infection are remarkably similar: 0.290 and 0.299. The prior probability that these two independent assessors are within 0.1 of each other is nearly 0, but the corresponding posterior probability is nearly 1. This demonstrates another feature of Bayesian methods: even investigators with wildly dissimilar prior beliefs can ultimately come to agreement once sufficient data have accumulated. ∎

2.2.6 Role of randomization

The random assignment of patients to either the treatment or control group in clinical trials is among the most important advances in the history of medical research. No other design gives a comparably high level of confidence in the trial's results. Randomization ensures that treatment assign-

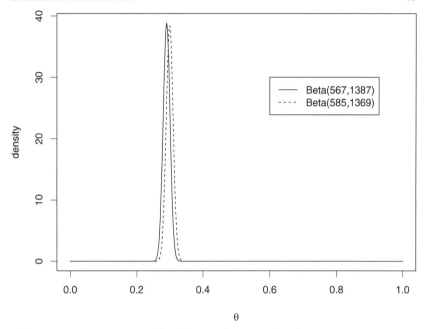

Figure 2.5 *Beta posterior distributions for prior distributions in Figure 2.4.*

ment is unbiased. In particular, randomization helps account for shifts in the patient population, changes in the standard of care, and competing treatment options over time. Without randomization, patient prognosis may be correlated with therapy assigned. While adjusting for covariates may help in parsing out treatment effect in a nonrandomized trial, the important covariates may not be known or assessable. A distinctly secondary advantage of randomization is that it serves to balance assignment among the various treatments, including within patient subgroups.

However, while randomization is a basis for frequentist inference, it plays no role in calculating posterior probabilities (except that a Bayesian may choose to discount data from nonrandomized trials as compared with randomized trials). This has led some Bayesians to suggest that randomization is not essential. We believe the ability to eliminate or minimize assignment bias makes randomization of utmost importance. If we could measure all the important covariates then randomization would not be necessary, but we cannot, or at least we cannot be sure that we know all the important covariates ahead of time.

That said, randomization in clinical trials has at least three disadvantages. First, physicians face ethical dilemmas in recommending a randomized trial to patients when their evaluation of the evidence is that the treatments are not equally effective and safe. Second, physicians worry that their relationship with patients will be adversely affected if they propose treatment by coin toss. Third, since not all patients and physicians are willing to participate in randomized trials, patients treated in a randomized trial may differ in important ways from those who might eventually be treated in a clinical setting with one of the competing treatments.

Examining clinical databases to compare therapeutic effects is wrought with bias. The major bias is the one solved by randomization: assignment to therapy may depend on prognosis. The Bayesian approach is ideal for analyzing such data because characteristics of the database – including the degree to which it is exchangeable with other databases and with data from clinical trials – can be assessed subjectively. Examples are discussed hereafter. To say that a Bayesian analysis is possible is not to say that the Bayesian approach makes up for imperfections in design. For some circumstances of poor data collection, the results can give no information about therapeutic comparisons *regardless* of the statistical approach.

2.2.7 Handling multiplicities

Multiplicities are among the most difficult of problems faced by statisticians and other researchers, and several types of multiplicities are discussed in this text, including metaanalysis, interim analysis, multiple comparisons, and subgroup analysis. Handling multiplicities is controversial in statistics and science. The standard frequentist approach is to condition on the null hypotheses of no effect in any of the comparisons or analyses, and this is the subject of much criticism (Carmer and Walker, 1982; O'Brien, 1983; Rothman, 1990). Some types of multiplicities (including metaanalysis, analysis of multicenter trials, and interim analysis) are not problematic for Bayesians. Other forms of multiplicities (including multiple comparisons, variable selection in regression, selecting transformations in regression, subset analyses, data dredging, and publication biases) are problematic for Bayesians as well as for frequentists.

Multiplicities are present in virtually every application of statistics. Most frequentist statisticians subscribe to the principle that adjustments in inferences must be made to account for multiplicities. A basic complaint against the frequentist attitude toward multiple comparisons is that it is inconsistent with what is perceived to be the scientific method, as the following simple example illustrates.

Example 2.6 Consider a scientist who collects data concerning the effectiveness of treatments A and B, and finds that the difference in treatment means is statistically significant, say based on a p-value of 0.03. Consider a second scientist who runs the same experiment except for the inclusion of a third treatment, treatment C, and on treatments A and B she obtains data identical to that of the first scientist. After adjusting for multiple comparisons the second scientist cannot claim statistical significance for the difference between treatments A and B. The second scientist ran a more informative experiment, yet is penalized for doing so by the increase in Type I error. This seems unscientific. To make matters worse, the second scientist may say that she had no intention of using the treatment C data for any inferential purpose; it was simply a control to ensure that the experiment was properly run. In this event, now she too can claim significance for treatment A vs. treatment B. Having conclusions depend on the mere *intentions* of the experimenter also seems unscientific. ∎

Conditioning on a null hypothesis is typically anathema to Bayesians. Therefore, the Bayesian approach seems to reject adjustments for multiple comparisons, and indeed this is the view of many Bayesians. However, Bayesian adjustments that are similar to frequentist adjustments are legitimate and appropriate in many applications; see e.g. Berry (1989), DuMouchel (1990), Gopalan and Berry (1997), or Berry and Hochberg (1999). Bayesian adjustments of posterior probabilities are similar to shrinkage adjustments mentioned above and will be discussed in Example 2.7. A distinction between the frequentist and Bayesian approaches is that, in the latter, the mere existence of a third treatment is irrelevant. Bayesian adjustments for comparing treatments A and B depend on the *results* that were actually observed on treatment C, as well as on A and B. An important caveat of posterior adjustment for multiplicities is that it is exactly that: only an adjustment of probabilities. But computation of posterior probabilities is only half the inference; the other half is making an actual decision (about rejecting H_0, etc.). For the latter, Bayesian inference is every bit as vulnerable to multiplicities as frequentist inference; see, for example, Berry and Berry (2004), as well as Section 6.3. In particular, Subsection 6.3.1 describes an extension of Berry and Berry (2004) and subsequent application to a real data set, while Subsection 6.3.2 further extends the thinking to the selection of significance thresholds in false discovery rate (FDR) estimation settings. Statistical adjustments necessary for realistic assessment of subgroup effects, discussed in Section 6.4, are also related to the multiplicity problem since they are often initially uncovered by "data dredging" after a trial fails to show a significant treatment effect in the overall patient population.

Rothman (1990) refers to the adoption of adjustments for multiple comparisons in the biomedical and social sciences as "half-hearted," and indeed it is. Rothman then concludes that such adjustments are never needed. As is clear from our foregoing comments, that is not our view. Science is subjective, and a standard adjustment for multiplicities is not possible. Sometimes adjustments are appropriate and sometimes they are not. When they *are* appropriate, the amount of adjustment depends on the available evidence, from both within and outside of the experiment in question. The lack of a consistent policy regarding adjustments in science may seem "half-hearted," but no routine policy is possible or desirable. Two scientists who analyze data from the same experiment may have different knowledge bases or they may interpret the available evidence differently. Statistical inference is not like calculating an amount of income tax owed: in our view, differences in conclusions from experimental results do not mean that one or both of the scientists' conclusions are wrong.

2.3 Bayesian computation

As mentioned above, in this section we provide a brief introduction to Bayesian computing, following the development in Chapter 3 of Carlin and Louis (2009). The explosion in Bayesian activity and computing power over the last decade or so has led to a similar explosion in the number of books in this area. The earliest comprehensive treatment was by Tanner (1998), with books by Gilks et al. (1996), Gamerman and Lopes (2006), and Chen et al. (2000) offering updated and expanded discussions that are primarily Bayesian in focus. Also significant are the computing books by Robert and Casella (2005) and Liu (2008), which, while not specifically Bayesian, still emphasize Markov chain Monte Carlo methods typically used in modern Bayesian analysis.

The presence of the integral in the denominator of Bayes' Theorem (2.1) means that, with a few exceptions, the history of real Bayesian data analysis goes back only as far as our ability to numerically evaluate integrals of dimension higher than 5 or 10 – that is, to the 1960s and 70s. In those days, most numerical integration routines did not use Monte Carlo methods, but rather more traditional *quadrature* methods. The most basic of these are the so-called *Newton-Cotes rules* that use a weighted sum of function values along a fixed partition in each dimension of the integrand. Examples of these rules include the trapezoidal and Simpson rules, familiar from elementary calculus textbooks since they are straightforward generalizations of the usual Riemann approximation to the integral. More complex rules, such as *Gaussian quadrature*, use fewer but irregularly spaced grid points, and can improve efficiency by strategically placing more function evaluations where the function is changing most dramatically.

While such approaches can be fast computationally, Bayesians largely abandoned them in the 1990s in favor of Monte Carlo integration for two reasons. First, quadrature methods suffer greatly from what numerical analysts call *the curse of dimensionality*, which essentially is the fact that the computational burden increases exponentially with the dimension of the integral. Since modern Bayesian data analysis often requires models with hundreds or even thousands of parameters, the curse often renders quadrature infeasible. Second, the tuning required to implement good quadrature methods is often rather high, compared to the Gibbs sampler and other Monte Carlo methods which (like the jackknife and the bootstrap) are often implemented straightforwardly by statisticians with relatively modest computing skills. Since the most prominent Bayesian software package, WinBUGS, also uses Monte Carlo methods, we focus on them throughout the rest of this section. However, we caution that quadrature methods still have a place in Bayesian clinical trials analysis, at least for those having relatively low-dimensional parameter spaces. In these settings, quadrature will be much more efficient, and thus possibly the best choice when simulating the operating characteristics of our procedures (see Subsection 2.5.4), a task that requires *repeated* integral evaluation over a large number of simulated data sets. Indeed, a simple normal approximation to the posterior (as provided by Theorem 2.1) will often suffice for such simulation studies; we provide examples in Chapters 3–5.

The current popularity of Markov chain Monte Carlo (MCMC) methods is due to their ability (in principle) to enable inference from posterior distributions of arbitrarily large dimension, essentially by reducing the problem to one of recursively solving a series of lower-dimensional (often unidimensional) problems. Like traditional Monte Carlo methods, MCMC methods work by producing not a closed form for the posterior in (2.1), but a *sample* of values $\{\boldsymbol{\theta}^{(g)}, g = 1, \ldots, G\}$ from this distribution. While this obviously does not carry as much information as the closed form itself, a histogram or kernel density estimate based on such a sample is typically sufficient for reliable inference; moreover such an estimate can be made arbitrarily accurate merely by increasing the Monte Carlo sample size G. However, unlike traditional Monte Carlo methods, MCMC algorithms produce *correlated* samples from this posterior, since they arise from recursive draws from a particular Markov chain, the stationary distribution of which is the same as the posterior.

The convergence of the Markov chain to the correct stationary distribution can be guaranteed for an enormously broad class of posteriors, explaining MCMC's popularity. But this convergence is also the source of most of the difficulty in actually implementing MCMC procedures, for two reasons. First, it forces us to make a decision about when it is safe to stop the sampling algorithm and summarize its output, an area known in the business as *convergence diagnosis*. Second, it clouds the determination of the quality of the estimates produced (since they are based not on i.i.d. draws from the posterior, but on correlated samples). This is sometimes called the *variance estimation* problem, since a common goal here is to estimate the Monte Carlo variances (equivalently standard errors) associated with our MCMC-based posterior estimates.

A great many useful MCMC algorithms have appeared in the last twenty or so years, many of which can offer significant advantages in certain specialized situations or model settings. For example, WinBUGS uses *slice sampling* (Neal, 2003) for nonconjugate settings over bounded parameter domains, partly because it turns out to be fairly natural here, and partly because these domains do not lend themselves to ordinary Metropolis sampling without transformation of the parameter space. Even more recent research has focused on *adaptive* MCMC methods (Haario et al., 2001; Roberts and Rosenthal, 2007) that attempt to accelerate convergence by using the early output of an MCMC chain to refine and improve the sampling as it progresses. In the remainder of this section, however, we restrict our attention to the two most popular and broadly applicable MCMC algorithms, the Gibbs sampler and the Metropolis-Hastings algorithm. We then return to the convergence diagnosis and variance estimation problems.

2.3.1 The Gibbs sampler

Suppose our model features k parameters, $\boldsymbol{\theta} = (\theta_1, \ldots, \theta_k)'$. To implement the Gibbs sampler, we must assume that samples can be generated from each of the *full* or *complete* conditional distributions $\{p(\theta_i \mid \boldsymbol{\theta}_{j \neq i}, \mathbf{y}), i = 1, \ldots, k\}$ in the model. Such samples might be available directly (say, if the full conditionals were familiar forms, like normals and gammas) or indirectly (say, via a rejection sampling approach). In this latter case two popular alternatives are the adaptive rejection sampling (ARS) algorithm of Gilks and Wild (1992), and the Metropolis algorithm described in the next subsection. In either case, under mild conditions, the collection of full conditional distributions uniquely determines the joint posterior distribution, $p(\boldsymbol{\theta}|\mathbf{y})$, and hence all marginal posterior distributions $p(\theta_i|\mathbf{y})$, $i = 1, \ldots, k$.

Given an arbitrary set of starting values $\{\theta_2^{(0)}, \ldots, \theta_k^{(0)}\}$, the algorithm proceeds as follows:

Algorithm 2.1 *(Gibbs Sampler)*.

For $(t \in 1 : T)$, repeat:

Step 1: Draw $\theta_1^{(t)}$ from $p\left(\theta_1 \mid \theta_2^{(t-1)}, \theta_3^{(t-1)}, \ldots, \theta_k^{(t-1)}, \mathbf{y}\right)$

Step 2: Draw $\theta_2^{(t)}$ from $p\left(\theta_2 \mid \theta_1^{(t)}, \theta_3^{(t-1)}, \ldots, \theta_k^{(t-1)}, \mathbf{y}\right)$

$$\vdots$$

Step k: Draw $\theta_k^{(t)}$ from $p\left(\theta_k \mid \theta_1^{(t)}, \theta_2^{(t)}, \ldots, \theta_{k-1}^{(t)}, \mathbf{y}\right)$

Then for t sufficiently large, $(\theta_1^{(t)}, \ldots, \theta_k^{(t)}) \overset{approx}{\sim} p(\theta_1, \ldots, \theta_k | \mathbf{y})$. ∎

The convergence of the k-tuple obtained at iteration t, $(\theta_1^{(t)}, \ldots, \theta_k^{(t)})$, to a draw from the true joint posterior distribution $p(\theta_1, \ldots, \theta_k | \mathbf{y})$ occurs under mild regulatory conditions that are generally satisified for most statistical models (see, e.g., Geman and Geman, 1984, or Roberts and Smith, 1993). This means that for t sufficiently large (say, bigger than t_0), $\{\boldsymbol{\theta}^{(t)}, t = t_0 + 1, \ldots, T\}$ is a (correlated) sample from the true posterior, from which any posterior quantities of interest may be estimated. For example, a histogram of the $\{\theta_i^{(t)}, \, t = t_0 + 1, \ldots, T\}$ themselves provides a simulation-consistent estimator of the marginal posterior distribution for θ_i, $p(\theta_i \,|\, \mathbf{y})$. We might also use a sample mean to estimate the posterior mean, i.e.,

$$\widehat{E}(\theta_i|\mathbf{y}) = \frac{1}{T - t_0} \sum_{t=t_0+1}^{T} \theta_i^{(t)} \, . \tag{2.16}$$

The time from $t = 0$ to $t = t_0$ is commonly known as the *burn-in* period; popular methods for selection of an appropriate t_0 are discussed below.

In practice, we may actually run m *parallel* Gibbs sampling chains, instead of only 1, for some modest m (say, $m = 3$). Parallel chains may be useful in assessing sampler convergence, and anyway can be produced with no extra time on a multiprocessor computer. In this case, we would again discard all samples from the burn-in period, obtaining the posterior mean estimate,

$$\widehat{E}(\theta_i|\mathbf{y}) = \frac{1}{m(T - t_0)} \sum_{j=1}^{m} \sum_{t=t_0+1}^{T} \theta_{i,j}^{(t)} \, , \tag{2.17}$$

where now the second subscript on $\theta_{i,j}$ indicates chain number. Again we defer comment on the issues of how to choose t_0 and how to assess the quality of (2.17) and related estimators to subsequent subsections.

2.3.2 The Metropolis-Hastings algorithm

The Gibbs sampler is easy to understand and implement, but requires the ability to readily sample from each of the full conditional distributions, $p(\theta_i \,|\, \boldsymbol{\theta}_{j \neq i}, \mathbf{y})$. Unfortunately, when the prior distribution $p(\boldsymbol{\theta})$ and the likelihood $f(\mathbf{y}|\boldsymbol{\theta})$ are not a conjugate pair, one or more of these full conditionals may not be available in closed form. Even in this setting, however, $p(\theta_i \,|\, \boldsymbol{\theta}_{j \neq i}, \mathbf{y})$ *will* be available up to a proportionality constant, since it is proportional to the portion of $f(\mathbf{y}|\boldsymbol{\theta}) \times p(\boldsymbol{\theta})$ that involves θ_i.

The *Metropolis algorithm* (or *Metropolis-Hastings algorithm*) is a rejection algorithm that attacks precisely this problem, since it requires only a function proportional to the distribution to be sampled, at the cost of requiring a rejection step from a particular *candidate* density. Like the Gibbs sampler, this algorithm was not developed by statistical data analysts for this purpose; the primary authors on the Metropolis et al. (1953) paper were computer scientists working on the Manhattan Project at Los Alamos National Laboratory in the 1940s.

While as mentioned above our main interest in the algorithm is for generation from (typically univariate) full conditionals, it is easily described (and theoretically supported) for the full multivariate $\boldsymbol{\theta}$ vector. Thus, suppose for now that we wish to generate from a joint posterior distribution

$p(\boldsymbol{\theta}|\mathbf{y}) \propto h(\boldsymbol{\theta}) \equiv f(\mathbf{y}|\boldsymbol{\theta})p(\boldsymbol{\theta})$. We begin by specifying a candidate density $q(\boldsymbol{\theta}^*|\boldsymbol{\theta}^{(t-1)})$ that is a valid density function for every possible value of the conditioning variable $\boldsymbol{\theta}^{(t-1)}$, and satisfies $q(\boldsymbol{\theta}^*|\boldsymbol{\theta}^{(t-1)}) = q(\boldsymbol{\theta}^{(t-1)}|\boldsymbol{\theta}^*)$, i.e., q is *symmetric* in its arguments. Given a starting value $\boldsymbol{\theta}^{(0)}$ at iteration $t = 0$, the algorithm proceeds as follows:

Algorithm 2.2 *(Metropolis Algorithm).*

  For $(t \in 1 : T)$, repeat:

  Step 1: Draw $\boldsymbol{\theta}^*$ from $q(\cdot|\boldsymbol{\theta}^{(t-1)})$

  Step 2: Compute the ratio $r = h(\boldsymbol{\theta}^*)/h(\boldsymbol{\theta}^{(t-1)}) = \exp[\log h(\boldsymbol{\theta}^*) - \log h(\boldsymbol{\theta}^{(t-1)})]$

  Step 3: If $r \geq 1$, set $\boldsymbol{\theta}^{(t)} = \boldsymbol{\theta}^*$;

  If $r < 1$, set $\boldsymbol{\theta}^{(t)} = \begin{cases} \boldsymbol{\theta}^* & \text{with probability } r \\ \boldsymbol{\theta}^{(t-1)} & \text{with probability } 1 - r \end{cases}$.

Then under generally the same mild conditions as those supporting the Gibbs sampler, $\boldsymbol{\theta}^{(t)} \overset{approx}{\sim} p(\boldsymbol{\theta}|\mathbf{y})$. ∎

Note that when the Metropolis algorithm (or the Metropolis-Hastings algorithm below) is used to update within a Gibbs sampler, it never samples from the full conditional distribution. Convergence using Metropolis steps, then, would be expected to be slower than that for a regular Gibbs sampler.

Recall that the steps of the Gibbs sampler were fully determined by the statistical model under consideration (since full conditional distributions for well-defined models are unique). By contrast, the Metropolis algorithm affords substantial flexibility through the selection of the candidate density q. This flexibility can be a blessing and a curse: while theoretically we are free to pick almost anything, in practice only a "good" choice will result in sufficiently many candidate acceptances. The usual approach (after $\boldsymbol{\theta}$ has been transformed to have support $\Re^k$, if necessary) is to set

$$q(\boldsymbol{\theta}^*|\boldsymbol{\theta}^{(t-1)}) = N(\boldsymbol{\theta}^*|\boldsymbol{\theta}^{(t-1)}, \widetilde{\Sigma}) , \tag{2.18}$$

since this distribution obviously satisfies the symmetry property, and is "self-correcting" (candidates are always centered around the current value of the chain). Specification of q then comes down to specification of $\widetilde{\Sigma}$. Here we might try to mimic the posterior variance by setting $\widetilde{\Sigma}$ equal to an empirical estimate of the true posterior variance, derived from a preliminary sampling run.

The reader might well imagine an optimal choice of q would produce an empirical acceptance ratio of 1, the same as the Gibbs sampler (and with no apparent "waste" of candidates). However, the issue is rather more subtle than this: accepting all or nearly all of the candidates is often the result of an overly narrow candidate density. Such a density will "baby-step" around the parameter space, leading to high acceptance but also high autocorrelation in the sampled chain. An overly wide candidate density will also struggle, proposing leaps to places far from the bulk of the posterior's support, leading to high rejection and, again, high autocorrelation. Thus the "folklore" here is to choose $\widetilde{\Sigma}$ so that roughly 50% of the candidates are accepted. Subsequent theoretical work (e.g., Gelman et al., 1996) indicates even lower acceptance rates (25 to 40%) are optimal, but this result varies with the dimension and true posterior correlation structure of $\boldsymbol{\theta}$.

As a result, the choice of $\widetilde{\Sigma}$ is often done adaptively. For instance, in one dimension (setting $\widetilde{\Sigma} = \widetilde{\sigma}$, and thus avoiding the issue of correlations among the elements of $\boldsymbol{\theta}$), a common trick is to simply pick some initial value of $\widetilde{\sigma}$, and then keep track of the empirical proportion of candidates that are accepted. If this fraction is too high (75 to 100%), we simply increase $\widetilde{\sigma}$; if it is too low (0 to 20%), we decrease it. Since certain kinds of adaptation can actually disturb the chain's convergence to its stationary distribution, the simplest approach is to allow this adaptation only during the burn-in period, a practice sometimes referred to as *pilot adaptation*. This is in fact the approach currently used by WinBUGS, where the default pilot period is 4000 iterations.

As mentioned above, in practice the Metropolis algorithm is often found as a substep in a larger Gibbs sampling algorithm, used to generate from awkward full conditionals. Such hybrid Gibbs-Metropolis applications were once known as "Metropolis within Gibbs" or "Metropolis substeps," and users would worry about how many such substeps should be used. Fortunately, it was soon realized that a single substep was sufficient to ensure convergence of the overall algorithm, and so this is now standard practice: when we encounter an awkward full conditional (say, for θ_i), we simply draw one Metropolis candidate, accept or reject it, and move on to θ_{i+1}. Further discussion of convergence properties and implementation of hybrid MCMC algorithms can be found in Tierney (1994) and Carlin and Louis (2009, Sec. 3.4.4).

We end this subsection with the important generalization of the Metropolis algorithm devised by Hastings (1970). In this variant we drop the requirement that q be symmetric in its arguments, which is often useful for bounded parameter spaces (say, $\theta > 0$) where Gaussian proposals as in (2.18) are not natural.

Algorithm 2.3 *(Metropolis-Hastings Algorithm).*

In **Step 2** of the Metropolis algorithm, replace the acceptance ratio r by

$$r = \frac{h(\boldsymbol{\theta}^*)q(\boldsymbol{\theta}^{(t-1)} \mid \boldsymbol{\theta}^*)}{h(\boldsymbol{\theta}^{(t-1)})q(\boldsymbol{\theta}^* \mid \boldsymbol{\theta}^{(t-1)})} . \qquad (2.19)$$

Then again under mild conditions, $\boldsymbol{\theta}^{(t)} \overset{approx}{\sim} p(\boldsymbol{\theta}|\mathbf{y})$ ∎

In practice we sometimes set $q(\boldsymbol{\theta}^* \mid \boldsymbol{\theta}^{(t-1)}) = q(\boldsymbol{\theta}^*)$, i.e., we use a proposal density that ignores the current value of the variable. This algorithm is sometimes referred to as a *Hastings independence chain*, so named because the proposals (though not the final $\boldsymbol{\theta}^{(t)}$ values) form an independent sequence. While easy to implement, this algorithm can be difficult to tune since it will converge slowly unless the chosen q is rather close to the true posterior (which is of course unknown in advance).

2.3.3 Convergence diagnosis

The most problematic part of MCMC computation is deciding when it is safe to stop the algorithm and summarize the output. This means we must make a guess as to the iteration t_0 after which all output may be thought of as coming from the true stationary distribution of the Markov chain (i.e., the true posterior distribution). The most common approach here is to run a few (say, $m = 3$ or 5) *parallel* sampling chains, initialized at widely disparate starting locations that are overdispersed with respect to the true posterior. These chains are then plotted on a common set of axes, and these *trace plots* are then viewed to see if there is an identifiable point t_0 after which all m chains seem to be "overlapping" (traversing the same part of the $\boldsymbol{\theta}$-space).

Sadly, there are obvious problems with this approach. First, since the posterior is unknown at the outset, there is no reliable way to ensure that the m chains are "initially overdispersed," as required for a convincing diagnostic. We might use extreme quantiles of the prior $p(\boldsymbol{\theta})$ and rely on the fact that the support of the posterior is typically a subset of that of the prior, but this requires a proper prior and in any event is perhaps doubtful in high-dimensional or otherwise difficult problems. Second, it is hard to see how to automate such a diagnosis procedure, since it requires a subjective judgment call by a human viewer. A great many papers have been written on various convergence diagnostic statistics that summarize MCMC output from one or many chains that may be useful when associated with various stopping rules; see Cowles and Carlin (1996) and Mengersen et al. (1999) for reviews of many such diagnostics.

Among the most popular diagnostic is that of Gelman and Rubin (1992). Here, we run a small number (m) of parallel chains with different starting points thought to be initially overdispersed with respect to the true posterior. (Of course, before beginning there is technically no way to ensure this; still, the rough location of the bulk of the posterior may be discernible from known ranges, the support of the (proper) prior, or perhaps a preliminary posterior mode-finding algorithm.) The diagnostic is then based on a comparison of the variance between the m chains and the variance within them, two quantities that should be comparable if the chains are in rough agreement regarding the location of the posterior. This approach is fairly intuitive and is applicable to output from any MCMC algorithm. However, it focuses only on detecting bias in the MCMC estimator; no information about the *accuracy* of the resulting posterior estimate is produced. It is also an inherently univariate quantity, meaning it must be applied to each parameter (or parametric function) of interest in turn, although Brooks and Gelman (1998) extend the Gelman and Rubin approach in three important ways, one of which is a multivariate generalization for simultaneous convergence diagnosis of every parameter in a model.

While the Gelman-Rubin-Brooks and other formal diagnostic approaches remain popular, in practice very simple checks often work just as well and may even be more robust against "pathologies" (e.g., multiple modes) in the posterior surface that may easily fool some diagnostics. For instance, sample autocorrelations in any of the observed chains can inform about whether slow traversing of the posterior surface is likely to impede convergence. Sample cross-correlations (i.e., correlations between two different parameters in the model) may identify ridges in the surface (say, due to collinearity between two predictors) that will again slow convergence; such parameters may need to be updated in multivariate blocks, or one of the parameters may need to be dropped from the model altogether. Combined with a visual inspection of a few sample trace plots, the user can at least get a good feeling for whether posterior estimates produced by the sampler are likely to be reliable.

2.3.4 Variance estimation

An obvious criticism of Monte Carlo methods generally is that no two analysts will obtain the same answer, since the components of the estimator are random. This makes assessment of the variance of these estimators crucial. Combined with a central limit theorem, the result would be an ability to test whether two Monte Carlo estimates were significantly different. For example, suppose we have a single chain of N post-burn-in samples of a parameter of interest λ, so that our basic posterior mean estimator (2.16) becomes $\hat{E}(\lambda|\mathbf{y}) = \hat{\lambda}_N = \frac{1}{N} \sum_{t=1}^{N} \lambda^{(t)}$. Assuming the samples comprising this estimator are independent, a variance estimate for it would be given by

$$\widehat{Var}_{iid}(\hat{\lambda}_N) = s_\lambda^2/N = \frac{1}{N(N-1)} \sum_{t=1}^{N} (\lambda^{(t)} - \hat{\lambda}_N)^2 , \qquad (2.20)$$

i.e., the sample variance, $s_\lambda^2 = \frac{1}{N-1} \sum_{t=1}^{N} (\lambda^{(t)} - \hat{\lambda}_N)^2$, divided by N. But while this estimate is easy to compute, it would very likely be an *underestimate* due to positive autocorrelation in the MCMC samples. One can resort to *thinning*, which is simply retaining only every kth sampled value, where k is the approximate lag at which the autocorrelations in the chain become insignificant. However, MacEachern and Berliner (1994) show that such thinning from a stationary Markov chain always increases the variance of sample mean estimators, and is thus suboptimal. This is intuitively reminiscent of Fisher's view of sufficiency: it is never a good idea to throw away information (in this case, $(k-1)/k$ of our MCMC samples) just to achieve approximate independence among those that remain.

A better alternative is to use all the samples, but in a more sophisticated way. One such alternative uses the notion of *effective sample size*, or *ESS* (Kass et al. 1998, p. 99). *ESS* is defined as

$$ESS = N/\kappa(\lambda) \, ,$$

where $\kappa(\lambda)$ is the *autocorrelation time* for λ, given by

$$\kappa(\lambda) = 1 + 2 \sum_{k=1}^{\infty} \rho_k(\lambda) \, , \tag{2.21}$$

where $\rho_k(\lambda)$ is the autocorrelation at lag k for the parameter of interest λ. We may estimate $\kappa(\lambda)$ using sample autocorrelations estimated from the MCMC chain. The variance estimate for $\hat{\lambda}_N$ is then

$$\widehat{Var}_{ESS}(\hat{\lambda}_N) = s_{\lambda}^2/ESS(\lambda) = \frac{\kappa(\lambda)}{N(N-1)} \sum_{t=1}^{N} (\lambda^{(t)} - \hat{\lambda}_N)^2 \, .$$

Note that unless the $\lambda^{(t)}$ are uncorrelated, $\kappa(\lambda) > 1$ and $ESS(\lambda) < N$, so that $\widehat{Var}_{ESS}(\hat{\lambda}_N) > \widehat{Var}_{iid}(\hat{\lambda}_N)$, in concert with intuition. That is, since we have fewer than N effective samples, we expect some inflation in the variance of our estimate.

In practice, the autocorrelation time $\kappa(\lambda)$ in (2.21) is often estimated simply by cutting off the summation when the magnitude of the terms first drops below some "small" value (say, 0.1). This procedure is simple but may lead to a biased estimate of $\kappa(\lambda)$. Gilks et al. (1996, pp. 50–51) recommend an *initial convex sequence estimator* mentioned by Geyer (1992) which, while still output-dependent and slightly more complicated, actually yields a consistent (asymptotically unbiased) estimate here.

A final and somewhat simpler (though also more naive) method of estimating $Var(\hat{\lambda}_N)$ is through *batching*. Here we divide our single long run of length N into m successive batches of length k (i.e., $N = mk$), with batch means $B_1, \ldots, B_m$. Clearly $\hat{\lambda}_N = \bar{B} = \frac{1}{m} \sum_{i=1}^{m} B_i$. We then have the variance estimate

$$\widehat{Var}_{batch}(\hat{\lambda}_N) = \frac{1}{m(m-1)} \sum_{i=1}^{m} (B_i - \hat{\lambda}_N)^2 \, , \tag{2.22}$$

provided that k is large enough so that the correlation between batches is negligible, and m is large enough to reliably estimate $Var(B_i)$. It is important to verify that the batch means are indeed roughly independent, say, by checking whether the lag 1 autocorrelation of the B_i is less than 0.1. If this is not the case, we must increase k (hence N, unless the current m is already quite large), and repeat the procedure.

Regardless of which of these estimates $\hat{V}$ is used to approximate $Var(\hat{\lambda}_N)$, a 95% confidence interval for $E(\lambda|\mathbf{y})$ is then given by

$$\hat{\lambda}_N \pm z_{.025}\sqrt{\hat{V}} \, ,$$

where $z_{.025} = 1.96$, the upper .025 point of a standard normal distribution. If the batching method is used with fewer than 30 batches, it is a good idea to replace $z_{.025}$ by $t_{m-1,.025}$, the upper .025 point of a t distribution with $m - 1$ degrees of freedom. `WinBUGS` offers both naive (2.20) and batched (2.22) variance estimates; this software is illustrated in the next section.

2.4 Hierarchical modeling and metaanalysis

This section has two purposes. One is to introduce the notions and methodologies of hierarchical modeling. Another is to give a rather detailed development of metaanalysis (Berry and Stangl, 2000) as an application of this methodology. The larger ideas of hierarchical modeling are developed in the context of this application. Other applications include the analysis of multicenter trials, multiple comparisons, variable selection in regression, subgroup or subset analyses, and pharmacokinetic modeling; see e.g. Section 4.5.

Metaanalysis is a single analysis of multiple studies. Different studies have different results. One reason is random variation. Other differences are inherent: different studies deal with different types of patients and different types of controls, they take place at different times and locations, etc. For example, some institutions may study healthier populations than others. But even when patient eligibility criteria are identical in two studies, the respective investigators may apply the criteria differently. For example, for two studies involving a particular device, both sets of eligibility criteria may include patients who have a left ventricular ejection fraction (LVEF) as low as 25%. However, one investigator may admit essentially every candidate patient who meets this criterion, while another worries that some patients with LVEF lower than 35% may be at unusual or unnecessary risk if treated with the experimental device. Therefore, the patients in the first study will tend to have a higher degree of heart failure, and the overall results in the first study may suggest that the device is less effective than in the second. Since LVEF is a rather obvious covariate, this circumstance is easy to address by accounting for LVEF in the analysis (Bayesian or frequentist). But there may be important covariates that differ in the two studies that have not been measured.

It is not uncommon for different studies to evince different treatment effects. Sometimes it is possible to account for patient differences using measurable covariates and sometimes it is not. In a Bayesian hierarchical approach, the study is one level of experimental unit, and patients within studies represent a second level of experimental unit. (Levels higher than study, such as country or study type, can also be included in a hierarchical model, but for the moment we do not consider more than two levels.) Characteristics of studies are unknown. In the Bayesian approach, all unknowns have probability distributions, so a Bayesian metaanalysis employs a random effects model.

Think of a study in a metaanalysis as having a distribution of patient responses that is specific to the study. Selecting a study means selecting one of these distributions. If the distribution of the selected study were to be revealed, this would give direct information about the study distributions, and result in a standard statistics problem. But since each study contributes only a finite number of patients, the selected study distributions are not completely revealed; instead, one can observe only a sample from each study's distribution. This gives indirect information about the distribution of study distributions. While it may seem strange to say "distribution of distributions," not only is this correct, it is an essential aspect of the approach.

Consider a simple analogy. A bag contains several thousand coins. These coins may have different propensities for producing heads. To get information about the distribution of these propensities among the coins in the bag, we select 10 coins at random, and toss each of them a total of 30 times. The data consist of 10 sample proportions of heads. If the observed proportions of heads are wildly different then it would seem that not all the coins in the bag have the same propensity for heads. However, because of sampling variability the sample proportions among the 10 coins tends to overestimate the dispersion in the population of coins. Further, if the sample proportions are quite similar then the coins in the bag may have similar propensities for heads. In any case, the sample proportions give information about the distribution of propensities of heads among the coins in the bag. Moreover, the results for one coin contain information about the propensity of heads for the other coins. This is because one coin's sample proportion gives information about the coins in the bag, and the other coins are themselves selected from the bag.

Example 2.7 *(metaanalysis for a single success proportion)*. Consider the case of a single treatment. Table 2.1 gives numbers of successes (x_i) and numbers of patients (n_i) for nine studies. A "success" is a response to an antidepressant drug (Janicak et al., 1988), but one could just as easily think of these as 9 studies (or 9 experiments) concerning the effectiveness of a medical device. Suppose that within study i the experimental units (patients, say) are exchangeable in the sense that all have the same propensity p_i of success. (For an example of a Bayesian analysis in the presence of differing prognoses, see Berry, 1989.)

study	x_i	n_i	$\hat{p}_i = x_i/n_i$
1	20	20	1.00
2	4	10	0.40
3	11	16	0.69
4	10	19	0.53
5	5	14	0.36
6	36	46	0.78
7	9	10	0.90
8	7	9	0.78
9	4	6	0.67
total	106	150	0.71

Table 2.1 *Successes and total numbers of patients in 9 studies.*

The likelihood function is

$$L(p_1, p_2, \ldots, p_9) \propto \prod_{i=1}^{9} p_i^{x_i}(1 - p_i)^{n_i - x_i} \ .$$

A combined analysis would assume that all 150 patients are exchangeable, so that the nine p_i are equal – say, with common value p. The likelihood function of p would then be

$$L(p) \propto p^{106}(1 - p)^{44} \ ,$$

which is shown in Figure 2.6. (The nine vertical bars in this figure correspond to the observed proportions for the nine studies, with bar heights proportional to sample sizes.) This figure shows that p is very likely to be between 0.6 and 0.8. This conclusion is somewhat curious since, as shown by the vertical bars on the p-axis in Figure 2.6, the observed success proportions in 5 of the 9 studies are outside this range. While sampling variability accounts for some of the differences among the sample proportions, the variability in Table 2.1 is greater than would be expected from sampling alone; this variability suggests that the p_i may not be equal.

Separate analysis of the 9 studies is even less satisfactory than combining all 9 studies. The effect of an experimental treatment is not well addressed by giving nine different likelihood functions, or by giving nine different confidence intervals. Consider the probability of success if the treatment were used with another patient, say one in a tenth study. How should the results from these 9 studies be weighed? Or, suppose that the focus is on a particular study, say study 9. How should the other 8 studies be weighed in estimating p_9?

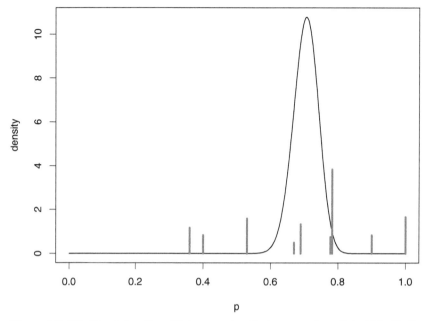

Figure 2.6 *Likelihood function $L(p)$ assuming that $p_i = p$ for all i. This likelihood, $p^{106}(1-p)^{44}$, is proportional to a $Beta(107, 45)$ density. The nine vertical bars correspond to the observed proportions for the nine studies, with bar heights proportional to sample sizes.*

From a hierarchical Bayesian perspective, each study's success propensity is viewed as having been selected from some larger population. Therefore, to use Bayes' Theorem requires a probability distribution of population distributions. Suppose $p_1, \ldots, p_9$ is a random sample from population distribution F which is itself random. Assume that F is a beta distribution with parameters a and b, where a and b are unknown. That is, assume that an observation p from F has beta density,

$$B(a, b)\, p^{a-1}(1-p)^{b-1},$$

where $a > 0$ and $b > 0$, and where

$$(B(a, b))^{-1} = \int_0^1 p^{a-1}(1-p)^{b-1} dp \ .$$

That is, $B(a, b)$ is the normalizing constant of the beta density. Referred to as the *beta function*, it can be constructed from the gamma function as

$$B(a, b) = \frac{\Gamma(a, b)}{\Gamma(a)\Gamma(b)} \ .$$

Assuming that F is a beta distribution is a restriction. This assumption

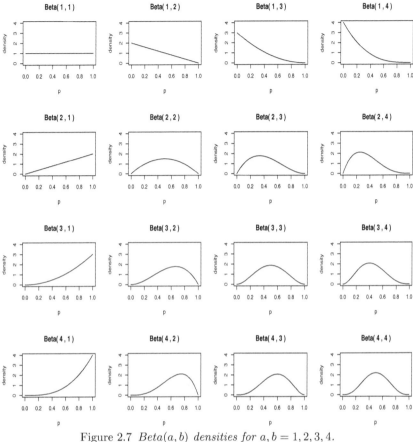

Figure 2.7 *Beta(a,b) densities for a, b = 1, 2, 3, 4.*

means a small number of parameters (two for the beta) index the distribution. Any other two-dimensional family would work as well computationally. The beta family has the pleasant characteristic that it represents a variety of types and shapes of distributions. However, beta distributions are either unimodal or bimodal, with the latter applying only if the two modes are 0 and 1 (the case with a and b both less than 1).

Another type of restriction made in this section is the assumption that $p_1, \ldots, p_9$ arise from the same distribution. More generally, studies may be more closely related to each other within subsets. For example, perhaps $p_1, \ldots, p_5$ might be viewed as arising from one distribution but $p_6, \ldots, p_9$ viewed as taken from a second distribution, with the relationship between the distributions being modeled.

Figure 2.7 shows several densities in the larger family of beta densities. The layout of the figure has increasing a from top to bottom and increasing

b from left to right. Beta densities not shown in this figure include those having a or b larger than 4, and those having fractional values of a and b. The mean of p for given a and b is $a/(a+b)$, and the variance is

$$\frac{ab}{(a+b)^2(a+b+1)} \; .$$

This tends to 0 as $a + b$ tends to infinity. So in a sense, $a + b$ measures *homogeneity* among studies. If $a + b$ is large then the distribution of the p_i will be highly concentrated (near the mean, $a/(a+b)$), and consequently the differences among studies will be slight. On the other hand, if $a + b$ is small then the p_i will vary from study to study, and there will be a large study effect.

As is the case for any unknown in the Bayesian approach, the user chooses a prior probability distribution for a and b; call it $\pi(a, b)$. If available information suggests homogeneity among studies then much of the probability under p can be concentrated on large values of a and b, whereas if this information allows for the possibility of heterogeneity then much of the probability under π can be placed on small values of a and b. If there is little information to suggest one or the other then both large and small values of $a + b$ should be assigned some prior probability, and indeed this will be the typical case.

Consider a generic observation, say p, from F. While it is not possible to observe p, temporarily suppose that this is possible. Call $\pi'(a, b|p)$ the posterior distribution of (a, b) given p. From Bayes' Theorem (2.1),

$$\pi'(a, b|p) \propto B(a, b)p^{a-1}(1 - p)^{b-1}\pi(a, b) \; .$$

Extending this to the observation of a sample $p_1, \ldots, p_9$ from F:

$$\pi'(a, b|p_1, \ldots, p_9) \propto \prod_{i=1}^{9} \left\{ B(a, b)p_i^{a-1}(1 - p_i)^{b-1} \right\} \pi(a, b) \; .$$

The more realistic case is that indirect information about $p_1, \ldots, p_9$ is available by observing $x_1, \ldots, x_9$, where the x_i are binomial variables with parameters n_i and p_i, respectively. Consider a single observation x having parameters n and p. Such an observation contains only indirect information about F. Call $\pi^*(a, b|x)$ the posterior distribution of a and b given x and n. From Bayes' Theorem,

$$\pi^*(a, b|x) \propto f(x|a, b)\pi(a, b),$$

where

$$\begin{aligned}
f(x|a, b) &= \int_0^1 \binom{n}{x} p^x(1 - p)^{n-x}B(a, b)p^{a-1}(1 - p)^{b-1}dp \\
&= \binom{n}{x}\frac{B(a, b)}{B(a + x, b + n - x)} \; .
\end{aligned}$$

Therefore,

$$\pi^*(a, b|x) \propto \frac{B(a, b)}{B(a + x, b + n - x)} \, \pi(a, b) \, .$$

Upon observing a sample $x_1, \ldots, x_9$, where $p_1, \ldots, p_9$ is a random sample from F, the joint posterior density of a and b is

$$\pi^*(a, b|x_1, \ldots, x_9) \propto \prod_{i=1}^{9} \left\{ \frac{B(a, b)}{B(a + x_i, b + n_i - x_i)} \right\} \pi(a, b) \, .$$

As each $n_i \to \infty$ the limit of this expression is π', setting p_i equal to x_i/n_i. This limiting equivalence is a law-of-large-numbers phenomenon and corresponds to the intuitive notion that an infinite amount of sample evidence about p_i is equivalent to observing p_i.

Now consider the response of an as yet untreated patient. First suppose the patient is treated at one of the 9 studies considered in Table 2.1. Given the results in that table, the probability of success for a patient treated in study i, for $i = 1, \ldots, 9$, is the posterior expected value of p_i,

$$E(p_i|x_1, \ldots, x_9) = E\left(\frac{a + x_i}{a + b + n_i} \,\Big|\, x_1, \ldots, x_9\right) \, .$$

This expectation is with respect to distribution π^*. That is, $(a + x_i)/(a + b + n_i)$ is calculated for the various possible values of a and b and weighed by the posterior distribution of a and b given the data. This formula applies as well for a patient treated in a new study, say study 10, by taking $i = 10$: the patient's probability of success is the expected posterior mean of p_{10},

$$E(p_{10}|x_1, \ldots, x_9) = E\left(\frac{a}{a + b} \,\Big|\, x_1, \ldots, x_9\right) \, . \tag{2.23}$$

To implement our Bayesian solution, we require a specific choice of the prior density $\pi(a, b)$. Applied Bayesians often attempt to choose the least informative prior available, at least in the initial phases of an analysis. This may be because it will typically produce answers that are not wildly inconsistent with those from traditional frequentist methods; note for instance that the posterior mode under a "flat" (uniform) prior is the same as the maximum likelihood estimate (MLE). Unfortunately, such priors are often *improper*, meaning that they do not themselves define a valid probability specification. An obvious example in our case is the bivariate uniform prior,

$$\pi(a, b) \propto 1 \text{ for } a, b > 0 \, . \tag{2.24}$$

This prior is "noninformative" in the sense that it does not favor any single pair of (a, b) values over any other; all receive the same *a priori* credibility. But this prior clearly does not integrate to 1 (or any finite number) over the entire domain for a and b. As mentioned above, such priors may still be acceptable if the resulting *posterior* distribution remains proper, but unfortunately that is not the case here: Hadjicostas (1998) shows that the joint posterior for (a, b) is improper under the unbounded flat prior (2.24). (See further discussion on this point below, as well as Natarajan and McCulloch, 1995, for similar difficulties with improper hyperpriors when the beta prior is replaced by a normal on the $\text{logit}(p_i)$.) A more sensible alternative is given by Gelman et al. (2004, p.128), who recommend reparametrizing from (a, b) to (μ, η) where $\mu = a/(a+b)$, the prior mean, and $\eta = 1/\sqrt{a + b}$, approximately the prior standard deviation, and placing independent uniform priors on both quantities.

In what follows, we simply *truncate* the range of the joint uniform prior (2.24) so it can be restandardized to a proper joint uniform distribution. That is, we suppose

$$\pi(a, b) \propto 1 \text{ for } 0 \leq a, b \leq 10 . \tag{2.25}$$

This distribution associates some probability with $a + b$ large and some with $a + b$ small, and it gives a moderate amount of probability to nearly equal a and b (meaning that there is a moderate amount of probability on p's near $1/2$).

This model is straightforwardly implemented via the WinBUGS package. WinBUGS is a freely available program developed by statisticians and probabilistic expert systems researchers at the Medical Research Council Biostatistics Unit at the University of Cambridge, England. In a nutshell, it allows us to draw samples from any posterior distribution, freeing us from having to worry overmuch about the integral in (2.1). This allows us instead to focus on the statistical modeling, which is after all our primary interest. WinBUGS uses syntax very similar to that of R, and in fact can now be called from R using the BRugs package, a subject to which we return below. As of the current writing, the latest version of WinBUGS may be downloaded from www.mrc-bsu.cam.ac.uk/bugs/welcome.shtml. Once installed, a good way to learn the basics of the language is to follow the tutorial: click on Help, pull down to User Manual, and then click on Tutorial. Perhaps even more easily, one can watch "WinBUGS – The Movie," a delightful Flash introduction to running the software available at www.statslab.cam.ac.uk/~krice/winbugsthemovie.html. To gain practice with the language, the reader may wish to turn to the ample collection of worked examples available within WinBUGS by clicking on Help and pulling down to Examples Vol I or Examples Vol II. See Carlin and Louis (2009, Chapter 2) for other step-by-step illustrations of various common statistical models implemented in WinBUGS.

WinBUGS solutions to Bayesian hierarchical modeling problems require three basic elements: (1) some BUGS code to specify the statistical model, (2) the data, and (3) initial values for the MCMC sampling algorithm. For our binomial-beta-uniform model, these three components can be specified in WinBUGS as follows:

BUGS code   `model{`

```
        for( i in 1:I) {
          x[i] ~ dbin(p[i] , n[i])
          p[i] ~ dbeta(a,b)
          }
        a ~ dunif(0,10)
        b ~ dunif(0,10)
    #    a ~ dgamma(2,2)
    #    b ~ dgamma(2,2)
    } #  end of BUGS code

    # Data:
    list(x = c(20, 4, 11, 10, 5, 36, 9, 7, 4, NA),
         n = c(20, 10, 16, 19, 14, 46, 10, 9, 6, 1), I=10)

    # Inits:
    list(a=4, b=2, p = c(.5, .5, .5, .5, .5, .5, .5, .5, .5, .5))
```

Everything after a # sign in WinBUGS is interpreted as a comment, so the $Gamma(2, 2)$ priors for a and b are not operative in this code. The data and inits are both being read in using list format (as also found in R), but this is not necessary; traditional columnar data stored in .txt files are also perfectly acceptable to WinBUGS. Note we deliberately expand the x vector with an extra, tenth entry that is set equal to NA (missing value). WinBUGS then treats this "missing data" value like another unknown in the model, and samples it according to its full conditional distribution, which in this case is simply the binomial likelihood given n_{10} (set to 1) and the also-imputed value of p_{10}. Finally, the initial values ("inits") are chosen to be "in the ballpark" but not really provide a convergence challenge for the model. Were this a more complicated and/or higher-dimensional model with correspondingly slower MCMC convergence, we would likely experiment with more extreme initial values (say, p_i closer to 0 and 1) that would provide a greater challenge to the algorithm.

WinBUGS features an intuitive point-and-click interface that is quite user friendly and perhaps best for initial runs and code testing. However, it becomes tedious once the model and its convergence are well understood, and we wish to investigate a significant number of different priors, models, etc. A useful tool in this regard is the BRugs function, which enables one to write a "script" of commands that are easily stored and then called (perhaps repeatedly) from R. We now offer a collection of BRugs commands to implement the WinBUGS analysis just described. We begin by loading the package, reading in the data, and writing it to disk for subsequent use by BUGS:

BRugs code
```
install.packages("BRugs")
library(BRugs)

x <- c(20, 4, 11, 10, 5, 36, 9, 7, 4, NA)
```

```
n <- c(20, 10, 16, 19, 14, 46, 10, 9, 6, 1)
I <- 10
dput(pairlist(x=x,n=n,I=I),"betabinHM_data.txt")
dput(pairlist(a=4,b=2,p=c(.5,.5,.5,.5,.5,.5,.5,.5,.5,.5)),
   "betabinHM_inits.txt")
```

Note the use of `dput` command to write out the data and inits files; these files can of course be created externally to R as well. Next we issue four BRugs commands corresponding to the Model - Specification menu in WinBUGS:

BRugs code
```
modelCheck("betabinHM_BUGS.txt")
modelData(paste("betabinHM_data.txt",sep=""))
modelCompile(numChains=1)
modelInits("betabinHM_inits.txt")
modelGenInits()    # generates an initial value for the missing x
```

Finally, we run a 1000-iteration burn-in period, set the parameters of interest into memory, run 10,000 more production iterations, and request histories, density estimates, and summary statistics for each:

BRugs code
```
modelUpdate(1000)
samplesSet(c("a","b","p"))

modelUpdate(10000)
samplesHistory("*", mfrow = c(3, 2))
samplesDensity("*")
samplesStats(c("a","b","p"))
```

The posterior samples of `p[10]` will be those from the predictive distribution of interest, $\pi(p_{10}|\mathbf{x})$.

Estimating the joint posterior of a and b is easily done via a plot of their matched Gibbs pairs:

BRugs code
```
par(mfrow=c(1,1))
plot(samplesSample("a"),samplesSample("b"),xlab="a",ylab="b")
```

Figure 2.8 shows the resulting plot of the 10,000 posterior sampled (a, b) pairs, providing a reasonably good idea of the joint posterior distribution. The posterior is "wedge-shaped" with increasing variability for larger a and b. The apparent truncation at $a = 10$ suggests that the data could support values of a even larger than 10. However, rerunning this model after expanding the upper bounds of the a and b domains to 100 or 1000 in prior (2.25) produces the same "truncated wedge" posterior. The implication is that the posterior would indeed be improper in the limiting case of the improper joint uniform prior (2.24). In what follows we carry on with the prior in (2.25), but emphasize that other proper priors (say, a and b assumed to be independent $Gamma(2, 2)$ variables, or the aforementioned Gelman et al. prior) may produce more defensible results. We also note that the posterior draws are centered near the line $a/(a+b) = 0.68$, corresponding to

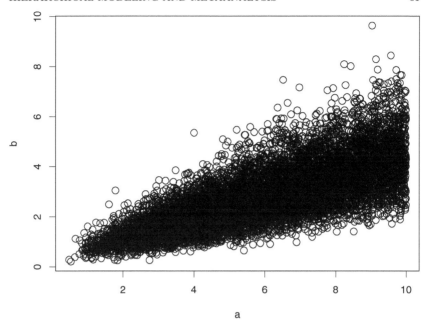

Figure 2.8 *Samples from the joint posterior distribution* $\pi^*(a, b|\mathbf{x})$ *for the data shown in Table 2.1.*

the posterior mean of the predictive probability (see Table 2.2). Densities with maximal posterior probabilities are essentially dispersed about this line.

The solid line in Figure 2.9 shows the mean posterior density of a generic p; the likelihood under the "all p_i's equal" assumption (dashed line) and study-specific estimates (vertical bars) from Figure 2.6 are repeated for easy comparison. **BRugs** code to draw this figure is as follows:

BRugs code
```
p <- seq(0,1,length=401)
phat <- c(1, .4, .69, .53, .36, .783, .9, .778, .67)
n <- n[1:9]
samp <- samplesSample("p[10]")

plot(p,dbeta(p,107,45),type="l",lty=2,lwd=2,ylab="density")
lines(density(samp,bw=.04,from=0,to=1),lty=1,lwd=2)
lines(phat,n/12, type = "h", col = "red", lwd=5)
legend(.1,10,c("posterior","likelihood (p_i's equal)"),lty=1:2)
```

Note the all-p_i's-equal likelihood is exactly a beta density, drawn using the **dbeta** command, but the posterior is a kernel density smooth (via **density**) of the p_{10} posterior samples produced earlier and stored in **samp**. Mathematically, the posterior is an *average* of beta densities, where the weights are $\pi^*(a, b)$. The mean of p for this density is 0.68, which can be found using

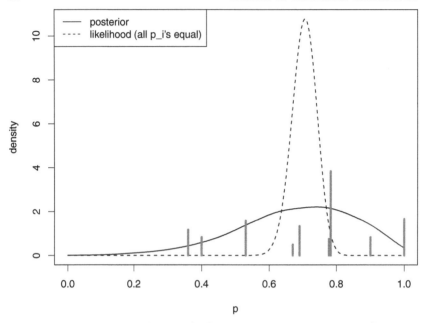

Figure 2.9 *Mean posterior density of p for the data shown in Table 2.1 (likelihood function from Figure 2.6 shown as dotted line).*

the formula for $E(p_{10}|\mathbf{x})$ as given in (2.23), or simply estimated by averaging all 10,000 Gibbs samples for p_{10}. Clearly, the variability suggested by this density estimate is greater than that in the all-p_i's-equal likelihood (dashed line; solid line in Figure 2.6). Again, we caution that restricting a and b to be no greater than 10 slightly overemphasizes heterogeneity, but replacing our truncated uniform hyperpriors with, say, gamma hyperpriors does not free us from having to think carefully *a priori* about the likely range and relative magnitudes of a and b.

Table 2.2 repeats Table 2.1, but with an extra column: the probability of success for the next patient in the corresponding study – including in a new, tenth study – which is the overall mean and is shown as the column total. The individual study probabilities are in effect shrunk toward the overall mean ("borrowing strength"), with greater shrinkage for smaller studies. For example, the estimated success probability for study 1 (0.90) is less than the observed success proportion (1.00) because the latter is relatively large. In the other direction, the estimated success proportion for study 5 (0.48) is larger than the observed proportion (0.36) because the latter is relatively small. In both cases the shrinkage toward the middle is an instance of the "regression effect" or "regression to the mean" (Berry, 1996, Sec. 14.3). The amount of shrinkage depends on the distances from

study	x_i	n_i	$\hat{p}_i = x_i/n_i$	pred. prob.
1	20	20	1.00	0.90
2	4	10	0.40	0.53
3	11	16	0.69	0.69
4	10	19	0.53	0.57
5	5	14	0.36	0.48
6	36	46	0.78	0.77
7	9	10	0.90	0.80
8	7	9	0.78	0.73
9	4	6	0.67	0.68
total	106	150	0.71	0.68

Table 2.2 *Predictive probability of success by study.*

the observed proportions to the mean and also on the sizes of the studies, with greater shrinkage for smaller studies. (The dependence on study size is not very clear in Table 2.2 because the study sample sizes are quite comparable.)

The predictive probability for study 10 (0.68 for "total" in Table 2.2) is different from the overall success proportion (0.71). The prior distribution is symmetric in a and b and so the prior probability of success is 0.50 (this being the average of $a/(a+b)$ over the various distributions considered in the prior). The overall predictive probability of success is an average of 0.71 and 0.50, although calculating this average is rather complicated. Just as for the case of normal sampling in Example 2.2 for which the posterior mean is an average of the prior and sample means, this shrinkage toward the prior mean wears off for larger numbers of studies. ∎

2.5 Principles of Bayesian clinical trial design

The use of Bayesian statistical methods is somewhat less controversial when matters turn to experimental design. This is because in order to carry out a sample size calculation, a trial designer must have and use some pre-existing knowledge (or what Bayesians would call *prior opinion*) regarding the likely effect of the treatment and its variability. More formally, all evaluations at the design stage are *preposterior*; i.e., they involve integrating over uncertainty in both the as-yet-unobserved data (a frequentist act) *and* the unobservable parameters (a Bayesian act). In the terminology of Rubin (1984), this double integration is a "Bayesianly justifiable frequentist calculation."

While the Bayesian advantages of flexibility and borrowing of strength (both from previous data and across subgroups) have been well-known to clinical trialists for some time, they have proven elusive to obtain in practice due to the difficulty in converting historical information into priors, and in computing the necessary posterior summaries. Still, pressure to minimize the financial and ethical cost of clinical trials encourages greater development and use of Bayesian thinking in their design and analysis. In the case of medical device trials, where data are often scanty and expensive, Bayesian methods already make up roughly 10% of new device approvals (Berry, 2006). While the area of drug trials has been slower to embrace the methods, even here they are gaining traction thanks to their ability to readily incorporate early stopping for safety or futility, as well as easily handle complications such as multiple endpoints or random effects. Bayes is also an especially natural approach for incorporating historical controls into the analysis (Section 6.1), an area for which the classical frequentist literature is very limited (though see Pocock, 1976; Prentice et al., 2006; and Neaton et al., 2007, for notable exceptions).

In this section, we outline the basics of Bayesian clinical trial design and analysis, and illustrate a general method for Bayesian sample size calculations using BRugs. This function's ability to call BUGS from R (as already seen in Example 2.7) allows us to repeatedly estimate the posterior given various artificial data samples, and hence simulate the Bayesian and frequentist operating characteristics (power and Type I error rates) of our Bayesian designs.

2.5.1 Bayesian predictive probability methods

The first two authors of this book have been strong and consistent advocates for the use of predictive probabilities in making decisions based on accumulating clinical trial data. Such an outlook is helpful in cases where, perhaps due to especially acute ethical concerns, we are under pressure to terminate trials of ineffective treatments early (say, because the treatment is especially toxic or expensive). The basic idea is to compute the probability that a treatment will *ever* emerge as superior given the patient recruitment outlook and the data accumulated so far; if this probability is too small, the trial is stopped. In the past, frequentists have sometimes referred to this as *stochastic curtailment*; applied Bayesians have instead tended to use the phrase *stopping for futility*. In this subsection we provide only the briefest outline of the main ideas; see Sections 4.2 and 5.2 for full details and illustrations.

To fix ideas, consider again the simple binomial case where each patient i is either a success on the study treatment ($Y_i = 1$) or a failure ($Y_i = 0$). Assuming the patients are independent with common success probability p, we obtain the familiar binomial likelihood for $X = \sum_i Y_i$. Now suppose

	No AE	AE	Total
Count	110	7	117
(%)	(94)	(6)	

Table 2.3 *Historical AE data, Safety Study A.*

we have observed n_1 patients to date, of which X_1 have been successes, so that $X_1 \sim Bin(n_1, p)$. Under a conjugate $Beta(a, b)$ prior for p, we of course obtain a $Beta(X_1 + a, n_1 - X_1 + b)$ posterior for p. Inference and decision making would now arise via the usual posterior summaries.

Now suppose that the trial has yet to reach a definitive conclusion, and we wish to decide whether or not to randomize an additional n_2 statistically independent patients into the protocol. Because we know Bayes' Rule may be used sequentially in this case, the current $Beta(X_1 + a, n_1 - X_1 + b)$ posterior now serves as the prior for p, to be combined with a $Bin(n_2, p)$ likelihood for X_2. Posterior inference would now focus on the resulting $Beta(X_1 + X_2 + a, n_1 + n_2 - X_1 - X_2 + b)$ updated posterior. The predictive point of view argues that the appropriate calculation at this point is to sample values p_j^* from the "prior" (actually, the interim posterior) $Beta(X_1 + a, n_1 - X_1 + b)$, followed by fake data values X_{2j}^* repeatedly from the $Bin(n_2, p_j^*)$ likelihood. Repeating this process for $j = 1, \ldots, N_{rep}$ produces the collection of *posterior predictive* distributions

$$p(\theta^* | X_1, X_{2j}^*) = Beta(X_1 + X_{2j}^* + a, n_1 + n_2 - X_1 - X_{2j}^* + b).$$

Inference is now based on an appropriate summary of these distributions.

Example 2.8 Suppose a medical device company wishes to run a safety study on one of its new cardiac pacemakers. Specifically, the company wishes to show that men receiving its new product will be very likely to be free from adverse events (AEs) during the three months immediately following implantation of the device. (Here, "adverse events" are limited to those for which the device is directly responsible, and which require additional action by the implanting physician.) Letting p be the probability a patient does *not* experience an AE in the first three months, we seek a 95% equal-tail Bayesian confidence interval for p, $(p_{.025}, p_{.975})$. Suppose our trial protocol uses the following decision rule:

Device is safe from AEs at 3 months $\Longleftrightarrow p_{.025} > 0.85$.

That is, if the lower confidence bound for the chance of freedom from AEs is at least 85%, the trial succeeds; otherwise it fails.

Now suppose we already have a preliminary study, Study A, whose results are given in Table 2.3. In our above notation, we have $X_1 = 110$ and

$n_1 = 117$. Our task is now to evaluate whether it is worth running a second study, Study B, which would enroll an additional n_2 patients. If we begin with a $Uniform(0,1) = Beta(1,1)$ prior for p, the interim posterior is then $Beta(X_1 + a, n_1 - X_1 + b) = Beta(111, 8)$. Sampling p_j^* values from this prior followed by potential Study B values X_{2j}^* from the $Bin(n_2, p_j^*)$ likelihood produces the necessary $Beta(111 + X_{2j}^*, 8 + n_2 - X_{2j}^*)$ posteriors and, hence, simulated lower confidence limits $p_{.025,j}^*$ from the posterior predictive distribution for $j = 1, \ldots, N_{rep}$. The empirical predictive probability of trial success is then

$$\widehat{P}(p_{.025} > 0.85) = \frac{\text{number of } p_{.025,j}^* > 0.85}{N_{rep}} . \tag{2.26}$$

If this number is less than some prespecified cutoff (say, 0.70), the trial would be declared *futile* at this point, and it would be abandoned without randomizing the additional n_2 patients. ∎

2.5.2 Bayesian indifference zone methods

Bayesian monitoring of clinical trials dates to the landmark but woefully underutilized work of Cornfield (1966a,b, 1969). These papers contained the basic framework for clinical trial decisionmaking based on posterior distributions, but in their era were regarded primarily as academic exercises, no doubt in part because they were so far ahead of their time (and ahead of the MCMC revolution in Bayesian statistics). Bayesian clinical trial methods did not begin to gain practical application until the 1980s, when the work of Freedman and Spiegelhalter (1983) saw implementation in a few large trials in the United Kingdom (see also Freedman and Spiegelhalter, 1989, 1992; Freedman et al., 1984; or the lovely review in Spiegelhalter et al., 2004, Ch. 6). These authors suggested implementation of Bayesian methodology through the use of an *indifference zone* (or *range of equivalence*) for a treatment effect parameter Δ. The basic idea is to replace the traditional but unrealistic point null hypothesis, $H_0 : \Delta = 0$, with a *range* of null Δ's, say $[\delta_L, \delta_U]$, over which we are *indifferent* between the intervention and the control. The upper bound, δ_U, represents the amount of improvement required by the intervention to suggest clinical superiority over control, while δ_L denotes the threshold below which the intervention would be considered clinically inferior.

Suppose positive values of Δ are indicative of an efficacious treatment. Then we might for example set $\delta_U = K > 0$ and $\delta_L = 0$, an additional benefit perhaps being required of the treatment in order to justify its higher cost in terms of resources, clinical effort, or potential toxicity. Bayesian stopping rules are then naturally based on the posterior probability of the tail areas determined by the indifference zone endpoints. For instance, we

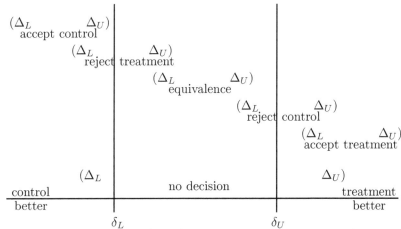

Figure 2.10 *Indifference zone* (δ_L, δ_U) *and corresponding conclusions for a clinical trial based on the location of the 95% posterior credible interval for* Δ.

might terminate the trial when

$$P(\Delta > \delta_U | \text{data}) \qquad (2.27)$$

is sufficiently small (deciding in favor of the control), *or* when

$$P(\Delta < \delta_L | \text{data}) \qquad (2.28)$$

is sufficiently small (deciding in favor of the treatment). Another rule would be to stop when one region's posterior probability is sufficiently *large*, or, failing this, when a predetermined total sample size is reached. Such a rule might be appropriately applied to the lower tail in a drug-placebo study, since clinicians would likely have very low prior belief in the placebo's superiority.

Trial stopping rules might also be based upon the location of the 95% posterior credible interval for Δ, (Δ_L, Δ_U), with respect to the indifference zone $[\delta_L, \delta_U]$, as demonstrated in Figure 2.10. Exactly six cases are possible, with stronger evidence required to "accept" one hypothesis than merely reject the other. Note that to conclude "equivalence," the 95% interval must lie entirely *within* the indifference zone; if the interval straddles *both* ends of the zone, posterior evidence is too weak to make a decision of any kind.

Consider a trial where increased Δ implies increased benefit associated with intervention. We sometimes take $\delta_L = 0$ and $\delta_U > 0$, but we might also center the indifference zone around 0, i.e., $\delta_L = -\xi$ and $\delta_U = \xi$. In the latter case, for a fixed n and under a proper prior on Δ, expanding the indifference zone by increasing ξ corresponds to a decrease in Type I error (since rejection of the control becomes more difficult) but also a decrease in power. On the other hand, decreasing ξ powers the trial for a more desirable effect difference, yet corresponds to an increase in Type I error. One often strives for an indifference zone with various appealing "symmetry" properties; however, note that symmetry within the indifference zone for regression coefficients in a logistic or Cox proportional hazards model does not yield corresponding symmetries on the (nonlinearly transformed) odds or hazard ratio scales.

Once the indifference zone is specified, the likelihood for the observed trial outcomes must be formulated. Consider again the case of a binary trial endpoint; say, whether the patient experiences progression of disease or not during the trial, for $i = 1, \ldots, N$. Then $Y_i \sim Bernoulli(p_i)$, where p_i is the probability of disease progression for the ith patient. Now let x_i be an indicator variable for the intervention group. One possible model for p_i assumes

$$logit(p_i) = \log\left(\frac{p_i}{1 - p_i}\right) = \lambda_0 + \lambda_1 x_i , \qquad (2.29)$$

where λ_0 and λ_1 are random hyperparameters. If $x_i = 0$ for control and 1 for treatment, then λ_1 captures the intervention effect. Inference is typically based on e^{λ_1}, the ratio of odds for disease progression between the two groups. Therefore, e^{λ_1} plays the role of Δ above.

Evaluating the posterior distribution of e^{λ_1} requires us to specify priors for the regression parameters. Because $\lambda_k \in \Re$ for $k = 0, 1$, normal priors could be used, with informative content added as indicated in the next subsection. Any important prognostic factor z_i may be added to $logit(p_i)$ as a $\lambda_2 z_i$ term, although e^{λ_1} would now need to be interpreted as the odds ratio of disease progression for individuals with identical z_i.

If instead of binary outcomes, we have continuous measurements (e.g., blood pressure, weight, etc.), then a normal likelihood may be more appropriate. Now Δ would be expressed as the difference in group means, prior knowledge on the likelihood mean would likely be incorporated using a normal prior, and the likelihood variance might use the standard inverse gamma prior. Time-to-event outcomes may also be of interest, and employ Weibull, gamma, or Cox partial likelihoods; Example 2.9 offers an illustration of the first case.

2.5.3 Prior determination

When determining the priors for crucial parameters such as λ_0 and λ_1 in (2.29), note that information may be plentiful for the former (since it is determined by the rate in the control group), but not the latter (since this parameter captures the improvement of the new therapy over control). Still, every prior determination strategy should begin with a review of all available historical evidence on both the treatment and control groups. This review helps to determine our *analysis priors*, the prior distributions that will be used when the data are ultimately collected and the posterior distribution computed. Even when not directed to do so by a regulatory agency, we will often wish to compare the results obtained under an informative analysis prior (i.e., one that incorporates available historical information) with those from a noninformative one, to see the impact the historical data have on the posterior.

We remark briefly that we may well be in need of *two* prior specifications: the aforementioned analysis prior, and also a *design prior*. This latter prior is the one we use when designing the trial, and would therefore typically use the full range of information gleaned from past data and literature review. The analysis prior, by contrast, might be somewhat less informative, especially if the goal of our trial is to win over skeptics whose faith in our review of the evidence is lower than ours, or who might simply want the results of the current trial to stand on their own. This is admittedly a confusing (and seemingly "illegal") distinction, and one we return to in greater detail later in this section.

Community of priors

Often, there will be a wide range of prior beliefs that could plausibly be derived from alternate readings of the available pre-trial information. In addition, subject matter experts consulted by trial designers may well contribute their own divergent opinions, based on their own clinical experience or other expertise. Since trial results may well be sensitive to the choice of prior (especially on the efficacy parameters that drive the outcome), Spiegelhalter et al. (1994) recommend using a *community* of several priors (c.f. Kass and Greenhouse, 1989) in order to represent the broadest possible audience. These priors might be broadly categorized as *skeptical, enthusiastic*, and *reference* (or *noninformative*). A *skeptical* prior is one that believes the treatment is likely no better than control (as might be believed by a regulatory agency). Such a prior might be centered around the clinical inferiority boundary, δ_L, which is often equal to 0. The spread of this prior will then determine the *a priori* chance of clinical superiority, $P(\Delta > \delta_U)$. An *enthusiastic* prior is one that believes the treatment will succeed. Since this viewpoint is typical of the one held by the clinicians running the trial, such a prior is sometimes known as a *clinical* prior. Here we might center the prior around the clinical superiority boundary, δ_U, and again determine the variance based on tail area considerations, or perhaps simply by matching to the skeptical prior variance. Finally, as already mentioned in Section 2.1, a *reference* prior is one that attempts to express no particular opinion about the treatment's merit. Since Δ is a mean parameter that is typically well-estimated by the data, an improper uniform ("flat") prior is often permissible.

Note that it may be sensible to match the prior to the decision one hopes to reach; the prior should represent "an adversary who will need to be disillusioned by the data to stop further experimentation" (Spiegelhalter et al., 1994). Thus, to conclude a treatment difference, we should use the skeptical prior, while to conclude *no* difference, we should use the enthusiastic prior.

Figure 2.11 illustrates the use of a community of priors in interim monitoring by looking at the marginal posterior probabilities of the two tail areas (2.27) and (2.28) for a particular trial with four monitoring points. This model is parametrized so that *negative* values of the treatment effect, β_1, indicate clinical superiority. The graph shows results for three priors: an enthusiastic, clinical prior (marked by "C" in the graphs), a skeptical prior ("S"), and a noninformative, flat prior ("L", indicating that only the likelihood is driving these results). Here the clinical inferiority boundary, $\beta_{1,U}$, is set to 0, while the clinical superiority boundary, $\beta_{1,L}$, is set to $\log(0.75) = -.288$, which in this model corresponds to a 25% reduction in hazard relative to control. In this particular example (see Carlin and Louis, 2009, Sec. 8.2 for full details), the accumulating data actually favor the placebo, with an excess of deaths gradually accumulating in the treatment group. Thus, in the upper panel we see the posterior probability of superiority steadily dropping over time, while the lower panel reveals the opposite trend in the posterior probability of inferiority. Notice from the upper panel that the skeptical and flat prior analyses are ready to stop and abandon the treatment by the third monitoring point (as its posterior probability has dropped below 0.1), but the enthusiastic clinical prior is not won over to this point of view until the fourth and final interim look. However, note also that the clinical prior is "unethical" in the sense that it is ready to stop for *superiority* at the very first monitoring point, when no data have yet accumulated. This illustrates a clear risk when using an overly optimistic prior, and one we shall adjust for by considering power and Type I error in Subsection 2.5.4.

2.5.4 Operating characteristics

Without doubt the most commonly asked question of biostatisticians working in the practice of clinical trials is, "How big a sample size do I need for this trial?" This *sample size* question is one that Bayesianism must have a ready answer for if it is to play a significant role in the practice of clinical trials. Fortunately, the Bayesian paradigm is quite natural for experimental design, and sample size calculation is a standard design problem. That is, we determine the sample size by finding the smallest number of patients that, for our chosen statistical model, will lead to a trial we know will have good *operating characteristics*, such as low Type I error and good power at "likely" alternatives. But "likely" here means "*a priori*," since at the design stage, no data are yet available (at least on the treatment group;

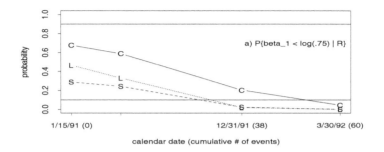

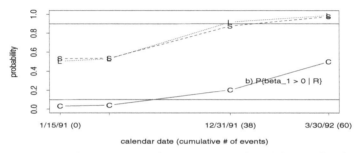

Figure 2.11 *Example monitoring plot: posterior tail probabilities for the treatment effect at four interim monitoring points. Top panel: probability of treatment superiority; bottom panel, probability of treatment inferiority.*

we may have historical controls, a subject to which we will return). So it makes sense that Bayesian methods might have something to offer here.

As has already been mentioned, the CDRH (Center for Devices and Radiological Health) branch of the FDA has been interested in Bayesian methods for quite some time. The initial impetus was to utilize prior information from previously approved medical devices in order to enhance data on new medical devices to be approved. Later on, the flexibility of Bayesian adaptive designs proved to be even more appealing to device companies. At present, the vast majority of Bayesian medical device clinical trials submitted to the FDA makes use of adaptive designs, even in the absence of prior information. Still, the FDA remains a regulatory agency whose fundamental mission is to protect the public from harmful products, and ensure that products billed as effective really are effective. Perhaps most significantly, they must do this "over the long haul;" when a product is judged "significantly better," it must mean averaging over all products that are tested over time. This is an inherently *frequentist* (not Bayesian) outlook.

So it is perhaps not surprising that FDA approval for Bayesian designs continues to depend on demonstration of controlled Type I and Type II error rates and acceptable frequentist power.

While it may seem odd to be adopting Bayesian methods if frequentist operating characteristics continue to be so important, keep in mind that the inherent advantages of the Bayesian paradigm (borrowing strength across similar but independent units, utilizing reliable historical information to supplement information in the data, etc.) will often permit well-designed Bayesian trials to have excellent frequentist properties. And of course, even if satisfying the FDA were not the primary goal, Bayesians still care about long-run behavior of their procedures; they would simply prefer a *prepos-terior* analysis – i.e., one that averaged over the variability in *both* the unknown parameters and the as-yet unobserved data. Adding in the averaging over the prior leads to obvious preposterior Bayesian analogs of Type I error and power, a subject on which we will elaborate.

To fix ideas, consider again the binary data setting, and the logistic response model of equation (2.29). Suppose we wish to power a study to deliver any of the six outcomes illustrated in Figure 2.10 (or combinations thereof) with a given probability. For any fixed, "true" values of the parameter vector λ_0 and λ_1 and proposed treatment allocation $\{x_i\}_{i=1}^{N}$, we can simulate the frequentist power of our Bayesian procedure by computing the p_i from equation (2.29), and then generating fake data values Y_{ij}^* repeatedly from the binomial likelihood for $j = 1, \ldots, N_{rep}$. Each fake data vector $\mathbf{Y}_j^* = (Y_{1j}^*, \ldots, Y_{Nj}^*)'$ leads to a 95% posterior interval for λ_1, and hence one of the six decisions in Figure 2.10. Repeating this for each of the N_{rep} datasets, we can compute the empirical probability of each of the six outcomes, and thus estimate any power we desire (a Type I error calculation arises by setting $\lambda_1 = 0$, the null value) in conjunction with the appropriate superiority hypothesis. Thus, our Bayesian sample size problem comes down to choosing a design (i.e., a sample size N and an indifference zone) that delivers some prespecified acceptable frequentist properties. The use of an informative fitting prior is likely to pay dividends in cases where the "truth" is congruent with this prior.

As alluded to above, a fully Bayesian version of this procedure would replace the fixed, true values (λ_0, λ_1) by draws $\{(\lambda_{0j}^*, \lambda_{1j}^*), j = 1, \ldots, N_{rep}\}$ from their prior distributions. This would acknowledge the uncertainty in these parameters; we will never know "the truth" at the design stage. However, note that the design prior (i.e., the prior used to generate the fake λ_{0j}^* and λ_{1j}^*) need *not* be the same as the analysis prior, with the latter typically being the vaguer of the two. That is, we would wish to use all available information at the design stage, but might prefer a vaguer, less risky prior once the data have accumulated, in order to improve our shot at good operating characteristics. Thus, in this text we will use the terms *design prior* and *analysis prior* (or *fitting prior*), and endeavor to clarify any differences between the two when they exist. Incidentally, these ideas were also appreciated by several previous authors, including O'Hagan and Stevens (2001); see Subsection 2.5.5.

Having selected design and analysis priors, all that remains is to summarize the (frequentist or Bayesian) power and Type I error, and select a sample size N that delivers satisfactory levels of each. Note that the posterior calculation for each fake data vector $\mathbf{Y}_j^*$ may be available in closed form, as in the beta-binomial setting of Example 2.8. However, many models in clinical trial design and analysis (especially survival models, using say the Weibull, gamma, or Cox partial likelihood) will require MCMC sampling, perhaps through N_{rep} calls to the BUGS software. A feasible solution here (and the one we recommend at least initially) is to write the outer, fake data-generating loop in R, and call BUGS repeatedly using commands from the BRugs package. Example 2.9 offers an illustration.

Example 2.9 *(simulating power and Type I error for a Weibull survival model)*. Let t_i be the time until death for subject i in a clinical trial, with corresponding treatment indicator x_i (set equal to 0 for control and 1 for treatment). Suppose the survival time t_i follows a $Weibull(r, \mu_i)$ distribution, where $r > 0$ and $\mu_i > 0$. Adopting BUGS' parametrization, this assumes a pdf of $f(t_i | r, \mu_i) = \mu_i r t_i^{r-1} \exp(-\mu_i t_i^r)$. To incorporate the treatment indicator into the model, we further parametrize $\mu_i = \mu_i(x_i) = e^{-(\beta_0 + \beta_1 x_i)}$. Then the baseline hazard function is $h_0(t_i) = r t_i^{r-1}$, and the median survival time for subject i is

$$m_i = [(\log 2)e^{\beta_0 + \beta_1 x_i}]^{1/r} .$$

Thus the relative change in median survival time in the treatment group is $\exp(\beta_1/r)$, and so $\beta_1 > 0$ indicates improved survival in the treatment group. Moreover, the value of β_1 corresponding to a 15% increase in median survival in the treatment group satisfies

$$e^{\beta_1/r} = 1.15 \iff \beta_1 = r \log(1.15) .$$

For humans older than age 1, we normally expect $r > 1$ (i.e., increasing baseline hazard over time). For the purpose of illustration, in this example we somewhat arbitrarily set $r = 2$, so our Weibull is equivalent to a *Rayleigh* distribution. This then helps us specify an indifference zone (δ_L, δ_U) as follows. First, we take δ_L, the clinical inferiority boundary, equal to 0, since we would never prefer a harmful treatment. However, in order to require a "clinically significant" improvement under the treatment (due to its cost, toxicity, and so on) we would prefer $\delta_U > 0$. Since we have selected $r = 2$, taking $\delta_U = 2 \log(1.15) \approx 0.28$ corresponds to requiring a 15% improvement in median survival. The outcome of the trial can then be based on the location of the 95% posterior confidence interval for β_1, say (β_{1L}, β_{1U}), relative to this indifference zone. The six possible outcomes and

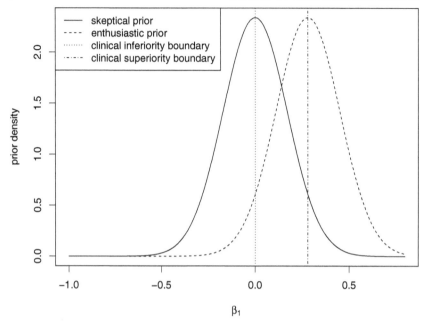

Figure 2.12 *Skeptical (solid line) and enthusiastic (dashed line) priors, Weibull survival model. Also shown (vertical lines) are the clinical inferiority boundary, $\delta_L = 0$, and the clinical superiority boundary, $\delta_U = 0.28$.*

decisions were previously shown in Figure 2.10; recall that a novel feature of this setup is that both "acceptance" and "rejection" are possible.

Next we need to select an appropriate prior distribution. Following the aforementioned "community of priors" idea, we select skeptical, enthusiastic, and reference priors for the treatment effect parameter, β_1. Beginning with the skeptical case, we simply set the prior mean equal to 0 (implying no change in survival in the treatment group relative to control) and then choose the variance so that $P(\beta_1 > \delta_U) = \epsilon$, for some small but positive probability ϵ. In our setting $\epsilon = 0.05$ delivers the $N(0, (0.17)^2)$ prior distribution, shown as a solid line in Figure 2.12. Turning to the enthusiastic prior, we raise the mean up to the clinical superiority boundary (0.28), but use the same standard deviation as the skeptical prior (0.17). This prior is shown as the dashed line in Figure 2.12. Finally, for our reference (noninformative) prior, we simply use an improper uniform ("flat") prior, since it will still lead to a proper posterior here.

In all three cases we use a $N(7.53, 0.2)$ prior for the intercept parameter, β_0. This prior is somewhat informative and centered near values that emerge as plausible for our data generation mechanism, explained below. We could certainly be less prescriptive regarding β_0, but since it is merely a "nuisance" parameter we prefer a fairly precise prior that will encourage the data's estimative power to focus on the parameter of interest, β_1.

As already mentioned, we simulate power or other operating characteristics within R, here also calling BUGS for each simulated data set since the marginal posterior for β_1 is not available in closed form. For example, to simulate Bayesian operating characteristics, we begin by sampling a "true" $\boldsymbol{\beta}$ from its design prior. Here this means sampling a β_0 value from its prior, followed by a β_1 value from one of our community of priors (here, skeptical or enthusiastic; the flat prior is improper and hence cannot be sampled). Given these, we then sample fake survival times t_i (say, N from each study group) from the Weibull likelihood. To add a bit of realism, we may also wish to sample fake *censoring* times c_i from a particular distribution (e.g., a normal distribution truncated below 0). Then for all individuals i for whom $t_i > c_i$, we replace t_i by "NA" (missing value), corresponding to the individuals who were still alive when the study ended. Next, we call BUGS to get the 95% equal-tail credible interval for β_1, which it obtains from a (sorted) collection of 1000 MCMC samples. We then determine the simulated trial's outcome based either on a posterior tail area (say, $P(\beta_1 < \delta_L | \mathbf{t}, \mathbf{x}, \mathbf{c})$ or $P(\beta_1 > \delta_U | \mathbf{t}, \mathbf{x}, \mathbf{c})$), or perhaps on the location of this interval relative to the indifference zone $(0, 0.28)$; once again, see Figure 2.10. After repeating this entire process some large number of times $Nrep$, we can report the appropriate summaries (e.g., the empirical frequencies of the six possible outcomes) as simulation-consistent estimates of the desired Bayesian trial operating characteristic.

A computer program to implement this solution is available online as "Example 3" at http://www.biostat.umn.edu/~brad/software/BRugs/. As in Example 2.7, we require two pieces of code: a piece of BUGS code to specify the Weibull model for any given dataset, and a piece of BRugs code to repeatedly generate the fake data values and send them to BUGS for analysis. Using our reference analysis prior, the BUGS code looks like this:

```
BUGS code    model {
                 for (i in 1:n) {
                   t[i] ~ dweib(2, mu[i]) I(t.cens[i], )
                   mu[i] <- exp(-beta0 - beta1*x[i])
                 }
                 beta0 ~ dnorm( 7.53, 25)
                 beta1 ~ dnorm(0,.0001)  # reference (noninformative) prior
             } #  end of BUGS code
```

This code is very simple, since (following the "mice" example in the WinBUGS manual) all that is necessary is the (censored) Weibull likelihood, an expression of the scale parameter μ_i in terms of the parameters and the treatment indicator, and priors for β_0 and β_1. The censoring aspect is handled rather ingeniously in BUGS using the I (indicator) function, which here specifies that the failure time t is restricted to being larger than the

N	analysis prior		
	Skeptical	Reference	Enthusiastic
25	.001	.053	.178
50	.009	.069	.213
75	.017	.110	.209
100	.034	.070	.214

Table 2.4 *Probability of rejecting the control under a skeptical design prior for four sample sizes N and three analysis priors, Weibull survival model.*

censoring time t.cens. Censored individuals will have t = NA and t.cens equal to their censoring times; individuals observed to fail will instead have t equal to these failure times and t.cens = 0 (i.e., no additional restriction on the usual Weibull distribution). BUGS then helpfully generates any missing t_i's, along with the unknown β parameters, ending up after convergence with the correct marginal posterior for β_1.

By contrast, the outer, BRugs code is fairly lengthy, and is relegated to the aforementioned website. This version of the code assumes a sample size of $N = 50$ in each group, a median survival of 36 days, and a $N(80, 20^2)$ censoring distribution. We also assume a (very optimistic) 50% improvement in the treatment group, and take the enthusiastic prior as the "truth" (i.e., our design prior is enthusiastic). However, we use the reference prior in our BUGS calls (i.e., our analysis prior is noninformative). For an admittedly too-small run of just $Nrep = 100$ replications, we obtained the following output:

```
Here are simulated outcome frequencies for N= 50
  accept control:     0
  reject treatment:  0.07
  equivalence:        0
  reject control:    0.87
  accept treatment:  0.06
  no decision:        0
End of BRugs power simulation
```

As expected in this optimistic design, we are able to reach the "reject control" decision 87% of the time, and in fact draw the even stonger "accept treatment" decision an additional 6% of the time. Grouping these two cases together, the estimated "Bayesian power" of our procedure is 93%. By contrast, the estimated "Bayesian Type II error rate" is 7%, since this is the empirical proportion of datasets for which the treatment was rejected despite its superiority.

For given design and analysis priors, we would repeat this process (i.e., rerun the **BRugs** program) for several different sample sizes N. We would then choose the smallest sample size that still delivers power and Type I error behavior we deem acceptable. Consider for instance the case of a skeptical design prior (i.e, the "truth" now is that the treatment is very similar to the control). Increasing $Nrep$ to 1000 (but still using 100 burn-in and 1000 production MCMC iterations per **BUGS** call), Table 2.4 shows the simulated probabilities of rejecting the control when the skeptical prior is true. The entries in this table are essentially Bayesian Type I error rates, since the "truth" here is that nothing much is going on. Unsurprisingly, error is lowest for the skeptical analysis prior, which has correctly guessed the truth in this case. The enthusiastic prior has what might be considered unacceptably high error rates, though they appear to have stabilized (up to simulation error) near 20% for the larger sample sizes. ∎

In the previous example, "true" parameter values were generated from a design prior, leading to Bayesian analogs of power and Type I and II error. But as mentioned previously, a fully *frequentist* Type I error calculation is also possible using our approach. For example, the frequentist Type I error of our Bayesian procedure could be simulated simply by *fixing* $\beta_1 = 0$ (rather than sampling it from a design prior), and generating only the t_i and c_i for each of the $Nrep$ iterations. Frequentist power and Type II error can be simulated similarly by fixing β_1 at nonzero values.

Finally, we remark that we have only considered stopping for a single endpoint (efficacy). But handling *multiple endpoints* is also straightforward within the Bayesian framework. For example, suppose we wish to power a study to evaluate both safety and long-term efficacy of a particular treatment. If the responses on both endpoints can be reasonably treated as discrete, a sensible and relatively simple Bayesian approach might use a *Dirichlet-multinomial* model, a straightforward extension of the beta-binomial model for binary responses. Specifically, once the joint distribution of the multiple endpoints is specified via cross-classification, the multinomial becomes the natural likelihood model. The Dirichlet distribution then offers a convenient conjugate prior whose specification is similar to that of the beta distribution and which is also available in both **R** and **BUGS**. More complex (e.g., survival) models would likely require MCMC sampling and the associated **BRugs** calls to **BUGS**. Early stopping for *futility* based on predictive distributions ("Bayesian stochastic curtailment") may also be of interest; see Berry and Berry (2004) and Section 4.3 below.

Interim analysis

The subject of interim analysis (or "multiple looks [at the data]") is a subject of constant worry in frequentist clinical trial analysis. The reason is clear: since frequentists make decisions based on p-values (i.e., Type I error levels) and other design-based summaries, if we decide to look at the accumulating data many times over the course of the study, we must account for this in the procedure or risk inflating its Type I error. Early solutions to this problem by Pocock (1977) and O'Brien and Fleming (1979) involve prespecifying the number of interim analyses and computing a stopping boundary for each that restricts overall Type I error. Lan and DeMets (1983) avoid prespecifying the number of interim looks by utilizing a Type I error "spending function." While an extremely clever tool, the spending function seems somewhat arbitrary and largely serves to rescue the frequentist from a tight mathematical spot without addressing the fundamental problems with p-values; see e.g. Subsection 2.2.7 and Carlin and Louis (2009, Sec. 2.3.3).

In principle, Bayesians do not face the "multiple looks problem" at all: their decisions are based on posterior summaries that do not depend on how the experiment was stopped; the posterior simply evolves (typically narrowing) as data accumulate. This is why Bayesians are free to "peek at their data" any time they wish, *provided* they really have no interest in the long-run frequency properties of their procedures. Of course, this is not the case in clinical trials, where we've already established the importance of the long run. And in any case, government regulators' ongoing interest in the subject forces the Bayesian's hand here.

Fortunately, simulation methods we have outlined once again come to the rescue. We simply incorporate whatever pre-ordained schedule of looks (say, every $N = 20$ patients, up to a maximum of 100) into the simulation program, and modify our empirical stopping proportions accordingly. Bookkeeping does become somewhat more complicated, since we are likely interested in the proportions of trials stopped for each reason *at each monitoring point*. At present this may begin to push the envelope of what is possible computationally with BRugs calling BUGS; at some point a normal or other approximation to the posterior may be necessary to avoid a BUGS call for every simulated fake dataset.

Finally, a potential concern when using sequential stopping extensively is that of "sampling to a foregone conclusion," the mathematical result that repeated calculation of Bayesian tail probabilities will ultimately lead to rejection of any null hypothesis. While the number of interim looks typically used in practice suggests this will rarely be a concern, see Spiegelhalter et al. (2004, Section 6.6.5) and references therein for more on this issue.

2.5.5 Incorporating costs

The methods discussed so far might be described as "probability only" methods, in that they base their decisions entirely on tail areas or confidence intervals derived from the posterior distributions of the model parameters of interest. No attempt is made to quantify any of the costs inherent in the process, or to have this information influence the decisionmaking.

Yet clearly there are many such costs inherent in the process: the monetary cost of enrolling and following each new patient, the cost to a company of continuing to develop a new drug (rather than abandon it and focus resources elsewhere), and of course the human cost of delaying a decision while patients in the trial (half of whom are by definition receiving an inferior treatment) are at risk for the trial's endpoint(s).

If they can be reliably quantified, Bayesian methods are well-suited to incorporating such costs, through the field of *Bayesian decision theory*. Whole textbooks (e.g. DeGroot, 1970; Berger, 1985) have been devoted to this topic, and whole journals (e.g., *Medical Decision Making*) are devoted to the use of Bayesian and non-Bayesian quantitative methods in medical cost-effectiveness studies. Still, statisticians have historically been somewhat reticent to use these methods, on the grounds that their results depend crucially on the precise costs selected, whose values are often easily criticized by potential readers of the analysis. The implementation of Bayesian decision-theoretic methods can also be complex, especially in the case where MCMC algorithms must be used to estimate posteriors. For our purposes, then, the primary use of these methods may be in internal studies where appropriate costs can be agreed upon, and where the final decision-makers are also "in house," rather than being some external reader whose opinions regarding costs and benefits cannot be known in advance. See Section 4.6 for more discussion, and Subsection 4.6.2 for a specific application of decision theoretic design to drug development.

A basic and computationally feasible framework for incorporating cost effectiveness was recently provided by O'Hagan and Stevens (2001). These authors laid out a Bayesian formulation of the sample size determination problem that generalizes a traditional frequentist sample size calculation based on hypothesis testing. They did this in the context of assessing the *cost effectiveness* of a particular treatment relative to control. Specifically, they let e_{ij} be the observed efficacy and c_{ij} be the cost of treatment i for patient j, $j = 1, \ldots, n_i$ and $i = 1, 2$, where $i = 1$ denotes control and $i = 2$ denotes treatment. These authors then assume the bivariate normal model

$$\begin{pmatrix} e_{ij} \\ c_{ij} \end{pmatrix} \sim N_2 \left(\begin{pmatrix} \mu_i \\ \gamma_i \end{pmatrix}, \Sigma \right),$$

where $\Sigma_{11} = \sigma_i^2, \Sigma_{22} = \tau_i^2$, and $\Sigma_{12} = \Sigma_{21} = \rho_i \sigma_i \tau_i$. Given the scale in which the costs c_{ij} are expressed (dollars, patient lives, etc.), suppose K is the maximum amount we are prepared to pay to obtain one unit of increase in efficacy e_{ij}. Then our cost effectiveness assessment must be based on the net benefit

$$\beta = K(\mu_2 - \mu_1) - (\gamma_2 - \gamma_1).$$

The treatment ($i = 2$) is cost effective if $\beta > 0$. Denoting all the data $\{e_{ij}, c_{ij}\}$ as $\mathbf{y}$, suppose we require $P(\beta > 0 | \mathbf{y}) > \omega$. Then this Bayesian analysis objective is analogous to rejecting $H_0 : \beta = 0$ in favor of the one-sided alternative $H_a : \beta > 0$ at a p-value of $\alpha = 1-\omega$. O'Hagan and Stevens (2001) refer to this as the *analysis objective*, and the prior used to calculate the posterior probability as the *analysis prior*.

Now, the sample sizes n_i in each group must be such that, averaging over all datasets we might see, the probability of a positive result is at least δ. That is, using subscripts to more clearly indicate the random variable with respect to which an expectation is taken, we require

$$P_{\mathbf{Y}}\left[P_{\boldsymbol{\xi}}(\mathbf{a}'\boldsymbol{\xi} > 0|\mathbf{y}) > \omega\right] > \delta , \qquad (2.30)$$

where $\boldsymbol{\xi} = (\mu_1, \gamma_1, \mu_2, \gamma_2)'$ and $\mathbf{a} = (-K, 1, K, -1)'$, so that $\beta = \mathbf{a}'\boldsymbol{\xi}$.

The authors refer to the left-hand side of (2.30) as the *Bayesian assurance*; note it is the Bayesian analogue of power, averaged with respect to the prior distribution used to calculate the marginal distribution of the data $\mathbf{Y}$. Like our treatment in Subsection 2.5.4, O'Hagan and Stevens (2001) observed that this prior distribution need *not* be the same as the one used to calculate the inner, posterior probability in (2.30). That is, they too recognized the need to allow for different priors at the design and analysis stages. In their notation, we would have

$$\text{design prior:} \qquad \boldsymbol{\xi} \sim N(\mathbf{m}_d, V_d) ,$$
$$\text{analysis prior:} \qquad \boldsymbol{\xi} \sim N(\mathbf{m}_a, V_a) ,$$

where $\mathbf{m}_d, V_d, \mathbf{m}_a$, and V_a are all assumed known. Note that $V_a^{-1} = 0$ produces a vague (zero precision) analysis prior, while $V_d = 0$ produces a point design prior. Under these two conditions, Bayesian assurance is equal to frequentist power at the proposed true $\mathbf{m}_a$ value. These fully specified, conjugate forms enable closed form posterior and marginal distributions for $\boldsymbol{\xi}$ and $\mathbf{Y}$, respectively, that in turn facilitate calculation of the assurance. For example, consider the frequentist setting of a flat analysis prior ($V_a^{-1} = 0$ in the limit) and a point design prior ($V_d = 0$). The former condition implies $V^* = S$, while the latter implies a precise specification of $\boldsymbol{\xi} = \mathbf{m}_d$. If we require $n = n_1 = n_2$, equal sample sizes in the treatment and control groups, then the common sample size in the frequentist case turns out to satisfy

$$n \geq \frac{(z_{1-\omega} + z_{1-\delta})^2 \mathbf{a}'S_1\mathbf{a}}{(\mathbf{a}'\mathbf{m}_d)^2} , \qquad (2.31)$$

where S_1 is the single-observation variance matrix obtained by setting $n_1 = n_2 = 1$ in the previous expression for S.

Obviously the results of this subsection depend heavily on the specific model used, which is somewhat artificial and specialized (normal distributions with known variance matrices). However, the principles involved, namely choosing design and analysis priors and using them to determine sample sizes through fixed definitions of trial success (analysis objective) and Bayesian power (design objective), are quite general. Given the increasing pressure to deliver therapies quickly and at low relative cost, along with the slowly but steadily emerging consensus on appropriate cost metrics (say, via *quality adjusted life years*, or QALYs), methods like these should find greater and greater application in clinical trials practice.

An important concept in cost effectiveness studies is the *incremental cost effectiveness ratio* (ICER), the incremental cost over incremental benefit for an experimental therapy compared to the standard of care. When the ICER for a new therapy is above a certain threshold, the therapy is judged to be cost effective. O'Hagan, Stevens, and Montmartin (2000) show that this rule can be justified as a decision theoretic optimal Bayes rule under a certain utility function.

Software note: In subsequent work (O'Hagan et al., 2001), these same three authors offer exemplification of the approach with a real dataset, with supporting `WinBUGS` code available at

`www.tonyohagan.co.uk/academic/Astradat.txt.`

2.5.6 Delayed response

Clinical studies often involve delayed responses, i.e., outcomes that are observed with a substantial time delay after assigning a treatment or enrolling a patient. Such lagged responses create challenges for clinical trial designs when a stopping decision or treatment allocation requires outcomes from earlier enrolled patients. Typical examples are phase II trials where the outcome might be an indicator for a certain change in tumor volume by a certain time, for example tumor response within 5 weeks after treatment. Another typical example is the occurrence of graft versus host disease (GVHD) within 100 days. In either case the outcome is observed with a substantial delay after treatment allocation. When the next patient is recruited, there would usually be several already enrolled patients who have been assigned treatments, but are still awaiting the final response. Such delays complicate clinical trial design when a decision for the next patient or patient cohort depends on responses from earlier patients.

For Bayesian designs, dependence on earlier outcomes is formalized by basing current decisions on the posterior distribution conditional on all previous outcomes. The principled nature of Bayesian inference offers an easy solution to the problem of delayed responses. The relevant posterior distribution simply includes the partial responses from already enrolled patients with missing final response. For example, when the response is an event time, this simply amounts to censoring. In general, the posterior conditional on the partially observed response is the expected posterior conditional on a hypothetical final response. The expectation is defined with respect to the posterior predictive distribution for the final response (see Subsection 2.5.1).

In many studies with delayed responses, it is possible to record early outcomes. For example, when the final response is progression-free survival, one could record shrinkage of tumor volume as an early outcome. Shrinkage of tumor volume is usually considered to be indicative of an improved survival outcome. Using the posterior predictive distribution conditional on such early responses can greatly improve efficiency of the clinical trial design. We defer further, more technical discussion of this issue to Subsection 4.4.4.

2.5.7 Noncompliance and causal modeling

While somewhat embarrassing to mention, everything we do in this book depends on the subjects' willingness to comply with the treatment they are (randomly) assigned by the trial protocol. But such *compliance* (or *adherence*) is far from given in most clinical trials. Acknowledging this reality forces a major reassessment of our theory: to what extent does failure to comply with the assigned treatment in a clinical trial alter the trial's fundamental findings?

Such considerations take us into the realm of *causal inference*, which attempts to estimate not the effect of being *assigned* to a particular treatment, but the "causal" effect of actually *receiving* such a treatment. It is often argued that this quantity is the real target of interest in a clinical trial, since we wish to estimate the actual effect of receiving the treatment, not merely the effect of being assigned to the group that was *supposed* to receive the treatment.

But even this modest intellectual leap is controversial. Many clinical trialists maintain that the effect of treatment assignment *is* what is relevant in every trial; after all, if the drug is approved and ends up being used by the general population, many patients assigned to receive the treatment by their physicians will not actually receive it, perhaps due to cost, unpleasant side effects, or any number of any other reasons. Such trialists would likely argue that since these problems are just as likely to appear in the trial as in post-trial practice, it is more appropriate to simply ignore the noncompliance problem at the trial stage and estimate the effect of treatment assignment. This viewpoint is extremely widespread and is captured by the phrase "intention to treat" (ITT): we attempt to estimate the effect of treatment *assignment* (rather than actual treatment received) since this is the effect we can expect if the drug is approved and utilized by the general population.

Still, the validity of the ITT approach clearly rests on the assumption that the nature and amount of noncompliance in the clinical trial will be the same as that emerging in the population at large. Clearly this may not be the case. For one thing, persons enrolling in a trial may be more likely to be concerned with their own well-being than an average person, and as such be more likely to comply with their treatment assignment. Second, the distribution of good compliers may not be the same in the treatment and control groups: if the treatment has unpleasant side effects, we might expect poorer compliance in that group. In any case, an informed person contemplating entering a drug regimen is more likely to wonder, "What is the likely benefit of this treatment given that I actually take it?" as opposed to, "What is the average treatment benefit for persons assigned to take this treatment in a clinical trial?" We face a classic case of needing to answer the right question, rather than the question that is easiest to pose and answer. In short, we have to think about causality.

The problem of noncompliance and its impact on causality has plagued Bayesians and frequentists alike. Both camps require extra model assumptions to advance beyond standard ITT approaches while still ensuring all model parameters are identifiable. A significant amount of the frequentist statistical literature in this area has arisen from the work of J.M. Robins and colleagues. For instance, Robins and Tsiatis (1991) extended the usual accelerated failure time model with time-dependent covariates to a class of semiparametric failure time models called *structural failure time* models, and proposed a rank-based estimation method. Robins (1998) broadened the set of models, focusing attention on several classes of what he termed *structural nested models*. This work assumes the decision whether or not to comply with treatment assignment is random conditional on the history of a collection of prognostic factors. Greenland, Lanes, and Jara (2008) explore the use of structural nested models and advocate what they call *g-estimation*, a form of test-based estimation adhering to the ITT principle and accommodating a semiparametric Cox partial likelihood. In these authors' data illustration, *g*-estimation does produce a slightly larger estimated treatment effect than ITT, but also a significantly wider confidence interval, reflecting what they argue is the true, higher level of uncertainty, the "statistical price" of noncompliance.

For the most part, the work is highly theoretical and notoriously difficult, though certainly not bereft of good data analysis; see e.g. Robins and Greenland (1994). A forthcoming textbook (Hernán and Robins, to appear) figures to shed substantial light on frequentist causal inference, both model-based and model-free. Of course, many good textbooks on the subject already exist; of these, Pearl (2000) is worthy of special mention.

On the Bayesian side, the literature is dominated by the work of D.B. Rubin and colleagues, and especially the "Rubin causal model" (Holland, 1986; Rubin, 2005). This framework, which is reminiscent of instrumental variables approaches in econometrics, also makes certain assumptions about the underlying state of nature in order to ensure identifiability. The usual reference is Imbens and Rubin (1997); here we follow the less technical summary in Mealli and Rubin (2002). These authors describe the basic two-arm randomized trial model, where we set $Z_i = 1$ if subject i is assigned to the active treatment arm, and $Z_i = 0$ if assigned to the control arm. The model imagines the existence of two *potential outcomes* $Y_i(1)$ and $Y_i(0)$, only one of which is observed for each individual, depending on their treatment assignment. In this basic model, compliance is assumed to be "all or nothing"; i.e., some subjects assigned to the new treatment will not take it, while some assigned to the control will take the new treatment. The latter case is possibly rare in many carefully controlled trials, but does occur in settings where randomization is not to a particular experimental drug but to "encouragement" of some sort, where patients in the treatment group are merely encouraged to take a treatment (say, a vaccine injection) to which patients assigned to control would also have access.

Next let $D_i(z)$ indicate the treatment actually received (again, 1 for treatment, 0 for control). These two indicators then partition the population into four groups:

- always takers (ATs), for whom $D_i(z) = 1$ regardless of z,
- never takers (NTs), for whom $D_i(z) = 0$ regardless of z,
- compliers (Cs), for whom $D_i(z) = z$, and
- defiers (Ds), for whom $D_i(z) = 1 - z$.

The model does not assume that exact group membership is observed; a subject assigned to treatment who actually receives control could be a defier or a never taker. However, thanks to randomization, the distribution across the four groups is at least roughly the same in each treatment arm.

As mentioned above, the problem with ITT analysis is that its interpretation is difficult when compliance differs across treatment group. In the language used above, we can write the ITT effect as

$$ITT = \eta_C ITT_C + \eta_{NT} ITT_{NT} + \eta_{AT} ITT_{AT} + \eta_D ITT_D , \qquad (2.32)$$

where the η's give the proportion of subjects in each of the four classes, and the ITTs give the effect of treatment assignment on subjects of that type. Since our data cannot identify all these ITT parameters, certain assumptions must be made. The first is the so-called *exclusion restriction*, which essentially argues that since treatment assignment does not alter the compliance behavior for ATs and NTs, it should not alter their outcomes either, and therefore we may set $ITT_{AT} = ITT_{NT} = 0$. Note there is no classical statistical estimate for either of these two quantities (since we never see ATs in the control group, nor NTs in the treatment group), so assuming them equal to 0 is certainly a convenient escape. A second common assumption is the so-called *monotonicity assumption*, which in this context is equivalent to assuming that there are no defiers (e.g., $\eta_D = 0$). Adding this to the exclusion restriction means that the effect of treatment assignment on compliers, ITT_C, can be consistently estimated via (2.32) provided both the $Y_i(Z_i)$ and $D_i(Z_i)$ are observed. In the presence of noncompliance ($\eta_C < 1$), it's easy to see that $ITT < ITT_C$, i.e., the usual ITT estimate is a conservative estimate of ITT_C. However, relaxing the exclusion restriction for NTs or ATs, this intuitive result may not manifest.

The Bayesian paradigm pays dividends in this setting by using proper priors. Combined with the (often weak) information in the data regarding the size of the effect in the four groups, we can often obtain improved estimates that better reflect the true effect of treatment assignment for noncompliers. Hirano et al. (2000) offer an example from a trial where one group of physicians were encouraged to remind their patients to receive flu shots, while another group received no such special encouragement. A standard ITT analysis suggests a 1.4% decrease in hospitalization rate in the encouragement group, suggesting a modest benefit arising from the treatment. However, in a reanalysis assuming monotonicity and fixing $ITT_{NT} = 0$ but allowing $ITT_{AT} \neq 0$, these authors find $ITT_C \approx ITT_{AT}$; the benefit arising from encouragement was roughly the same for the compliers as for subjects who would have gotten the flu shot no matter what. This in turn suggests the shot itself is *not* very effective, a counterintuitive result that the authors suggest may be due to some encouraged ATs getting their flu shots a bit *earlier* than normal, which in turn provided as much benefit as the flu shot itself did for the compliers.

Mealli and Rubin (2002) go on to outline further enhancements to the model to accommodate missing outcomes in the presence of noncompliance. The most recent work in this area builds on (and uses the dataset of) Efron and Feldman (1991): Jin and Rubin (2008) use principal stratification to extend to the case of *partial* compliance, where each patient may only take some portion of the assigned dose. This paper also allows differential compliance levels in the treatment and control groups. Again, the work is technical, but guided by Bayesian principles that at least permit a fair comparison across models and informative priors.

While a full description of the technical issues involved in Bayesian causal inference is well beyond the scope of this book, in the remainder of this subsection we do provide some flavor for the complexity of the modeling as practiced today by describing the approach of Chib and Jacobi (2008). This work is technically challenging, even for a model slightly simpler than that of Imbens and Rubin (1997), which to us only reemphasizes the necessity of being Bayesian, at least formally, just to make sense of such causal models and provide a framework for judging performance. Chib and Jacobi (2008) consider the case of an *eligibility trial*, where

$$D_i(Z_i) = \begin{cases} 0 & \text{if } Z_i = 0 \\ 0 \text{ or } 1 & \text{if } Z_i = 1 \end{cases}.$$

That is, persons assigned to control do not have access to the drug and must therefore comply; there are no ATs. Chib and Jacobi (2008) assume that $x_i \equiv D_i(z_i)$ is observed for every subject, as is $\mathbf{w}_i$, a p-vector of observed confounders that simultaneously affect both the outcome and the intake in the treatment arm. Writing the two potential outcomes as Y_{0i} and Y_{1i}, these authors go on to model the joint density of each with drug intake given the treatment assignment and the confounders,

$$p(y_i, x_i = 0 | \mathbf{w}_i, z_i = \ell) = p(y_{0i}, x_i = 0 | \mathbf{w}_i, z_i = \ell)$$
$$\text{and } p(y_i, x_i = 1 | \mathbf{w}_i, z_i = \ell) = p(y_{1i}, x_i = 1 | \mathbf{w}_i, z_i = \ell),$$

for $\ell = 0, 1$. To specify these joint distributions, we first define $I_{\ell j} = \{i : z_i = \ell \text{ and } x_i = j\}$, and note that only I_{00}, I_{10}, and I_{11} are non-empty ($I_{01} = \emptyset$ since in this trial, those assigned the control cannot take the treatment). If we further define $s_i = 0$ or 1 for never-takers and compliers, respectively, then we can write

$$p(y_i, x_i = j | \mathbf{w}_i, z_i = \ell) = \begin{cases} (1 - q_i)p_0(y_i | \mathbf{w}_i, s_i = 0) \\ \qquad + q_i p_0(y_i | \mathbf{w}_i, s_i = 1) & \text{if } i \in I_{00} \\ (1 - q_i)p_0(y_i | \mathbf{w}_i, s_i = 0) & \text{if } i \in I_{10} \\ q_i p_1(y_i | \mathbf{w}_i, s_i = 1) & \text{if } i \in I_{11} \end{cases},$$

where $q_i = P(s_i = 1 | \mathbf{v}_i, \alpha) = \Phi(\mathbf{v}_i' \alpha)$, and $\Phi(\cdot)$ is the standard normal cdf. Chib and Jacobi (2008) go on to specify all the components in the above expression, choosing Student t densities with means that involve linear regressions on the $\mathbf{w}_i$ for the conditional densities of the y_i. Normal and inverse gamma hyperpriors complete the model specification. The authors then provide a Gibbs-Metropolis algorithm for estimating the posterior distributions of the model parameters, which in turn enables predictive inference for compliers, and hence a natural estimate of the causal effect.

This approach, while fairly involved, clarifies some previous literature by making more explicit assumptions that can be debated and checked. Future work in this area likely involves extending the approach to partial compliance, clustered outcomes, binary response, and other more challenging model settings. From a practical viewpoint, adoption of all of these strategies awaits user-friendly software, and perhaps more importantly, greater agreement among trialists that making the sorts of subjective assumptions about compliance required by these models is preferable to simply living with an ITT analysis that, while undoubtedly imperfect, at least offers an interpretable and typically conservative option.

2.6 Appendix: R Macros

The online supplement to this chapter

www.biostat.umn.edu/~brad/software/BCLM_ch2.html

provides the R and BUGS code that was used in this chapter, including that for the basic clinical trial operating characteristic simulation program described in Example 2.9 of Subsection 2.5.4.

## CHAPTER 3

Phase I studies

In this chapter we tackle "early phase" problems, specifically those associated with phase I trials for safety and appropriate dosing of a new treatment. Representing the first application of a new drug to humans, early phase trials are typically small – say, 20 to 50 patients. The main goal in the early phases is to establish the safety of a proposed drug, and to study what the body does to the drug as it moves through the body (*pharmacokinetics*), and what the drug in turn does to the body (*pharmacodynamics*). Determining an appropriate dosing schedule for a drug, or *dose-finding*, is a major component of phase I studies. For relatively nontoxic agents, phase I trials may start with healthy volunteers. For agents with known toxicity, such as cytotoxic agents in cancer therapy, phase I trials are conducted among cancer patients for whom standard therapies have failed. We will use drug development in cancer therapy as our main example in this and subsequent chapters to demonstrate the application of adaptive Bayesian methods, but stress that the methods are equally applicable in a wide variety of non-cancer drug and device settings.

For developing a cytotoxic agent, the highest possible dose is sought, since the benefit of the new treatment is believed to increase with dose. Unfortunately, the severity of toxicity is also expected to increase with dose, so the challenge is to increase the dose without causing an unacceptable amount of toxicity in the patients. Thus the primary goal of a phase I study is to identify this dose, the *maximum tolerated dose (MTD)* in a dose-escalation fashion.

Key elements of phase I studies include (a) defining the starting dose, (b) defining the toxicity profile and *dose-limiting toxicity* (DLT), (c) defining an acceptable level of toxicity, the *target toxicity level* (TTL), and (d) defining a dose escalation scheme. For the first study in humans, the starting dose is often chosen as one tenth of the LD_{10} (a lethal dose for 10% of the animals) in mice, or one third of the lowest toxic dose in dogs, as these doses have been shown to be safe in humans for cytotoxic agents (Collins et al., 1986). While starting with a safe and low dose is important, investigators must balance the risk of toxicity with the risk of treating patients with drugs at ineffective doses. For most drugs, we assume that as the dose increases, the probability of toxicity and the probability of efficacy will both increase. Hence, the goal is to define the MTD or the *recommended phase II dose* (RP2D) which yields an acceptable TTL – typically between 20% and 33%.

The dose escalation scheme contains three components: (i) a dose increment, (ii) a dose assignment, and (iii) a cohort size. Many studies use pre-determined dose increments at fixed doses, such as 10 mg, 20 mg, 30 mg, and so on. Alternatively, we may specify a general scheme for setting the doses, such as doubling the current dose when no toxicities are observed, reducing to a 50% dose increment when non-dose-limiting toxicities are observed, and reducing to a 25% dose increment when a DLT is observed. In the examples of this chapter, we assume that all the dose levels are specified in advance. We also generally assume that new patients are treated in cohorts of a prespecified size (say, 1, 3, or 6).

Dose assignment refers to how to new patients enrolled in the trial are assigned to dose levels. Based on dose assignment, phase I trials can be classified into *rule-based methods* and *model-based methods*. The next two sections consider each of these broad areas in turn.

3.1 Rule-based designs for determining the MTD

Standard rule-based designs assign new patients to dose levels according to prespecified rules and without stipulating any assumption regarding the dose-toxicity curve. These designs belong to the class of "up-and-down" designs (Dixon and Mood, 1948; Storer, 1989), as they allow dose escalation and de-escalation based on the absence or presence of toxicity in the previous cohort. The simple up-and-down design converges to a dose corresponding to a probability of DLT around 50%. The traditional *3+3 design* is a rule-based design which remains widely used in clinical practice. Variations of the 3+3 design, such as the pharmacologically guided dose escalation method (Collins et al., 1990) and accelerated titration designs (Simon et al., 1997), have also been applied in clinical trials.

3.1.1 Traditional 3+3 design

The traditional 3+3 design involves no modeling of the dose-toxicity curve beyond assuming that toxicity increases with dose. The design proceeds in cohorts of three patients, the first cohort being treated at a starting dose, and the next cohorts being treated at increasing dose levels that have been fixed in advance. Dose levels have historically been chosen according to some variation of a *Fibonacci sequence*. A Fibonacci sequence is a sequence of numbers where each number is the sum of the two previous numbers in the sequence; an example is {1,1,2,3,5,8,...}. The doses are increased according to the percentage increase between successive numbers in the Fibonacci sequence; for this example {100,50,67,60,...}. Often, a modified

1. Cohort	Dose Level 1	2	3	4	5
1	0/3				
2		0/3			
3			1/3		
4			0/3		
5				2/3	
MTD			***		

2. Cohort	Dose Level 1	2	3	4	5
1	0/3				
2		0/3			
3			0/3		
4				2/3	
5			0/3		
MTD			***		

Figure 3.1 *Example of the traditional 3+3 design; entries are (number of DLTs/number of patients treated) by cohort and dose level.*

sequence such as {100,67,50,40,33} is used so that the increments decrease as the dose level increases.

There are slight variations on the traditional 3+3 design, but a commonly used version is as follows. If none of the three patients in a cohort experiences a DLT, another three patients will be treated at the next higher dose level. If one of the first three patients experiences a DLT, three more patients will be treated at the same dose level. The dose escalation continues but stops as soon as at least two patients experience DLTs, among a total of up to six patients (i.e. probability of DLT at the dose$\geq$ 33%). The MTD is typically defined as the highest dose level in which at least 6 patients are treated and where no more than 33% of the patients experience DLT. Thus, a summary of one common version of the approach is as follows:

Algorithm 3.1 *(3+3 design)*
    Step 1: Enter 3 patients at the lowest dose level
    Step 2: Observe the toxicity outcome
        0/3 DLT $\Rightarrow$ Treat next 3 patients at next higher dose
        1/3 DLT $\Rightarrow$ Treat next 3 patients at the same dose
            1/3 + 0/3 DLT $\Rightarrow$ Treat next 3 patients at next higher dose
            1/3 + 1/3 DLT $\Rightarrow$ Define this dose as MTD
            1/3 + 2/3 or 3/3 DLT $\Rightarrow$ dose exceeds MTD
        2/3 or 3/3 DLT $\Rightarrow$ dose exceeds MTD
    Step 3: Repeat Step 2 until MTD is reached. If the last dose exceeds MTD, define the previous dose level as MTD if 6 or more patients were treated at that level. Otherwise, treat more patients at the previous dose level.
    Step 4: MTD is defined as a dose with $\leq$ 2/6 DLT ∎

Figure 3.1 depicts two simple idealized illustrations of the 3+3 design. In the first panel of the figure, five cohorts of patients were treated sequentially

Dose Level (mg/m^2/day x 5 days)

Cohort	1	4[a]	8	12[c]	14[c]	16
1	0/3					
2		0/3				
3			0/3			
4						6/12[b]
5				2/10		
6					2/8	
MTD					***	

Figure 3.2 *Result of the taxotere trial applying the traditional 3+3 design; entries are (number of DLTs/number of patients treated) by cohort and dose level. Notes: (a) the 2 mg/m^2/day x 5 days dose was skipped when another study reported no toxicities at a total dose level greater than 10 mg/m^2 just after this trial began; (b) after observing DLTs, the study was expanded to include a heavily pretreated group and a non-heavily pretreated group; (c) these intermediate doses were added after the trial began.*

in four dose levels. Dose level 3 is chosen as the MTD with an estimated DLT rate of 16.7%. Similarly, in the second panel of Figure 3.1, dose 3 was chosen as the MTD but the estimated DLT rate is 0%. Had one or two DLTs been observed in the three patients in Cohort 5, dose 3 would still have been chosen as the MTD in this case, with a DLT rate of 33%. The examples show that the choice of the MTD in the traditional 3+3 design is *ad hoc* and fairly imprecise.

We now give two examples showing how the traditional 3+3 design is used in practice.

Example 3.1 Figure 3.2 shows the results from the taxotere trial reported by Pazdur et al. (1992). In this trial, a total of 39 patients were treated. The first DLT was observed at the dose level of 16 mg/m^2. The initial toxicities were seen in heavily pretreated patients and the investigators decided to expand the cohort to include non-heavily pretreated patients as well. The dose was eventually shown to be too toxic; hence, two intermediate doses were added to the trial. The MTD was defined as the 14 mg/m^2/day level, for which the estimated DLT rate was 0.25. ∎

Example 3.2 Figure 3.3 shows the results of a second trial employing a 3+3 design, the gemcitabine trial reported by Abbruzzese et al. (1991). The starting dose level, 10 mg/m^2 was chosen as 1/20 of the rat LD_{10}. This trial took 12 dose escalations to determine the MTD as 790 mg/m^2, a dose level 79 times the starting dose. This trial illustrates that the traditional 3+3

Dose Level (mg/m^2)

	10	15	22.5	35	53	80	120	180	225[a]	350	525	790	1000[a]
Cohort													
1	0/3												
2		0/3											
3			0/3										
4				0/3									
5					0/3								
6						0/3							
7							0/3						
8								0/3					
9									1/4				
10										0/3			
11											1/3		
12												1/7	
13													3/6
MTD												***	

Figure 3.3 *Result of the gemcitabine trial applying the traditional 3+3 design; entries are (number of DLTs/number of patients treated) by cohort and dose level.*

design can be very inefficient when the starting dose is too low and the dose increment is moderate. In a recent report (Le Tourneau et al., 2009), 19 anticancer agents were approved by the US Food and Drug Administration (FDA) in solid tumors using the traditional 3+3 design. Among them, more than half involved *six or more* dose levels. ■

3.1.2 Pharmacologically guided dose escalation

To more efficiently identify the dose region containing the MTD, the *pharmacologically guided dose escalation* (PGDE) method assumes that DLTs can be predicted by drug plasma concentrations, based on animal data (Collins et al., 1990). The PGDE method is carried out in two stages. In the first stage, pharmacokinetic data are measured for each patient in real time to determine the subsequent dose level. As long as a pre-specified plasma exposure defined by the area under the concentration-time curve (AUC), extrapolated from preclinical data, is not reached, dose escalation proceeds with one patient per dose level, typically at 100% dose increments. Once the target AUC is reached or if DLTs occur, dose escalation switches to the traditional 3+3 design with smaller dose increments (usually around 40%). In clinical practice, the PGDE method has achieved good results with some cytotoxic agents such as certain anthracyclines and platinum compounds, while the method has been found to be inappropriate for other classes of agents such as antifolates that display a high interpatient pharmacokinetic heterogeneity. The logistical difficulties in obtaining real-time pharmacokinetic results and in extrapolating preclinical pharmacokinetic data to phase I studies also impedes the success of the PGDE method.

3.1.3 Accelerated titration designs

The *accelerated titration design* (ATD; Simon et al., 1997) is a commonly used variation of the traditional 3+3 design in which intrapatient dose escalation is allowed in multiple cycles of the same patient. Although the dose escalation scheme is rule-based, all the observed data can be used to provide further modeling of the dose-toxicity curves. Two-stage designs with an accelerated phase used in ATD theoretically help to reduce the number of patients treated at subtherapeutic doses. Permitting intrapatient dose escalation is also appealing because it gives some patients the opportunity to be treated at higher, presumably more effective doses. The main drawback of intrapatient dose escalation is that it may mask any cumulative effects of treatment, and would certainly make them less obvious and difficult to differentiate from chronic or delayed toxicity.

3.1.4 Other rule-based designs

Alternative rule-based designs besides the 3+3 have been proposed, including the "2+4", "3+3+3" and "3+1+1" (also referred to as "best of five" rule) designs; see Storer (2001). In the 2+4 design, an additional cohort of four patients is added if one DLT is observed in a first cohort of two patients. The stopping rule is the same as with the traditional "3+3" design. In the 3+3+3 design, a third cohort of three patients is added if two of six patients experienced a DLT at a certain dose level. The trial terminates if at least three of nine patients experience a DLT. Finally, the "best of five" design is more aggressive, as one additional patient can be added if one or two DLTs are observed among the first three patients. Another patient will be added if two DLTs are observed among the four treated patients. Dose escalation is allowed if 0/3, 1/4 or 2/5 DLTs are observed, while the trial will terminate if three or more DLTs are observed.

3.1.5 Summary of rule-based designs

The advantages of the rule-based methods are that they are easy to implement and do not require specialized software. Their performance (operating characteristics), however, may not be particularly attractive. For example, their target toxicity levels are implicit, and fixed after the rule is specified. The methods may also be inefficient in getting to a drug's "action zone." As a result, in a review of studies at M.D. Anderson Cancer Center, only

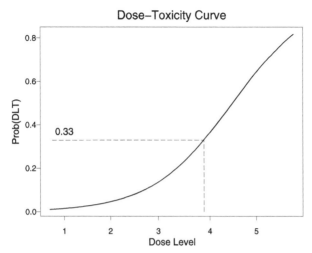

Figure 3.4 *Illustration of a dose-toxicity curve for a model-based design. If the target toxicity level (TTL) is 33%, dose level 4 is the MTD, since it comes closest to yielding the desired TTL.*

about 3% of the patients responded to the assigned treatment in phase I trials (Smith et al., 1996). The decision on dose allocation for future patients, as well as the definition of MTD or RP2D, is "memoryless" in that it relies on information from the current dose level only, and thus does not use all available information. As such, the MTD is then selected from the pre-specified dose levels depending on which one best fits the definition set *a priori*. In addition, the target toxicity level is fixed and implicitly specified once the rule is set. Although the implicit TTL can be calculated (Lin and Shih, 2001), the design is rigid and the rule often needs to be "bent" to target a particular TTL.

3.2 Model-based designs for determining the MTD

An alternative to the rule-based methods for finding the MTD is to assume that there is a monotonic dose-response relationship between the dose and the probability of DLT for patients treated at that dose; see Figure 3.4. In this approach, a dose-toxicity curve as well as the TTL are explicitly defined. The goal for the phase I clinical trial is, through treating patients in a dose escalation fashion, to seek a suitable quantile of the dose-toxicity curve; specifically, a dose that will induce a probability of DLT at a specified target toxicity level. This method is most conveniently carried out under the Bayesian framework. Simple one- or two- parameter parametric models are often used to characterize the dose-toxicity relationship, with the Bayesian

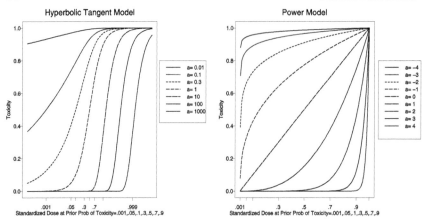

Figure 3.5 *Typical CRM dose-toxicity response curves: left, hyperbolic tangent; right, power.*

posterior distribution used to estimate the parameters. These designs use all the data to model the dose-toxicity curve, and provide a credible interval for the MTD at the end of the trial.

3.2.1 Continual reassessment method (CRM)

The *continual reassessment method* (CRM) seems to have been the first Bayesian model-based phase I design introduced in the literature (O'Quigley et al., 1990). In its most basic form, this method characterizes the dose-toxicity relationship by simple one-parameter parametric models, such as the hyperbolic tangent model, logistic model, or the power model. Specifically, letting $p(d)$ be the probability of DLT at dose d, these three parametric models are given by

$$\text{Hyperbolic tangent: } p(d) \;=\; [(tanh(d) + 1)/2]^a = \left[\frac{\exp(d)}{\exp(d) + \exp(-d)}\right]^a$$

$$\text{Logistic: } p(d) \;=\; \frac{\exp(3 + ad)}{1 + \exp(3 + ad)}$$

$$\text{Power: } p(d) \;=\; d^{\exp(a)}$$

Figure 3.5 shows the different shapes of the dose-toxicity curves for two of these models for varying values of the parameter a.

The original CRM is carried out using the following algorithm:

Algorithm 3.2 *(CRM design)*

Step 1: Assume a vague or fully non-informative prior for a.

Step 2: Treat 1 patient at the level closest to the current estimate of the MTD.

Step 3: Observe the toxicity outcome.

Step 4: Update a by computing its posterior distribution. This is of course obtained by multiplying the prior chosen in Step 1 by the likelihood, which after treating n patients is given by

$$L(a; \mathbf{d}, \mathbf{y}) \propto \prod_{i=1}^{n} p(d_i)^{y_i} [1 - p(d_i)]^{1-y_i} ,$$

where d_i and y_i are the dose level and toxicity outcome for patient i, and where $y_i = 1$ if a DLT is observed and $y_i = 0$ if not. In this simple one-parameter setting, the posterior arising from (2.1) might be most easily computed by a standard numerical quadrature method (e.g., trapezoidal rule), but of course MCMC methods (say, as implemented in WinBUGS) can also be used.

Step 5: Treat the next patient at the level closest to the updated estimate of MTD based on the posterior distribution of a.

Step 6: Repeat Steps 1–5 until a sufficiently precise estimate of a is achieved or the maximum sample size is reached.

∎

The choice of the dose-toxicity curve and the initial estimate of a will generally be elicited from experts familiar with drug development. Although this initial estimate may be inaccurate, it should provide an adequate starting point for dose escalation. As the trial moves along, a more accurate estimate of a is obtained; hence, more patients are treated at the dose thought to be closest to the MTD, which corresponds to the dose at the target toxicity level that maximizes the treatment effect while controlling toxicity. The original CRM allows jumping over multiple dose levels if so indicated in Step 5 above.

The CRM was not well-accepted in its original format due to safety considerations, as it could expose patients to unacceptably toxic doses if the prespecified model were incorrect. Consequently, modifications to the CRM were proposed to add additional safety measures which include (1) treating the first patient at the lowest starting dose level based on animal toxicology and conventional criteria, (2) increasing the dose by only one pre-specified level at a time, (3) not allowing dose escalation for the immediate next patient if a patient experienced a DLT, and (4) treating more than one patient at the same dose level, especially at higher dose levels. For more on these and other CRM modifications, see Korn et al. (1994), Faries (1994), Goodman et al. (1995), Piantadosi et al. (1998), and Heyd and Carlin (1999).

	Dose Level					
	1	2	3	4	5	6
Dose (mg/m^2)	10	20	40	60	75	90
Prob(toxicity)	0.05	0.10	0.20	0.30	0.50	0.70
Standardized dose	−1.47	−1.1	−0.69	−0.42	0	0.42

Table 3.1 *Dose levels, standardized doses, and prior probabilities of toxicity, CRM example.*

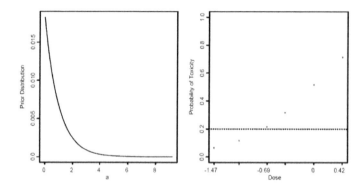

Figure 3.6 *Plots of the posterior distribution of a and the corresponding dose-toxicity curve for a CRM trial, Step 0: based only on the prior information; current MTD = dose 3.*

We now offer a simple example to illustrate how CRM is implemented in practice.

Example 3.3 Suppose that in developing a new agent, six dose levels are to be studied. We assume a hyperbolic tangent dose-toxicity curve with target toxicity level set at 20%. Note that the actual dose level is not important in the calculation. For convenience, the standardized dose can be calculated as $tanh^{-1}(2p-1)$ assuming $a = 1$. This is legitimate since, due to the one-to-one correspondence between a and d when p is given, we can set a at any fixed value to calculate the standardized dose. We assume the prior distribution for a follows an exponential distribution with mean 1. As a result, the prior probability of DLT at each dose will center around the initial estimate of p with a fairly wide credible interval. The dose levels and our prior beliefs regarding the probability of toxicity at each dose level are given in Table 3.1.

Figures 3.6–3.11 show a realization of one such trial applying the original

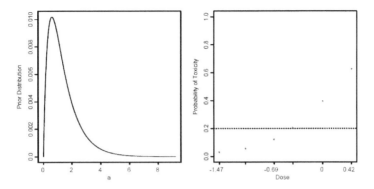

Figure 3.7 *Plots of the posterior distribution of a and the corresponding dose-toxicity curve for a CRM trial after Step 1: treat first patient at dose 3; result = no DLT; updated MTD = dose 4.*

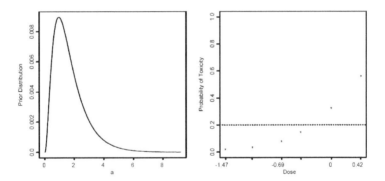

Figure 3.8 *Plots of the posterior distribution of a and the corresponding dose-toxicity curve for a CRM trial after Step 2: treat second patient at dose 4; result = no DLT; updated MTD = dose 4.*

CRM. The left panel of Figure 3.6 shows the prior distribution of a following the unit exponential distribution. The right panel shows the dose toxicity curve at the posterior mean of a. From the dose-toxicity curve, we find that dose level 3 is the dose closest to the current estimate of the MTD which yields a TTL of 0.2. Figure 3.7 shows the result (no DLT) after the first patient is treated at dose 3. With this information, the posterior distribution of a is calculated. The resulting dose-toxicity curve shows that the updated estimate of MTD is now dose level 4.

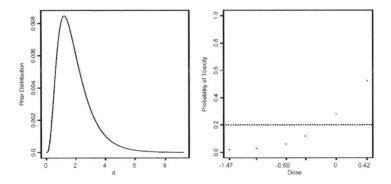

Figure 3.9 *Plots of the posterior distribution of a and the corresponding dose-toxicity curve for a CRM trial after Step 3: treat third patient at dose 4; result = no DLT; updated MTD = dose 5.*

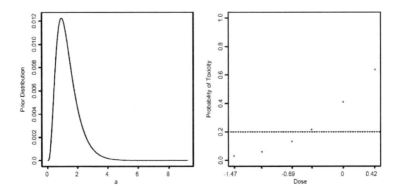

Figure 3.10 *Plots of the posterior distribution of a and the corresponding dose-toxicity curve for a CRM trial after Step 4: treat fourth patient at dose 5; result = DLT; updated MTD = dose 4.*

Suppose the second patient treated is treated at dose level 4 and results in no DLT. Figure 3.8 shows that the dose-toxicity curve continues to move downward because no DLT is found. At this point, the current estimate of MTD remains at dose level 4. The third patient is treated at dose level 4 and again no DLT is observed. Figure 3.9 shows that the new estimated MTD moves up to dose level 5. Patient 4 is treated at dose 5 and develops the first DLT. The posterior of a is updated again (Figure 3.10, left panel), and the resulting MTD now moves back to dose level 4.

To bring this example to a close, suppose the trial terminates at this

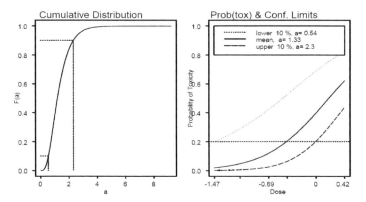

Figure 3.11 *CRM trial, Step 5: stop the trial now; the final posterior cdf of a and corresponding dose-toxicity curve (with 80% confidence bounds) are as shown.*

point. Then the final cumulative distribution of a is shown in the left panel of Figure 3.11, with the corresponding dose-toxicity curve and its 80% credible interval boundaries shown in the right panel. At the end of the trial, the posterior mean of a is 1.33. Thus dose level 4 is chosen as the final MTD because it is the dose which yields a probability of DLT closest to the targeted toxicity level. ∎

In the previous example, all necessary calculations were carried out in R. This code can be nested within a simulation program in order to evaluate and compare the operating characteristics of the 3+3 and CRM designs. Specifically, Table 3.2 compares the performance of the 3+3 and two CRM designs using 10,000 simulated trials over three scenarios, each of which operate over five dose levels. In all cases, we set the target toxicity level to 0.30. In Scenario 1, the true probabilities of DLT at dose levels 1 to 5 are 0.05, 0.15, 0.30, 0.45, and 0.60, respectively. Therefore, dose level 3 is the true MTD. The percentages of patients treated at the five dose levels using the 3+3 design are 26.0, 32.5, 27.2, 12.1, and 2.3, respectively. Alternatively, using the CRM design with a cohort size of 1 (CRM 1), the corresponding percentages are 15.6, 24.1, 34.7, 19.0, and 6.7. Thus more patients are treated at the true MTD level, but more are also treated at dose levels above the MTD. The overall percent of DLT for the 3+3 and CRM 1 designs are 21.1 and 27.0, respectively. However, by increasing the CRM cohort size from 1 to 3, this new design (CRM 3) treats fewer patients at levels above the MTD. At the end of the trial, the percentages of trials recommending dose level 3 as the MTD are 27.5, 52.4, and 49.8 for the 3+3, CRM 1, and CRM 3, respectively. Thus, compared to the 3+3 design, CRM designs are much more likely to identify the correct MTD level.

Scenario 2 depicts the case when the probabilities of DLT at dose levels

				Dose			Ave	%
		1	2	3	4	5	N	DLT
Scenario 1	P(DLT):	0.05	0.15	0.30	0.45	0.60		
3+3	% patients	26.0	32.5	**27.2**	12.1	2.3	15.2	21.1
	% MTD	20.5	42.7	**27.5**	5.7	0		
CRM 1	% patients	15.6	24.1	**34.7**	19.0	6.7	18.5	27.0
	% MTD	1.0	21.4	**52.4**	23.0	2.2		
CRM 3	% patients	21.3	31.4	**29.1**	15.8	2.5	19.0	23.3
	% MTD	1.5	22.6	**49.8**	23.7	2.4		
Scenario 2	P(DLT):	0.05	0.10	0.20	0.30	0.50		
3+3	% patients	21.6	25.7	26.4	**18.9**	7.3	16.9	18.3
	% MTD	9.5	28.5	33	**21.1**	0		
CRM 1	% patients	13.0	13.2	23.3	**30.4**	20.2	18.6	25.7
	% MTD	0.1	6.4	25.6	**49.4**	18.5		
CRM 3	% patients	19.3	19.8	25.2	**25.2**	10.5	19.1	20.8
	% MTD	0.2	5.5	25.4	**48.3**	20.5		
Scenario 3	P(DLT):	0.15	0.30	0.45	0.60	0.85		
3+3	% patients	43.9	**36.4**	16.3	3.2	0.2	11.6	27.0
	% MTD	***65.4***	**27.9**	6.3	0.4	0.0		
CRM 1	% patients	40.5	**35.4**	17.7	6.1	0.3	18.5	28.7
	% MTD	24.5	**52.8**	19.9	2.8	0.1		
CRM 3	% patients	41.5	**39.0**	15.3	4.1	0.1	18.5	27.3
	% MTD	23.6	**53.7**	19.6	3.0	0.1		

Table 3.2 *Simulation studies for comparing the operating characteristics of the 3+3 design versus the CRM designs. Abbreviations: CRM 1, CRM with cohort size 1; CRM 3, CRM with cohort size 3; P(DLT), probability of DLT at each dose level; % patients, % of patients treated at each dose level; % MTD, % of dose level selected as the MTD; Ave N, average sample size in the trial; % DLT: percentage of patients developing DLT. Values corresponding to the true MTD (0.30) are shown in* **boldface type***; value in* **slanted bold** *includes a 21.3% chance that the recommended MTD is* below *Dose 1.*

1 to 5 are 0.05, 0.10, 0.20, 0.30, and 0.50, respectively, a case where the assigned doses are somewhat less toxic than anticipated. Again targeting 30% DLT, this means that dose level 4 is the true MTD in this scenario. For the 3+3, CRM 1, and CRM 3 designs, the percentages of patients treated at dose 4 are 18.9, 30.4, and 25.2, respectively. The corresponding percentages for choosing dose 4 as the MTD are 21.1, 49.4, and 48.3, respectively.

Again, the CRM designs are much more likely to identify the correct MTD compared to the 3+3 design. The overall percentages of DLT for each of the three designs are 18.3, 25.7, and 20.8, respectively, showing that CRM 1 has the highest proportion of patients developing DLT, but one that is still below the 30% target level. CRM 3 again offers some protection in this regard relative to CRM 1, and for only a fractionally higher average sample size ("Ave N" in the table).

Scenario 3 illustrates a high-toxcity case, with DLT probabilities at dose levels 1 to 5 of 0.15, 0.30, 0.45, 0.60, and 0.85. In this scenario, the second dose is now the true MTD. The percentages of patients treated at dose level 2 for the 3+3, CRM 1, and CRM 3 designs are 36.4, 35.4, and 39.0, respectively. The percentages correctly identifying dose 2 as the MTD are 27.9, 52.8, and 53.7, respectively, As before, the CRM methods have a much better chance of correctly identifying the MTD. However, the percentages of patients treated at high dose levels (say, level 3 and above) are slightly higher for the CRM methods, as are the percentages of DLT (28.7 and 27.3 for CRM 1 and CRM 3, compared to 27.0 for the 3+3). So while the CRM methods are slightly more aggressive, the price paid in terms of higher risk of DLT (a few percent) seems small relative to the much more dramatic (roughly 25%) rise in correct selection probability, relative to the overly conservative 3+3 method. We also note that the 65.4% chance of selecting the lowest dose as the MTD actually includes a 21.3% chance that the method will determine the MTD to be *below* even this initial dose, which occurs with 3+3 when the first dose is determined to be too toxic.

In summary, CRM designs can identify the MTD level much more accurately compared to the 3+3 design. On the other hand, CRM designs treat more patients at the MTD level and above. Choosing a CRM cohort size of 3 instead of 1 offers some protection, reducing the number of patients treated at levels above the DLT.

Software note: The M.D. Anderson website,

$$\text{http} : //\text{biostatistics.mdanderson.org/SoftwareDownload/}$$

offers a freely downloadable stand-alone program called CRMSimulator. This program has a friendly user interface, and can do simulations and be used to run trials for a modest set of settings (e.g., only the power model is implemented).

Alternatively, this book's software page for this chapter,

$$\text{www.biostat.umn.edu/~brad/software/BCLM\_ch3.html}$$

contains an R program called phaseIsim.R that was used to produce the results above. This program can run both 3+3 and CRM, and permits the hyperbolic tangent, logistic, and power models for the latter. This page also offers two other programs, CRMexplore and CRMinteractive, that allow users to draw the families of dose toxicity curves and interactively conduct CRM trials.

Finally, since R (actually BRugs) source code is available, users can easily modify the code to fit their own purposes. For example, the R commands

R code
```
p.tox0 <- c(.05,.15,.3,.45,.6)
s.dose  <- log(p.tox0/(1-p.tox0)) - 3
phaseIsim(nsim=10000, npat=30, sdose=s.dose, prob.tox=p.tox0,
    design=30, outfile='sc1aout.txt')
```

will carry out a simulation using the 3+3 method for the five standardized doses (s.dose) in Scenario 1 above. The alternate use of the program,

R code
```
phaseIsim(nsim=10000, npat=30, sdose=s.dose, prob.tox=p.tox0,
    design=2, outfile='sc1bout.txt')
```

instead illustrates the case of CRM with a cohort size of 1, while

R code
```
phaseIsim(nsim=10000, npat=30, sdose=s.dose, prob.tox=p.tox0,
    crm.group.size=3, design=2, outfile='sc1cout.txt')
```

handles the case of a cohort size of 3.

3.2.2 Escalation with overdose control (EWOC)

As we mentioned, the CRM method's greatest virtue (its efficient use of all available information) also leads to its greatest weakness (its potential for exposing patients to overly toxic doses if the first few patient responses are atypical or the model is misspecified). The mechanistic modifications of Goodman et al. (1995) and others mentioned just prior to Example 3.3 are attempts to limit wild swings in the MTD estimates as data accumulate. Babb, Rogatko, and Zacks (1998) introduced an alternative approach that directly seeks to reduce the risk of overdose; see also Zacks et al. (1998). Called *escalation with overdose control* (EWOC), the method is the same as CRM *except* in the way that it selects each successive new dose. While CRM always uses the middle (say, the mean or the mode) of the MTD's posterior distribution as the next dose, EWOC instead selects the αth quantile, where α, called the *feasibility bound*, is taken to be less than or equal to 0.5. The "overdose control" then comes from the fact that the predicted probability that each successive patient's dose exceeds the MTD is only α; Babb et al. suggest $\alpha = 0.25$.

To be more specific, denote the target toxicity level (TTL) by θ, and the dose by x, so that $P(DLT|x = MTD) = \theta$. Let $d_1, \ldots, d_r$ be the ordered dose levels available for experimentation, where we assume that d_1 is safe for humans and $d_1 < \gamma < d_r$. The EWOC algorithm proceeds as follows:

Algorithm 3.3 *(EWOC design)*

Step 1: Start with the lowest dose level, i.e., set $x_1 = d_1$.

Step 2: For any patient k, let $\pi_k(\gamma)$ be the posterior cumulative distribution function (CDF) of the MTD, i.e.

$$\pi_k(\gamma) = P(MTD \leq \gamma \,|\, \mathbf{y}_k) ,$$

where $\mathbf{y}_k$ denotes the data available at the time of treatment for patient k. EWOC selects the dose level x_k such that

$$\pi_k(x_k) = \alpha .$$

Since this x_k will almost surely not be identical to any of our prespecified dose levels d_i, we would instead choose dose

$$x_k^* = \max\{d_1, \ldots, d_r : d_i - x_k \leq T_1 \text{ and } \pi_k(x_k) - \alpha \leq T_2\}$$

for prespecified nonnegative tolerances T_1 and T_2. This permits treatment of patients at doses only slightly above the optimal dose x_k.

Step 3: As in CRM, we repeat Step 2 until a sufficiently precise estimate of the MTD is achieved, or the maximum sample size n is reached. In either case we estimate the MTD by the middle (mean, mode, or median) of its posterior distribution.

∎

The EWOC doses x_k have an attractive decision-theoretic interpretation: they minimize risk with respect to the asymmetric loss function

$$L(x, \gamma) = \begin{cases} \alpha(\gamma - x) & \text{for } x \leq \gamma \text{ (i.e., } x \text{ is an underdose)} \\ (1 - \alpha)(x - \gamma) & \text{for } x > \gamma \text{ (i.e., } x \text{ is an overdose)} \end{cases} .$$

Note that choosing the feasibility bound $\alpha < 0.5$ corresponds to placing a higher penalty on overdosing than on underdosing; adminstration of a dose δ units above the MTD is judged $(1 - \alpha)/\alpha$ times worse than treating a patient δ units below the MTD. Choosing $\alpha = 0.5$ implies a symmetric loss function, and indeed leads to the posterior median of the MTD as the new dose; see e.g. Carlin and Louis (2009, Appendix B, Section B.3.1).

A somewhat unusual feature of the basic EWOC method is that when $\alpha << 0.5$, the final dose recommended for phase II study (say, the median of the MTD posterior distribution) may be significantly larger than the dose *any* phase I patient has received (say, the 25th percentile of the same distribution). For this reason, the possibility of a *varying* feasibility bound has been discussed by Babb and Rogatko (2001, 2004), as well as other authors. Chu et al. (2009) propose a hybrid method that begins with EWOC using $\alpha = 0.1$, then gradually increases α according to a fixed schedule up to $\alpha = 0.5$ near the end of the trial (thus concluding with a posterior median version of CRM).

Current research in EWOC methods focuses on the incorporation of patient-specific covariates, so that the dose assigned at each stage can be "individualized." For example, Babb and Rogatko (2001) consider the case of a single continuous covariate, while current work by these and other authors deals with the case of a binary covariate, as well as multiple covariates.

Software note: Software for some basic EWOC design formulations is available; see Rogatko, Tighiouart, and Xu (2008) as well as the website of the biostatistics group at the Winship Cancer Institute at Emory University,

$$\mathtt{http://www.sph.emory.edu/BRI-WCI/ewoc.html} \, .$$

The current version, EWOC 2.0, is a free standalone Windows XP/Vista package, and features a complete and easy-to-follow online user's guide.

Of course, Algorithm 3.3 may be implemented in general purpose Bayesian packages as well. The next example provides a sample WinBUGS implementation of EWOC, courtesy of Prof. Brani Vidakovic of Georgia Institute of Technology and Emory University.

Example 3.4 Consider an EWOC implementation using the logistic model,

$$Prob(DLT|dose = x) \equiv p(x) = \frac{\exp(\beta_0 + \beta_1 x)}{1 + \exp(\beta_0 + \beta_1 x)} \, .$$

Because it is difficult to specify prior distributions on regression β's, we instead follow the advice of Kadane et al. (1980) and reparameterize from (β_0, β_1) to (ρ_0, γ), where $\rho_0 = p(X_{min})$, the probability of DLT at the minimum dose, X_{min}, and γ is the MTD. This reparameterization is easy since

$$\begin{aligned} \text{logit}(\rho_0) &= \beta_0 + \beta_1 X_{min} \\ \text{and} \quad \text{logit}(\theta) &= \beta_0 + \beta_1 \gamma \, , \end{aligned}$$

where θ is the TTL. Subtracting these two equations, we can easily solve for β_1 and then for β_0 as

$$\begin{aligned} \beta_0 &= \frac{1}{\gamma - X_{min}} [\gamma \, \text{logit}(\rho_0) - X_{min} \text{logit}(\theta)] \\ \text{and} \quad \beta_1 &= \frac{1}{\gamma - X_{min}} [\text{logit}(\theta) - \text{logit}(\rho_0)] \, . \end{aligned}$$

Here we are assuming that γ lies in (X_{min}, X_{max}) with probability 1; we would typically take the starting dose $d_1 = X_{min}$.

The following WinBUGS code specifies the priors on γ and ρ_0 simply as independent uniforms on the ranges (X_{min}, X_{max}) and $(0, \theta)$, respectively.

```
BUGS code  model{
            for (i in 1:N){
        # Likelihood
            Y[i]~dbern(p[i])
            logit(p[i])<- (1/(gamma - Xmin))*(gamma*logit(rho0)
                - Xmin*logit(theta)+(logit(theta)-logit(rho0))*X[i])
            } #  end of for loop
        # Priors
            gamma ~ dunif(Xmin, Xmax)
            rho0 ~ dunif(0,theta)
            } #  end of BUGS code
```

```
# Data (1st patient 140, no tox):
list(Y=c(0), X=c(140), Xmin=140, Xmax =425, theta=0.333, N=1)

# Data (1st patient 140, no tox; 2nd patient 210, no tox):
list(Y=c(0,0), X=c(140,210), Xmin=140, Xmax=425, theta=0.333, N=2)

# Data (1st patient 140, no tox; 2nd patient 210, tox):
list(Y=c(0,1), X=c(140,210), Xmin=140, Xmax=425, theta=0.333, N=2)

# Data (1st patient 140, no tox; 2nd patient 210, no tox;
#   3rd patient 300, no response yet):
list(Y=c(0,0,NA),X=c(140,210,300),Xmin=140,Xmax=425,theta=0.333,N=3)

#Inits:
  list(rho0=0.05, gamma=160)
```

The first two accumulating datasets shown in this code are the same as those used in the illustration in the EWOC 2.0 user's guide. Note this code assumes $d_1 = X_{min} = 140$, $X_{max} = 425$, and $\theta = 1/3$. The $10^{th}, 25^{th}$, and 50th percentiles of the MTD γ, which can be taken as the next dose, are available in WinBUGS by choosing the appropriate percentile from the percentile selection box in the Sample monitoring tool.

Running the code above using two parallel MCMC chains and the first dataset for 1000 burn-in MCMC iterations followed by 10,000 production iterations yields a 25th percentile for γ of 212, which rounded to the nearest 10 is 210. This is the dose for the second patient added to the subsequent datasets. Running the second dataset in the same way produces a 25th percentile for γ of 242 and a 50th percentile of 304. The final dataset shows the third patient receiving this higher dose, illustrating the case of increasing α from 0.25 to 0.50 as the trial wears on. Running this final dataset produces 25th and 50th percentiles for γ of 240 and 304 — very similar to the previous results since Y_3 is assumed still to be unknown by this code. The posterior predictive mean of Y_3 in this case emerges as about 0.40, slightly less than 0.50, indicating WinBUGS expects even this higher dose (300, rounded from 304) to produce no toxicity. ∎

The EWOC algorithm is readily modified to handle the case of patient-specific *covariates*; see the book's website for the case of a single binary covariate case. Subsequent extension to continuous and multiple covariates is forthcoming.

3.2.3 Time-to-event (TITE) monitoring

One key feature of the CRM method is its reliance on binary outcomes only. The advantage here is increased model robustness, but an important disadvantage is the limited information contained in the binary outcome. In many trials this outcome is defined as an indicator for some adverse event happening within a certain time horizon. There are several directions to generalize the basic CRM to the case of time-to-event (TITE) outcomes. One reasonable choice is to base the design on a parametric event time model. This is the approach chosen in Thall, Wooten, and Tannir (2005) and Cheung, Inoue, Wathen, and Thall (2006). Of course, a concern with any parametric model is robustness with respect to the chosen parametric family. The problem is far more important in design than in data analysis. Good statistical inference always includes a critical look at the model assumptions using residual analysis, appropriate plots, and formal tests to critically evaluate the model. If need be, we can revise the model assumptions as indicated. But this is not possible in design. When available, historical data permits model criticism, and operating characteristics can be used to investigate robustness with respect to possible model violations. Alternatively, one proceeds with a minimal set of model assumptions.

This is the approach of Cheung and Chappell (2000), who introduce the TITE-CRM as an extension of the CRM to TITE outcomes. Let $p(d, a)$ denote the probability of a toxicity for a patient assigned to dose d. We use models $p(d, a)$ as in the usual CRM setup (see Subsection 3.2.1). There the response is assumed to be a binary outcome $y_i \in \{0, 1\}$, with $y_i = 1$ indicating that the toxicity outcome was observed for the i-th patient. Let d_i denote the dose assigned to the i-th patient, and let $\mathbf{y} = (y_1, \ldots, y_n)$. The likelihood conditional on the data from the first n patients is

$$L(a; \mathbf{y}) = \prod_{i=1}^{n} p(d_i, a)^{y_i} \{1 - p(d_i, a)\}^{1-y_i} .$$

The TITE-CRM replaces $p(d_i, a)$ by $g(d_i, a) \equiv w_i p(d_i, a)$. The factor w_i, $0 \leq w_i \leq 1$, is a weight for the i-th patient. For example, we might let $w_i = U_i/T$ for a horizon T and time to toxicity U_i (truncated by T) for patient i. Except for replacing p by g, the design proceeds as in the basic CRM.

The use of $g(\cdot)$ is justified as an approximation. Assume that a binary toxicity event is defined as toxicity by some (large) time T. Then $P(U_i \leq t) = P(U_i \leq T \mid d_i, a) \, P(U_i \leq t \mid U_i \leq T, d_i, a) = p(d_i, a) \, P(U_i \leq t \mid U_i \leq T, d_i, a)$. Approximating the last factor by w_i justifies the use of $g(\cdot)$ in the likelihood. Cheung and Chappell (2000) show that the recommended dose under the TITE-CRM converges to the correct dose (under certain conditions).

Software note: The TITE-CRM is implemented in the R package `titecrm` (http://cran.r-project.org/web/packages/titecrm/index.html).
A basic implementation in R is shown in this chapter's software page,

www.biostat.umn.edu/~brad/software/BCLM_ch3.html

The following steps summarize the proposed TITE-CRM of Cheung and

Chappell (2000). For this and all other algorithms in this section we give the algorithm to simulate a single trial realization. To compute the next dose in an actual trial we would start with Step 2 and drop the loop over patient cohorts. To compute operating characteristics, we would instead embed the algorithm in an additional outer loop over repeated artificial datasets.

Algorithm 3.4 *(TITE-CRM).*

Step 0. Initialization: Fix an assumed truth, $p_j^o = Pr$(toxicity at dose j). Set the initial starting dose $d = 1$ and initialize calendar time (months) $t = 0$ and sample size $n = 0$.

Step 1. Initial dose escalation: Repeat Step 1.1 until the first toxicity response is observed or the maximum sample size is reached. Set batch size $k = 3$.

Step 1.1. Simulate next cohort: Simulate U_i, $i = n + 1, \ldots, n + k$. Record the recruitment times $t_{0i} = t$, and thus calendar event time $t_{0i} + U_i$.

Step 1.2. Stopping the initial escalation: If $U_i \leq T$ is observed or $d = 6$ is reached, stop escalation. Otherwise, increment d to $d + 1$, n to $n + k$, t to $t + 6$, and repeat from Step 1.1.

At the end of the initial escalation change the cohort size to $k = 1$.

Step 2. Posterior update: Compute $\bar{a} = E(a \mid y_1, d_1, \ldots, y_n, d_n)$ based on the pseudo likelihood

$$p(y^n \mid a) = \prod_{i=1}^{n} g(d_i, a)^{y_i} \{1 - g(d_i, a)\}^{1-y_i}.$$

The (univariate) integral is easily carried out as a summation over a grid (approximating the integral by a Riemann sum). Let $(a_1, \ldots, a_M)$ denote an equispaced grid covering the range of possible a values; we used $M = 50$, $a_1 = 0.01$ and $a_M = 7.0$.

Log likelihood and prior: Let $w_{ti} = \min\{1, (t - t_{0i})/T\}$, and let $y_{ti} = I\{(U_i < T) \cap (t > t_{0i} + U_i)\}$ denote the current weight and outcome indicator for the ith observation at time t.

For $m = 1, \ldots, M$, evaluate $\ell(a_m) \equiv \log p(y^n \mid a = a_m)$, given by

$$\sum_{i:y_i=1} \log[w_{ni} p(d_i; a = a_m)] + \sum_{i:y_i=0} \log[1 - w_{ni} p(d_i; a = a_m)],$$

and $\log p(a_m) = -a_m$.

Posterior: Evaluate the pointwise posterior

$$p(a_m \mid y^n) \propto exp(\ell(a_m) + \log p(a_m))$$

and compute $\bar{a} = \sum_m a_m p(a_m \mid y^n) / \sum_m p(a_m \mid y^n)$.

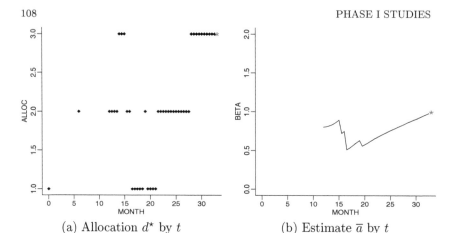

(a) Allocation $d^\star$ by t (b) Estimate $\bar{a}$ by t

Figure 3.12 *TITE CRM: The left panel plots the allocated dose against calendar time. The initial $d = 1$ is chosen by definition, to start the initial dose escalation. The right panel shows the estimated parameter $\bar{a}$ against calendar time t. The star shows the final reported posterior estimate.*

Step 3. Next dose: Evaluate the estimated toxicity probabilities $\hat{p}(d, \bar{a}) = d^{\bar{a}}$, and select the dose $d^\star = \arg\min |\hat{p}(d, \bar{a}) - p^\star|$ with estimated toxicity closest to the desired level $p^\star$. The next cohort is assigned to dose $d^\star$.

Step 4. Next cohort: Simulate U_{n+1} corresponding to $k = 1$ new patient allocated at $d^\star$. Record the recruitment times $t_{0i} = t$ (and thus calendar event time $t_{0i} + U_i$). Increment $n \equiv n+1$ and advance the calendar time $t = t + 0.5$.

Step 5. Stopping: if $n \geq n_{max}$, stop and report posterior estimated toxicity probabilities (computed as in Step 2); else repeat from Step 2.

■

Example 3.5 *(Simulation study).* We implemented the proposed method for the simulation study reported in Cheung and Chappell (2000, Section 5). We used an assumed simulation truth $p^o = (0.05, 0.1, 0.2, 0.3, 0.5, 0.7)$ for a dose grid $d \in \{0.05, 0.1, 0.2, 0.3, 0.5, 0.7\}$; i.e., the assumed toxicity probabilities follow the CRM model with $a = 1$. The target toxicity is $p^\star = 20\%$.

Figure 3.12 summarizes a simulated trial history. We use the CRM power model, $p(d, a) = d^a$ (recall that the doses are scaled between 0 and 1). For the first two cohorts, at $t = 0$ and 6 months, the dose assignment is determined by the initial dose escalation of Step 1. After $t = 6$ the first toxicity was observed and the dose assignment switches to the allocation described in Step 3. Note how the cohort size switches from $k = 3$ to $k = 1$ after the initial escalation. Panel (b) plots the posterior means $\bar{a}$ computed in Step 2. The plot starts only after the first toxicity is observed and the algorithm leaves the initial dose escalation loop of step 1. The see-saw pattern of the posterior mean trajectory is typical. Each time a toxicity is observed the posterior mean drops, and then raises again slowly while no toxicities occur. The final star indicates the posterior mean $\bar{a} = E(a \mid y)$ upon conclusion of the trial in Step 5. In this case the simulation truth was $a^o = 1.0$. The fact that the posterior estimate so closely matches the simulation truth is coincidental. In general, with only 25 binary responses the posterior mean could still be a biased estimate, far from asymptotic posterior consistency. ■

Bekele et al. (2008) propose an extension of the TITE-CRM. The method is based on a discretization of the time to event. The discretized variable y_i is an ordinal outcome. These authors assume a probit regression for the conditional probabilities $P(y_i = j \mid y_i \geq j, d_i)$. The basic model does not include monotonicity constraints, which can be awkward to impose within an MCMC algorithm. Instead, monotonicity across doses is enforced by post-processing of the posterior estimated probabilities of toxicity using an isotonic regression. The adjusted posterior probabilities are then used to define rules for dose escalation, de-escalation, suspension of accrual, and early stopping for excessive toxicity.

Braun et al. (2005) go a step further and assume a sampling model for the time to event. The probability model for time to toxicity is defined by piecewise linear hazards. Based on posterior probabilities under this model, the proposed trial conduct is then again analogous to the CRM design. Alternative methods based on fully parametric models for the event times are proposed in Cheung et al. (2006) and Thall et al. (2005).

3.2.4 Toxicity intervals

As already seen, many phase I designs require the specification of a target level of toxicity. The implicit assumption that such a single target toxicity exists and can be reliably identified by the investigator is probably unrealistic. It is more likely that the investigator might have a *range* of acceptable toxicity levels in mind. This idea is formalized by several approaches that are based on toxicity probability *intervals*, rather than target levels.

Ji, Li, and Bekele (2007) define a target toxicity interval relative to the current precision of posterior estimated toxicities. Let s_i denote the posterior standard deviation of the mean toxicity at dose d_i and let $p^\star$ denote a nominal target toxicity level. These authors define a toxicity interval as $p^\star$ plus or minus s_i. For each dose d_i let n_i, x_i and p_i denote the number of patients enrolled at dose d_i, the number of observed toxicities, and the unknown probability of toxicity at that dose. Posterior probabilities are defined with respect to a binomial sampling model $x_i \sim \text{Bin}(n_i, p_i)$, and independent beta priors for p_i.

Assume that the current patient cohort is assigned to dose d_i. After adding each patient cohort, one computes the posterior probabilities of p_i being below, within, and above the target interval. Let Y denote the currently available data, and let $d = d_i$ denote the currently assigned dose. We define

$$
\begin{aligned}
q_D &= Pr(p_i > p^\star + K_1 s_i \mid Y) \\
q_E &= Pr(p_i < p^\star - K_2 s_i \mid Y) \\
\text{and } q_S &= Pr(p^\star - K_2 s_i < p_i < p^\star + K_1 s_i \mid Y) = 1 - (q_D + q_E),
\end{aligned}
\tag{3.1}
$$

where K_1 and K_2 are user-selected design constants (in our code below, we chose $K_1 = 1$ and $K_2 = 1.5$). Depending on which of these probabilities is largest, the design recommends dose escalation (when q_E is largest), remaining with the current dose (q_S), or dose de-escalation (q_D), respectively. The design does not skip doses, and stops early for excessive toxicity if the lowest dose is found to be excessively toxic. At the end of the trial the maximum tolerated dose is reported as the dose with estimated p_i closest to $p^\star$. The estimate of p_i that is used for this decision is an isotonic regression of posterior mean toxicities $E(p_i \mid data)$ (Ji, Li, and Yin, 2007).

Software note: An implementation as a spreadsheet application is available at http://odin.mdacc.tmc.edu/~yuanj/software.htm. An implementation in R, used in the example below, is listed in this chapter's software page,

www.biostat.umn.edu/~brad/software/BCLM_ch3.html

The following outline shows a step-by-step implementation of the Ji, Li, and Bekele (2007) method. We illustrate the simulation of a possible trial realization. First, let $d = 1, \ldots, J$ denote the set of doses. We assume independent priors $p_i \sim Beta(a_0, b_0)$, $i = 1, \ldots, J$. Let $\mathbf{y}^{(n)}$ denote all data up to and including the n-th patient.

Algorithm 3.5 *(Toxicity Intervals).*

Step 0. Initialization: Fix an assumed scenario, i.e., a simulation truth p_i^o for the true toxicity probabilities $p_i = Pr(\text{toxicity at dose i})$. Fix cohort size $k = 3$ and sample size $n = 0$. Start with dose $d = 1$.

Step 1. Next cohort: Record responses $y \sim Bin(k, p_d^o)$. Increment $n \equiv n + k$.

Step 2. Posterior updating: The posterior distributions are given by $p(p_i \mid \mathbf{y}^{(n)}) = Be(a_0 + x_i, b_0 + n_i - x_i)$. Evaluate the posterior probabilities q_D, q_E and q_S as in (3.2).

Step 3. Utilities: We define utilities for the actions $a \in \{E, D, S\}$, where E, D, and S indicate escalation, de-escalation, and remaining at the current dose, respectively, as follows:

- When $d = 1$, then $u(D) = 0$.
- When $d = J$ then $u(E) = 0$.

- We fix a threshold ξ for unacceptably high probability of toxicity. If $p(p_{d+1} > p^\star \mid Y) > \xi$, then $u(E) = 0$.
- Subject to these constraints $u(a) = q_a$, $a \in \{E, D, S\}$. In other words, the probabilities q_a are used to define utilities.

Step 4. Next dose: The next dose is defined by maximizing the utilities $u(a)$

$$
d \equiv \begin{cases} d - 1 & \text{if } u(D) = \max_a u(a) \\ d + 1 & \text{if } u(E) = \max_a u(a) \\ d & \text{otherwise} \end{cases}
$$

Step 5. Stopping: If $n \geq n_{\max}$ we stop for maximum sample size. If $p(p_1 > p^\star \mid Y) > \xi$ we stop early for excessive toxicity. Otherwise repeat starting from Step 1. Early stopping for excessive toxicity is atypical; the trial is expected to run to $n_{\max}$.

Step 6. Recommended dose: Let $\bar{p}_i = E(p_i \mid Y)$ denote the estimated toxicity probabilities. Let $\tilde{p}_i$ denote an isotonic regression of the $\bar{p}_i$. The final recommended dose is

$$
\arg\min_i |\tilde{p}_i - p^\star| \, .
$$

◼

The isotonic regression in step 6 above is implemented via *iterative pooling of adjacent violators* (Robertson et al., 1988). "Adjacent violators" are two consecutive doses whose responses violate monotonicity. We use the following simple ad hoc implementation of this algorithm:

Algorithm 3.6 *(Pooling adjacent violators).* We work with a set of indices $c = (c_1, \dots, c_J)$ that indicate pooling of adjacent values. Any doses with matching indices c_j are pooled.

Step 0. Initialization: Let $\tilde{p} = \bar{p}$ and $c = (1, 2, \dots, J)$.

Step 1. Find adjacent violators: Let $V = \{i : \tilde{p}_i > \tilde{p}_{i+1}, i < J\}$ denote the set of adjacent violators.

Step 2. Stopping the iteration: If $V = \emptyset$ then stop the iteration. Otherwise select the first violator $v = c_{V_1}$. Let $W = \{i : c_i = v \text{ or } c_i = v + 1\}$. Let $m_W = mean(\tilde{p}_W)$ denote the average value over W.

Step 3. Pool adjacent violators: Set $c_i \equiv v$, $i \in W$ and replace $\tilde{p}_i \equiv m_w$, $i \in W$. Repeat from Step 1.

◼

As always, to carry out an actual trial, one would replace the simulation in Step 1 with a simple recording of the actual response.

Example 3.6 *(Dose escalation).* We implement the proposed algorithm for an example used in Ji, Li, and Bekele (2007). The example is based on

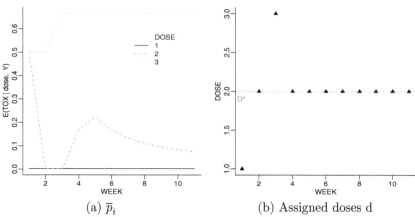

(a) $\bar{p}_i$ (b) Assigned doses d

Figure 3.13 *Toxicity intervals: The left panel plots posterior estimated toxicity probabilities $\bar{p}_i$ for doses $i = 1, 2, 3$ against cohort. The right panel shows the assigned dose (vertical axis) by cohort (horizontal axis).*

a trial described in Goodman, Zahurak, and Piantadosi (1995). There are eight allowable dose levels, $d \in \{1, \ldots, 8\}$. For the simulation study we assume a scenario with toxicity probabilities $p_i^o = 5, 25, 50, 60, 70, 80, 90$, and 95%. We use $p^\star = 20\%$ and $n_{\max} = 100$, and assume Beta(0.005, 0.005) priors for all eight toxicity probabilities p_i. This prior is chosen to reflect little prior information, and essentially corresponds to equal masses of 0.5 at both 0 and 1.

Figure 3.13 summarizes the simulation output. Panel (a) plots the estimated toxicity probabilities for the three lowest doses $i = 1, 2, 3$ against week. Initially, at $t = 0$ all three toxicity probabilities are centered at $E(p_i) = 0.5$. The plot starts at $t = 1$. The first cohort is assigned to dose $d = 1$ (step 0) and we observe $x_1 = 0$ toxicities. This shifts the posterior distribution $p(p_1 \mid \mathbf{y}^{(1)})$ down to $E(p_1 \mid \mathbf{y}^{(1)}) \approx 0$. The Be(0.005, 0.005) prior provides only negligible shrinkage toward the prior mean 0.5. For the next cohort the dose is escalated to $d = 2$, and again $x_2 = 0$ toxicities are observed. This shifts the posterior mean for p_2 to approximately 0. In the third cohort we continue dose escalation to $d = 3$, but now observe toxicities. This leads to a dose de-escalation. For the rest of the trial we never leave $d = 2$ anymore. The implication is that the posterior distributions for p_1 and p_3 remain unchanged for the rest of the trial. Note, however, that the figures only show one trial simulation. For the evaluation of operating characteristics we would carry out massive repeat simulations. Design evaluation is then based on the average of many such simulations. ∎

The design proposed by Ji, Li, and Bekele (2007) introduces the toxicity intervals based on the uncertainty in estimating mean toxicities. In other words, the use of intervals is motivated by the lack of precise estimates.

3.2.5 Ordinal toxicity intervals

Neuenschwander et al. (2008) go a step further and acknowledge that it is impossible to define a single precise target toxicity $p^\star$. They extend the traditional binary classification into acceptable versus unacceptable toxicity to an ordinal scale over four sub-intervals of toxicity probabilities. Let $\bar{p}_i$ denote the posterior probability of a dose limiting toxicity (DLT) at dose d_i. Neuenschwander et al. (2008) partition the range of toxicity probabilties into $\bar{p}_i \in (0, 0.20]$ ("under-dosing"), $\bar{p}_i \in (0.20, 0.35]$ ("targeted toxicity"), $\bar{p}_i \in (0.35, 0.60]$ ("excessive toxicity"), and $\bar{p}_i \in (0.60, 1.00]$ ("unacceptable toxicity"). On the basis of this classification, the authors propose to proceed with a pragmatic design that prescribes de-escalation, escalation, and continued enrollment at the current dose depending on these four probabilities. Alternatively, they note that one could define a loss function as a linear combination of the four interval probabilities and proceed with a decision theoretic design.

Software note: The paper includes WinBUGS code to evaluate posterior probabilities and posterior expected losses under a logistic regression model with normal priors (Neuenschwander et al., 2008, Appendix II). A basic implementation in R is given in the book's website.

The following steps implement the design proposed in Neuenschwander et al. (2008). We describe one simulation of a possible trial history. To compute the next dose in an actual trial realization, start at Step 1, dropping the loop over patient cohorts. To compute operating characteristics one would embed the algorithm in an additional outer loop over repeat simulations. We assume a dose grid $d = (d_1, \ldots, d_7)$ with $d^o \equiv d_7$ as a reference dose (used in the algorithm below). Letting $\Phi(z)$ denote the standard normal c.d.f. as usual, the algorithm assumes a probit sampling model

$$p(y_i = 1 \mid d_i = d) = \pi(d) \text{ with } \pi(d) = 1 - \Phi\left[-\log a - b\log(d/d^o)\right]. \quad (3.2)$$

This model allows an easy interpretation of the parameters, with a being approximately the prior odds at the reference dose d^o, and b being a shift in log odds for doses away from d^o. The interpretation would be exact for a logistic regression model, as used in Neuenschwander et al. (2008). We use the probit model instead, in order to use the built-in posterior simulation in the R package Bayesm. The model is completed with a bivariate normal prior, namely $(\log a, b) \sim N(\mu, \Sigma)$.

Algorithm 3.7 (Ordinal Toxicity Intervals).

Step 0. Initialization: Fix an assumed scenario, i.e., a simulation truth p_i^o for the true toxicity probabilities $p_i = Pr(\text{toxicity at dose i})$. Fix cohort size $k = 3$ and sample size $n = 0$. Start with dose $d = 1$.

Step 1. Next cohort: Record responses $y \sim \text{Bin}(k, p_d^o)$. Increment $n \equiv n + k$.

Step 2. Posterior updating: Let $\theta = (\log a, b)$. The posterior distribution is given by $p(\theta \mid y) \propto p(\theta) \cdot p(y \mid \theta)$, with the bivariate normal prior and the probit regression likelihood (3.2). Use the R package bayesm (Rossi et al., 2005) to generate a posterior MCMC sample $\Theta \equiv \{\theta^m; \ m = 1, \ldots, M\}$ where $\theta^m \sim p(\theta \mid y)$.

Use the posterior MCMC sample Θ to evaluate posterior probabilities of under, target, excess and unacceptable toxicity at each dose. Let $P_i(under)$ denote the probability of under-dosing at dose $d = d_i$. Let $\theta^m = (\log a^m, b^m)$, and evaluate

$$P_i(under \mid y) = \frac{1}{M} \sum_{m=1}^{M} I \{lo \leq 1 - \Phi \left[-\log(a^m) - b^m \log(d_i/d^o) \right] \leq hi \} ,$$

where $lo = 0$ and $hi = 0.20$. Repeat similarly for $P_i(target \mid y)$, $P_i(excess \mid y)$ and $P_i(unacc \mid y)$, each using appropriate boundaries (lo, hi).

Step 3. Next dose: Let $\mathcal{D} = \{i : \ P_i(excess) + P_i(unacc) < 0.25\}$. The next dose is $d^\star = d_{i^\star}$ with

$$i^\star = \arg \max_{\mathcal{D}} \{i : P_i(target)\}$$

and $i^\star = \emptyset$ if no dose is found with probability of excessive or unacceptable toxicity < 0.25.

If $i^\star \neq \emptyset$ then set $d = d^\star \equiv d_{i^\star}$ and continue with step 1.

Step 4. Stopping: If $n \geq n_{\max}$ or if no dose satisfies the constraint, i.e., $i^\star = \emptyset$, then stop and report the last assigned dose $d = d^\star$ as optimal dose. Otherwise continue with Step 1.

∎

Example 3.7 *(Phase I trial).* We implemented the algorithm for an example reported in Neuenschwander et al. (2008). They consider a phase I dose escalation study to characterize safety and tolerability of a drug and to determine the maximum tolerable dose (MTD).

We assume a dose grid $d = (12.5, 25, 50, 100, 150, 200, 250)$ with $d^o = 250$ as a reference dose. Neuenschwander et al. (2008) use a bivariate normal prior $(\log a, \log b) \sim N(\mu, \Sigma)$. The covariance matrix Σ is determined by $\text{Var}(\log a) = 0.84^2$, $\text{Var}(\log b) = 0.8^2$ and correlation $\text{Corr}(\log a, \log b) = 0.2$. The mean is $\mu = (2.15, 0.52)$. The moments are chosen to best match the 2.5%, 50%, and 97.5% quantiles for the toxicity probabilities that are implied by a one-parameter CRM model (see Neuenschwander et al., 2008, for details). We find the implied prior moments $m = E(\theta)$ and $S = \text{Var}(\theta)$ for $\theta = (\log a, b)$ and use a bivariate normal prior $p(\theta) = N(m, S)$. The maximum sample size was set to $n_{\max} = 30$.

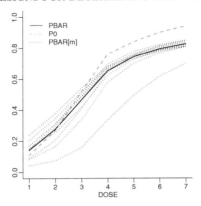

Figure 3.14 *Ordinal toxicity intervals: assumed truth p^o (dashed line) and posterior estimated toxicities $E(p_i \mid y)$ after each of 10 cohorts (dotted lines) and after cohort 11 (solid line).*

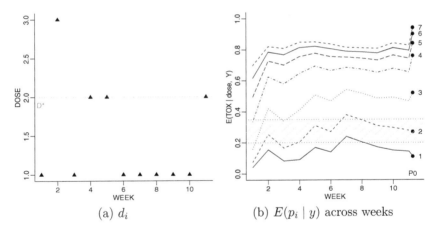

Figure 3.15 *Ordinal toxicity intervals: assigned doses d_i (left panel) and estimated toxicity probabilities $\bar{p}_i = E(p_i \mid y)$ against weeks (panel b). For comparison, the final point on each curve (Week 11, labeled "P0") shows the simulation truth.*

Figure 3.14 shows the assumed simulation assumed truth

$$p^o = (0.11, 0.27, 0.52, 0.76, 0.84, 0.90, 0.94).$$

Under the assumed truth p^o, dose d_2 is the maximum dose with true toxicity within the target toxicity interval $[0.20, 0.35]$. The figure shows p^o, together with the posterior mean toxicity probabilities $\bar{p}_i = E(p_i \mid y)$ after each of 10 patient cohorts.

Figure 3.15 summarizes one trial simulation. The initial dose assignment at is fixed at $d = 1$ by the algorithm. The simulated toxicity responses for the first patient cohort were $(0, 0, 1)$, shifting the posterior distribution on $(p_i, i = 1, \ldots, 7)$ to low estimated toxicities. However, notice how the prior prevents inference from over-reacting and pushing the recommended dose too high. The corresponding trajectory of posterior estimates is shown in panel (b). For each week t (cohort), the figure shows the posterior means $E(p_i \mid y)$ conditional on data up to and including week t. The plot starts at week $t = 1$, thus prior means are not shown. Starting with week 6 posterior estimates settle down to recommend $d^\star = 1$, until eventually switching to the correct $d^\star = 2$ after week 11. ∎

3.3 Efficacy versus toxicity

In recent years, there has been increasing interest and effort in developing dose finding methods incorporating both toxicity and efficacy endpoints (e.g., Zohar and Chevret, 2007). After all, drug doses are acceptable only if they are safe and efficacious. One such method, *EffTox* developed by Thall and Cook (2004) and later extended by Thall, Cook, and Estey (2006) takes the approach of efficacy-toxicity trade-offs. As mentioned before, it is commonly accepted that the drug's toxicity increases with dose. Efficacy also increases with dose in general. However, for some biological agents it is possible that efficacy may plateau, or increase and then decrease, as the dose is increased. Our goal is then to find the best dose which provides the highest efficacy and lowest toxicity, and to treat most patients at that dose. Since it is rare to find drugs that are both effective and nontoxic, it is typically necessary to make a trade-off between efficacy and toxicity. This type of study can be considered as a "phase I-II" trial, since it combines the goals of conventional phase I and II studies. Later, in Subsection 4.3.2 we will provide a purely phase II joint efficacy-toxicity approach, where a single dose is chosen for further evaluation, and where requirements on false positive and false negative rates are more stringent.

EffTox is a Bayesian outcome-based adaptive method featuring four key statistical tasks:

- choose the trial parameters, including the definition of binary efficacy and toxicity outcomes, dose levels, cohort size, and maximum sample size,

- specify the joint probability model for efficacy and toxicity and prior distributions of model parameters,

- define the acceptable doses based on the efficacy and toxicity criteria, and

- elicit and define the parameters for efficacy-toxicity trade-offs.

Patients are treated in cohorts. After observing the efficacy and toxicity outcomes, the posterior mean of the joint efficacy-toxicity distribution for each dose is computed. Then, the most desirable dose level based on the efficacy-toxicity trade-off is identified to treat the next cohort of patients. We now provide details for each of the four tasks above.

3.3.1 Trial parameters

Binary efficacy and toxicity outcomes should be defined according to the context of disease. For example, major response (defined as complete or partial response) or disease control (major response or stable disease) are useful efficacy endpoints, while dose-limiting toxicity can be used for the toxicity endpoint. Typically, there are only a few (e.g., 3 to 6) dose levels to evaluate, and the cohort size is taken as 3 or larger. Too small a cohort size is not recommended due to the instability of parameter estimates, and potentially longer trial duration due to suspension of study enrollment before the outcomes of the current cohort are observed. A large cohort size is also not recommended because it limits adaptation and learning from the trial's interim results. The maximum sample size can be from 30 to 100, depending on number of doses, the accrual rate, and the precision of the estimates at the end of the trial.

3.3.2 Joint probability model for efficacy and toxicity

Thall and Cook (2004) specified the following joint model. Let $Y = (Y_E, Y_T)$ be the binary indicators of efficacy (E) and toxicity (T). The bivariate probabilities for $a, b \in \{0,1\}$ at dose x,

$$\pi_{a,b}(x, \theta) = \Pr(Y_E = a, Y_T = b \mid x, \theta),$$

are formulated in terms of the marginal toxicity probability $\pi_T(x, \theta)$, efficacy probability $\pi_E(x, \theta)$, and an association parameter ψ. Specifically, $\pi_T(x, \theta) = \pi_{0,1}(x, \theta) + \pi_{1,1}(x, \theta) = \text{logit}^{-1}\{\eta_T(x, \theta)\}$ where $\eta_T(x, \theta) = \mu_T + x\beta_T$ and $\pi_E(x, \theta) = \pi_{1,0}(x, \theta) + \pi_{1,1}(x, \theta) = \text{logit}^{-1}\{\eta_E(x, \theta)\}$ where $\eta_E(x, \theta) = \mu_E + x\beta_{E,1} + x^2\beta_{E,2}$. Note that the toxicity is assumed to be monotone in x, but a more general form of efficacy $\eta_E(x, \theta)$ is assumed to allow quadratic non-monotonicity in x. Therefore, the full parameter vector is $\theta = (\mu_T, \beta_T, \mu_E, \beta_{E,1}, \beta_{E,2}, \psi)'$. The bivariate distribution for efficacy and toxicity (suppressing x and θ in the notation) is

$$\pi_{a,b} = \pi_E^a(1-\pi_E)^{1-a}\pi_T^b(1-\pi_T)^{1-b} + (-1)^{a+b}\pi_E(1-\pi_E)\pi_T(1-\pi_T)\frac{e^\psi - 1}{e^\psi + 1}.$$

Consequently, the likelihood for a patient treated at dose x, $L(Y, x|\theta)$, is

$$\pi_{1,1}(x, \theta)^{Y_E Y_T}\pi_{1,0}(x, \theta)^{Y_E(1-Y_T)}\pi_{0,1}(x, \theta)^{(1-Y_E)Y_T}\pi_{0,0}(x, \theta)^{(1-Y_E)(1-Y_T)}.$$

Given dose-outcome data $D_n = \{(Y_1, x_1), ..., (Y_n, x_n)\}$ from the first n patients in the trial, the full likelihood is $L_n(D_n|\theta) = \prod_{i=1}^n L_i(Y_i, x_i|\theta)$.

An appropriate prior distribution can then be chosen to reflect the physician's overall assessment and uncertainty before the trial starts. It must be sufficiently uninformative such that the cumulative data will dominate in calculating the posteriors for decisionmaking. Thall and Cook (2004) recommended the use of normal distributions for each of the six components in θ.

3.3.3 Defining the acceptable dose levels

A dose is deemed *acceptable* if it meets both minimum efficacy and maximum toxicity requirements. Let $\underline{\pi}_E$ be the lower limit of desirable efficacy, and $\bar{\pi}_T$ be an upper limit of the tolerable toxicity, both elicited from the physician. For example, in treating a certain cancer, a lower limit of 20% on efficacy and an upper limit 50% on toxicity might be desired. Given the current data D_n, a dose x is considered acceptable if

$$\Pr\{\pi_E(x,\theta) > \underline{\pi}_E | D_n\} > p_E ,$$

and

$$\Pr\{\pi_T(x,\theta) < \bar{\pi}_T | D_n\} > p_T ,$$

where p_E and p_T are fixed design parameters, typically chosen between 0.05 and 0.20. These are considered the "lower bars" or "gatekeepers" for meeting the minimum efficacy and maximum toxicity criteria. As p_E increases, the method is more likely to exclude doses due to lack of efficacy. As p_T increases, the method is more likely to exclude doses due to excessive toxicity. These two parameters can be "tuned" via simulations to include clinically viable doses as acceptable doses. Based on the posterior probability, patients can be assigned only to the acceptable doses, denoted as $A(D_n)$.

3.3.4 Efficacy-toxicity trade-off contours

Any point $(\pi_E(x,\theta), \pi_T(x,\theta))$ treated with dose x lies in a two-dimensional space $\pi = (\pi_E, \pi_T)$ that spans $[0,1]^2$. Our goal is to define an efficacy-toxicity trade-off contour C such that all the points on C are equally desirable. One thought is to use the Euclidean distance from the point of interest to the most desirable point, $\pi = (1, 0)$. Doing this, however, puts equal weight on efficacy and toxicity, which may not reflect real-life clinical desires. A more sensible and general approach is to use the distance based on the L^P norm. To find the contour C, one needs to elicit from the physician three equally desirable design points $\{\pi_1^*, \pi_2^*, \pi_3^*\}$, where $\pi_1^* = (\pi_E^*, 0)$, $\pi_2^* = (1, \pi_T^*)$, and $\pi_3^* = (\pi_E', \pi_T^*)$. π_E^* defines the smallest response rate that the physician would consider acceptable if the treatment has no toxicity. π_T^* reflects the highest toxicity level that the physician

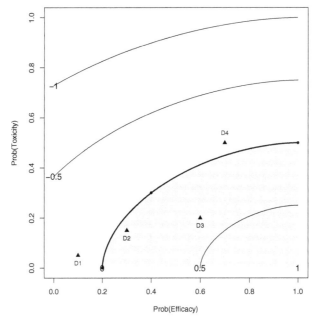

Figure 3.16 *Contour plot of the desirability measure by probabilities of toxicity and efficacy. The three design points are shown as circles, while the four doses are shown as triangles. The shaded area has desirability measure greater than 0, and is thus the "acceptable" dose region.*

is willing to accept if the treatment is 100% efficacious. The intermediate point π_3^* depicts an efficacy-toxicity trade-off that is more realistic but equally desirable as the previous two extreme settings. The desirability measure for point (π_E, π_T) is defined as $\delta = 1 - r$, with r obtained from

$$\left(\frac{1 - \pi_E}{1 - \pi_E^*}\right)^p + \left(\frac{\pi_T}{\pi_T^*}\right)^p = r^p .$$

Before calculating δ or r, we must first find p. We do this by plugging (π_E', π_T') in for (π_E, π_T) and setting $r = 1$ in the above equation. After solving for p, the desirability measure can be computed for any point (π_E, π_T) by re-solving the equation for r, hence δ. A larger desirability measure indicates a more favorable efficacy-toxicity profile. Note that the contours are concave, straight-line, and convex for p less than, equal to, and greater than 1, respectively. R code is available (see this chapter's software page) to compute p and plot the contour lines given the three design points.

Figure 3.16 shows the contour plot for the design points $\pi_1^* = (0.2, 0)$, $\pi_2^* = (1, 0.5)$, and $\pi_3^* = (0.4, 0.3)$ on the probability of toxicity versus probability of efficacy plane. The resulting contour passing through the

design points (shown as solid dots) is shown in a thick curve with $\delta = 0$
or $r = 1$. Points "inside" this contour line (i.e., toward the lower right,
the shaded area) have positive δ and are more desirable. Conversely, points
"outside" this contour line (i.e., to the upper left) have negative δ and are
less desirable.

The algorithm for trial conduct is as follows:

Algorithm 3.8 *(EffTox design)*

Step 1: Treat the first cohort of patients at the starting dose specified by
the physician. Typically, the first (lowest) dose level is chosen.

Step 2: For subsequent cohorts, no untried dose may be skipped, either
when escalating or de-escalating.

Step 3: Observe the efficacy and toxicity outcomes, then, compute the
posterior probability and posterior means, $E\{\pi(x_i, \theta)|D_n\}$ for each dose
x_i given the cumulative data D_n.

Step 4: Determine the acceptable dose(s) $A(D_n)$.

Step 5: Compute the desirability measure δ for each dose x_i in $A(D_n)$.

Step 6a: If there are no acceptable doses, the trial is terminated and no
doses are selected for further evaluation.

Step 6b: Otherwise, there is at least one acceptable dose. Treat the next
cohort of patients at the dose with maximum desirability. Return to Step
2 until the maximum sample size is reached.

Step 7: When the trial reaches the maximum sample size and there is at
least one acceptable dose, select the dose with maximum desirability for
further evaluation.

∎

Software note: The EffTox program can be used for both trial design (via simulations) and trial conduct, and can be downloaded from the M.D. Anderson
software page, biostatistics.mdanderson.org/SoftwareDownload/.

Example 3.8 We illustrate the design properties in a simulation study.
Suppose that we are interested in finding the best dose of a new agent.
There are four doses to be studied with the true probabities $\pi_1 = (0.10, 0.05)$,
$\pi_2 = (0.30, 0.15)$, $\pi_3 = (0.60, 0.20)$, and $\pi_4 = (0.70, 0.50)$. The four doses
are shown as solid triangles labeled as D1 through D4 in Figure 3.16. Assume the maximum sample size is 60 with a cohort size of 3; the starting
dose is dose level 1. The results of 1000 simulation studies are summarized
in Table 3.3. The first three lines in the table list the true probabilities of
outcomes for characterizing the underlying joint probability model at each
dose. The desirability measures for dose 1, 2, 3, and 4 are –0.133, 0.055,
0.333, and –0.094, respectively. Based on the assumption, dose 3 has the
highest desirability measure and is the best dose among the four. The results show that 56.7% of the patients are treated at dose 3. At the end of

	Dose			
	1	2	3	4
true Pr(efficacy)	0.10	0.30	0.60	0.70
true Pr(toxicity)	0.05	0.15	0.20	0.50
true Pr(efficacy w/o toxicity)	0.05	0.10	0.20	0.30
desirability measure	-0.133	0.055	0.333	-0.094
ave # patients treated	3.4	12.0	34.0	10.6
(% of patients treated)	(5.7%)	(20.0%)	(56.7%)	(17.7%)
selection probability	0.001	0.133	0.756	0.110

Table 3.3 *Operating characteristics of the EffTox design with four doses, maximum sample size of 60, and cohort size of 3 based on 1000 simulations.*

the trial, about 76% of the time, dose 3 will be chosen as the best dose. For the two adjacent doses, 12% and 10.6% of the patients are treated at doses 2 and 4 with selection probabilities of 0.133 and 0.110, respectively. The results illustrate that the *EffTox* method performs well in this setting. ■

3.4 Combination therapy

Up until now in this chapter, we have addressed dose-finding for a single drug. But increasingly, clinicians wish to investigate the therapeutic effect of *multiple* drugs used in combination, either sequentially or concurrently. In many fields, two agents (say, A and B) may be more effective than either one used alone due to synergistic effects. In such cases, clinicians may know the MTDs for each drug used separately, but now need to discover the dose *combination* (A_j, B_k) having probability of dose-limiting toxicity (DLT) no larger than some prespecified limit $\pi^* \in (0, 1)$.

Although this field of research is fairly recent, several authors have already tackled this problem. For example, Thall et al. (2003) proposed a six-parameter model for the toxicity probabilities arising from the various dose combinations. The approach is reminiscent of the CRM of Section 3.2.1, in that the authors specify two-parameter logistic models relating dose and toxicity for each of the two agents separately, and then add two more parameters to control the correlation in the (now-bivariate) dose-response space (note it will typically be inappropriate to assume the two agents operate independently). Thall et al. (2003) also point out that, rather than there being a single MTD as in the univariate case, we will now have a contour of MTD values in two-dimensional dose space, all of which will

		Drug A	
		p_j^{α}	$1 - p_j^{\alpha}$
Drug B	q_k^{β}	$\pi_{jk}^{(11)}$	$\pi_{jk}^{(01)}$
	$1 - q_k^{\beta}$	$\pi_{jk}^{(10)}$	$\pi_{jk}^{(00)}$

Table 3.4 *Joint (π) and marginal (p, q) probabilities of toxicity, latent contingency table approach to combination therapy problem.*

have the desired target toxicity π^*. Thus, in their dose-finding algorithm, the authors recommend slowly increasing the dose in a diagonal direction by increasing the dose of both agents, and then identifying two additional dose combinations "off the diagonal" by randomly venturing out in opposite directions along the current estimate of the toxicity equivalence contour.

While dose can often be thought of as continuous, in practice clinicians typically prefer to establish a finite number of doses of each drug, say J for Drug A and K for Drug B. This then determines a finite number (JK) of dose combinations, perhaps none of which will have toxicity exactly equal to π^*. As such, one often takes the combination with toxicity *closest* to π^* as the MTD.

3.4.1 Basic Gumbel model

In this section, we follow the basic setup of Yin and Yuan (2009a), who let A_j be the jth dose for drug A, $A_1 < \cdots < A_J$, and B_k be the kth dose for Drug B, $B_1 < \cdots < B_K$. For a patient treated with dose combination (A_j, B_k), these authors assume $X_{jk} = 1$ if the patient experiences toxicity from Drug A, with $X_{jk} = 0$ otherwise, and $Y_{jk} = 1$ if the patient experiences toxicity from Drug B, with $Y_{jk} = 0$ otherwise. Next, suppose we have physician-specified marginal probabilities of toxicity p_j and q_k associated with doses A_j and B_k, respectively. These may be available from previous studies of the two drugs separately. At the very least, p_J and q_K will be available since the highest doses A_J and B_K will typically be equal to the marginal MTDs, after which the p_j and q_k for the remaining, lower doses can be guessed. To allow for uncertainty in this assessment, reminiscent of the CRM we incorporate two unknown, positive parameters α and β, so that the marginal toxicity probabilities when (A_j, B_k) is given in combination are p_j^{α} and q_k^{β}.

Assuming the p_j^{α} and q_k^{β} are strictly increasing in j and k, respectively, Table 3.4 gives the probability model for the resulting 2×2 table. That is, the table gives $\pi_{jk}^{(xy)}$ for $x = 0, 1$, $y = 0, 1$, the *joint* probabilities associated with the bivariate binary outcomes. To model the $\pi_{jk}^{(xy)}$ as functions of the marginal probabilities, similar to the approach of the previous section, Yin and Yuan (2009a) suggest a Gumbel model,

$$\pi_{jk}^{(xy)} = p_j^{\alpha x}(1-p_j^{\alpha})^{1-x}q_k^{\beta y}(1-q_k^{\beta})^{1-y}+(-1)^{x+y}p_j^{\alpha}(1-p_j^{\alpha})q_k^{\beta}(1-q_k^{\beta})\frac{e^{\gamma}-1}{e^{\gamma}+1}, \tag{3.3}$$

for dose jk where $X_{jk} = x$ and $Y_{jk} = y$. Notice that setting the association parameter $\gamma = 0$ produces the case where the drugs produce toxicities independently.

As usual, we require a likelihood and a prior to carry out the Bayesian analysis. For the former, suppose that of the n_{jk} patients treated at combination dose jk, we observe $n_{jk}^{(00)}$ experiencing no toxicities, $n_{jk}^{(10)}$ experiencing toxicities only from Drug A, $n_{jk}^{(01)}$ experiencing toxicities only from Drug B, and $n_{jk}^{(11)}$ experiencing toxicities from both agents. Then the likelihood is a simple multinomial,

$$L(\alpha,\beta,\gamma|Data) \propto \prod_{j=1}^{J}\prod_{k=1}^{K}[\pi_{jk}^{(00)}]^{n_{jk}^{(00)}}[\pi_{jk}^{(01)}]^{n_{jk}^{(01)}}[\pi_{jk}^{(10)}]^{n_{jk}^{(10)}}[\pi_{jk}^{(11)}]^{n_{jk}^{(11)}}. \tag{3.4}$$

Note that this likelihood assumes that data correponding to all four cells in Table 3.4 are observable. This is actually not unreasonable in some cancer studies, where two chemotherapeutic agents having nonoverlapping dose-limiting toxicities (DLTs) can sometimes be identified, perhaps with the help of chemoprotective agents that prevent patients from experiencing any toxicities common to both agents. In such cases, any remaining toxicities can be immediately identified as being the result of either one drug or the other. However, in most cases, toxicities from the two drugs will be at least partially overlapping, precluding the matching of toxicities to drugs. In this setting, Yin and Yuan (2009a) proceed simply by assuming the contingency table in Table 3.4 is *latent*, with the observed data corresponding to the lower right cell (no toxicity) and the *sum* of the other three cells (toxicity arising from one or both drugs). This alters likelihood (3.4) to

$$L(\alpha,\beta,\gamma|Data) \propto \prod_{j=1}^{J}\prod_{k=1}^{K}[\pi_{jk}^{(00)}]^{n_{jk}^{(00)}}[1-\pi_{jk}^{(00)}]^{n_{jk}-n_{jk}^{(00)}}.$$

In a subsequent, closely related paper, Yin and Yuan (2009b) replace this latent 2×2 table approach with a direct specification of π_{jk}, now defined as the joint probability of *any* toxicity arising from dose jk. They continue to assume the availability of the marginal guesses p_j and q_k, but now construct the joint from the marginals using *copula* models (Shih and Louis, 1995; Nelsen, 1999). For instance, using what they term the "Clayton copula"

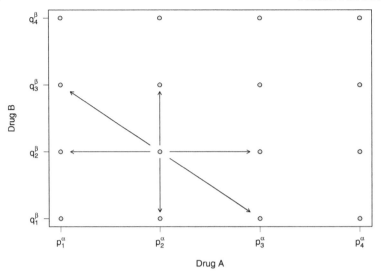

Figure 3.17 *Sample dose escalation/de-escalation scheme, combination therapy trial with 4 × 4 levels. From the current dose (A_2, B_2), only changes to dose combinations indicated by the arrows are permitted.*

enables replacing (3.3) with

$$\pi_{jk} = 1 - \left[(1 - p_j^\alpha)^{-\gamma} + (1 - q_k^\beta)^{-\gamma} - 1 \right]^{-1/\gamma},$$

while the "Gumbel-Hougaard copula" instead produces

$$\pi_{jk} = 1 - \exp\left(-\{[-\log(1 - p_j^\alpha)]^{1/\gamma} + [-\log(1 - q_k^\beta)]^{1/\gamma}\}^\gamma \right).$$

Returning to the 2 × 2 table model setting, Yin and Yuan (2009a) recommend a vague $Gamma(0.1, 0.1)$ prior for γ, and moderately informative, independent $Unif(0.2, 2)$ priors for α and β. We note that the former insists on $\gamma > 0$, which in our Gumbel model means positive association (synergy between the two drugs), while the latter is roughly centered around $\alpha = \beta = 1$, i.e., fully accurate initial prediction of the marginal toxicity probabilities p_j and q_k.

MCMC can be easily used to obtain the posterior for the parameter vector (α, β, γ), from which posterior distributions for the $\pi_{jk}^{(xy)}$ can be obtained from (3.3), which in turn determine the progression of our dose-finding algorithm. Suppose c_e and c_d are predetermined probability thresholds for dose escalation and de-escalation, respectively. We might choose c_e and c_d so that the trial has acceptable operating characteristics, subject to the constraint that $c_e + c_d > 1$. Following common practice by treating small groups of patients in cohorts (say, of size 3, thus mimicking the classic

3+3 design), Yin and Yuan (2009a,b) recommend restricting to one-level dose changes, and also not allowing moves along the diagonal (i.e., where the doses of both drugs are escalated or de-escalated simultaneously). That is, the only dose changes permitted are of the sort indicated by the arrows in Figure 3.17, which illustrates the case of a trial having $J = K = 4$ dose levels for each drug, and where the current dose is (A_2, B_2).

The basic dose-finding algorithm is as follows:

Algorithm 3.9 *(Yin-Yuan combination dose-finding design)*

Step 1: Treat patients in the first cohort at the lowest dose combination, (A_1, B_1).

Step 2: If for the current dose (jk) we have

$$P(\pi_{jk} < \pi^* | Data) > c_e \ ,$$

then escalate to an adjacent dose combination whose probability of toxicity is higher than that of the current dose and as close as possible to the target π^*. If the current dose is already the highest possible, (A_J, B_K), do not change the dose.

Step 3: If for the current dose (jk) we have

$$P(\pi_{jk} > \pi^* | Data) > c_d \ ,$$

then de-escalate to an adjacent dose combination whose probability of toxicity is lower than that of the current dose and as close as possible to π^*. If the current dose is already the lowest possible, (A_1, B_1), the trial is terminated.

Step 4: Otherwise, treat the next cohort at the current dose combination, (A_j, B_k).

Step 5: Once the maximum sample size has been reached, take the dose combination having probability of toxicity closest to π^* as the MTD.

∎

Note that, as with any dose-finding algorithm, there is a certain amount of "ad hockery" here, and apparently sensible and subtle changes to this algorithm can have marked impacts on how the design performs. However, and also as seen before, sufficient tinkering with any design after repeated simulation of operating characteristics should enable sensible choice of design parameters, such as c_e and c_d. In particular, Yin and Yuan (2009a,b) compare their designs to a "restricted CRM" method that first fixes Drug B at each given dose and then searches over the doses of Drug A, essentially reducing the bivariate search problem to a series of univariate searches. As one might expect, the true combination methods emerge with superior overall Type I error and power performance.

3.4.2 Bivariate CRM

It is tempting to refer to the approach just described as "bivariate CRM," since it employs a CRM-type Bayesian algorithm, but with two drugs instead of one. However, in the literature that moniker has become associated with the related problem of dose-finding with two competing *outcomes* observed from various doses of a *single* agent. The first reference appears to be Braun (2002), who considered the case of competing 0-1 outcomes for toxicity, Y_i, and disease progression, Z_i. Conditional on the dose of a (single) drug x_j, the bivariate CRM method specifies probability models

$$
\begin{aligned}
p_{1j} &= h_1(x_j, \boldsymbol{\beta}_1) = P(\text{toxicity seen at dose } j), \text{ and} \\
p_{2j} &= h_2(x_j, \boldsymbol{\beta}_2) = P(\text{progression seen at dose } j)
\end{aligned}
\tag{3.5}
$$

where h_1 and h_2 are monotonic, and possibly parameterized so as to ensure a low probability of toxicity and high probability of disease progression at the lowest dose. The choice recommended and used by Braun (2002) is

$$
\log\left(\frac{p_{1j}}{1 - p_{1j}}\right) = -3 + \beta_1 x_j, \quad \text{and} \quad \log\left(\frac{p_{2j}}{1 - p_{2j}}\right) = 3 - \beta_2 x_j,
$$

which is computationally convenient, and assumes additivity of the dose effects on the log-odds scale.

To specify the bivariate distribution of Y and Z, Braun (2002) assumes that conditional on dose x, this distribution can be constructed using a copula approach as

$$
f(y, z | x) = k(p_1, p_2, \psi) p_1^y q_1^{1-y} p_2^z (1 - p_2)^{1-z} \psi^{yz} (1 - \psi)^{1-yz}
$$

for $y, z \in \{0, 1\}$ and $0 < \psi < 1$, where p_1 is the probability of toxicity at dose x, p_2 is the probability of progression, $q_i = 1 - p_i$, ψ is an association parameter, and k is a normalizing constant. Since $\psi/(1-\psi)$ is the odds ratio between Y and Z, we have that Y and Z are independent if $\psi = 1/2$, are positively associated if $\psi > 1/2$, and are negatively associated if $\psi < 1/2$.

For a prior on the parameter vector $\boldsymbol{\theta} = (\beta_1, \beta_2, \psi)'$, Braun (2002) recommends

$$
p(\boldsymbol{\theta}) = 6\psi(1 - \psi)e^{-(\beta_1 + \beta_2)},
$$

i.e., independent *Exponential*(1) priors on the β_i, and an independent *Beta*(2, 2), a minimally informative prior having mean $1/2$, on ψ. We then do the usual prior-to-posterior updating for $\boldsymbol{\theta}$, and in turn obtain the posteriors for the toxicity and progression probabilities p_{1j} and p_{2j}.

Regarding the dosing algorithm, Braun suggests randomizing patients in cohorts of size c (typically 3), obtaining the posterior means $E[p_{1j}|\mathbf{y}, \mathbf{z}]$ and $E[p_{2j}|\mathbf{y}, \mathbf{z}]$, and then choosing the next dose by minimizing

$$
\sqrt{\sum_{\ell=1}^{2} (E[p_{\ell j}|\mathbf{y}, \mathbf{z}] - p_\ell^*)^2},
$$

the Euclidean distance between our current estimates and some desired rates of toxicity and progression p_1^* and p_2^*, respectively. A weighted version of this metric may be useful when we wish to place more emphasis on toxicity or progression; other, non-Euclidean metrics may also be sensible.

Software note: A program called bCRM to implement the bivariate continual reassessment method can be downloaded from biostatistics.mdanderson.org/ SoftwareDownload/SingleSoftware.aspx?Software_Id=15.

3.4.3 Combination therapy with bivariate response

The obvious question at this point is how to merge the two major ideas of this section, in order to handle bivariate responses (say, toxicity and disease progression) with more than one therapy. That is, returning to the case of a combination dose (A_j, B_k) indexed as jk, in the notation of Braun (2002) used in (3.5), we would now need to specify

$$p_{1jk} = h_1(A_j, B_k, \boldsymbol{\alpha}_1, \boldsymbol{\beta}_1) = P(\text{toxicity seen at dose } jk), \text{ and}$$
$$p_{2jk} = h_2(A_j, B_k, \boldsymbol{\alpha}_2, \boldsymbol{\beta}_2) = P(\text{progression seen at dose } jk) \tag{3.6}$$

where h_1 and h_2 are again parametric functions, possibly monotonic in both dose levels. The building blocks for such an approach (copula modeling, dose-finding algorithm, and so on) are found in our work so far; here we briefly outline a few published references in this rapidly emerging area.

Mandrekar et al. (2007) give an adaptive phase I design for dual-agent dose finding where both toxicity and efficacy are considered as responses. However, the authors do not use the full bivariate response setting indicated in (3.6), but rather a "TriCRM" approach (Zhang et al., 2006; Fan and Chaloner, 2004). Here, a continuation ratio (CR) model is utilized to turn the bivariate toxicity-efficacy response into a univariate combined endpoint with three mutually exclusive and exhaustive outcomes: "no response" (no efficacy and acceptable toxicity), "success" (efficacy and acceptable toxicity), and "toxicity" (unacceptable toxicity, regardless of efficacy outcome). Letting $\psi_0(x, \boldsymbol{\theta}), \psi_1(x, \boldsymbol{\theta})$, and $\psi_2(x, \boldsymbol{\theta})$ denote the probabilities of these three outcomes, respectively, the CR model for the single-agent TriCRM design is given by

$$\log(\psi_1/\psi_0) = \alpha_1 + \beta_1 x \text{ and } logit(\psi_2) = \alpha_2 + \beta_2 x, \tag{3.7}$$

where x is the dose and $\boldsymbol{\theta} = (\alpha_1, \alpha_2, \beta_1, \beta_2)$ and $\beta_1, \beta_2 > 0$. The dual-agent generalization of Mandrekar et al. (2007) employs a dual dose vector $\mathbf{x} = (x_1, x_2)$, and replaces (3.7) with

$$\log(\psi_1/\psi_0) = \alpha_1 + \beta_1 x_1 + \beta_3 x_2 \text{ and } logit(\psi_2) = \alpha_2 + \beta_2 x_1 + \beta_4 x_2,$$

where now we have $\boldsymbol{\theta} = (\alpha_1, \alpha_2, \beta_1, \beta_2, \beta_3, \beta_4)$ and $\beta_i > 0$ for $i = 1, \ldots, 4$.

Adding the constraint that the three probabilities must sum to 1, we obtain

$$\psi_2(\mathbf{x}, \boldsymbol{\theta}) = \frac{e^{\alpha_2 + \beta_2 x_1 + \beta_4 x_2}}{1 + e^{\alpha_2 + \beta_2 x_1 + \beta_4 x_2}} ,$$

$$\psi_1(\mathbf{x}, \boldsymbol{\theta}) = \frac{e^{\alpha_1 + \beta_1 x_1 + \beta_3 x_2}}{(1 + e^{\alpha_1 + \beta_1 x_1 + \beta_3 x_2})(1 + e^{\alpha_2 + \beta_2 x_1 + \beta_4 x_2})} ,$$

$$\text{and} \quad \psi_0(\mathbf{x}, \boldsymbol{\theta}) = \frac{1}{(1 + e^{\alpha_1 + \beta_1 x_1 + \beta_3 x_2})(1 + e^{\alpha_2 + \beta_2 x_1 + \beta_4 x_2})} .$$

These three probabilities readily determine the likelihood,

$$L(\boldsymbol{\theta}; \mathbf{x}, \mathbf{y}) \propto \prod_{i=1}^{n} \psi_0(\mathbf{x}_i, \boldsymbol{\theta})^{y_{0i}} \psi_1(\mathbf{x}_i, \boldsymbol{\theta})^{y_{1i}} \psi_2(\mathbf{x}_i, \boldsymbol{\theta})^{y_{2i}} ,$$

where $\mathbf{x}_i$ is the dose assigned to the ith cohort and $\mathbf{y}_i = (y_{0i}, y_{1i}, y_{2i})'$ is the trinomial outcome arising from this cohort. Mandrekar et al. (2007) specify flat priors (albeit over a bounded version of the parameter space), and then estimate all parameters using a quasi-Bayesian (psuedo-likelihood) CRM approach. The authors use a dose-finding algorithm similar to Algorithm 3.9, and investigate their design's performance across a broad range of true efficacy-toxicity scenarios, including one where the efficacy of one of the two drugs is *not* monotone in dose, as assumed by the model.

Huang et al. (2007) offer a design for a combination therapy trial in the presence of two binary responses (in their case, efficacy and toxicity) that maintains the full complexity of model (3.6). This design also incorporates ideas from seamless (but two-stage) phase I-II designs, beginning with a dose escalation phase that uses a modified 3+3 design to choose admissible joint dose levels (A_j, B_k). In the second stage, patients are randomized adaptively to the various admissible doses with probabilities proportional to the current posterior probability that each dose is the best; see equation (4.5) in Section 4.4.

The design also compares the benefit of giving the two drugs sequentially versus concurrently, adding yet another level of complication. However, the design is not particularly sophisticated in terms of the modeling of the two response probabilities. For instance, letting p_{2jk} denote the probability of efficacy (complete remission, in the authors' example) for a patient assigned dose jk, a simple logistic link function h_2 is selected for use with (3.6), i.e.,

$$logit(p_{2jk}) = \begin{cases} \gamma_s + \alpha_2 A_j + \beta_2 B_k & \text{if therapies assigned sequentially} \\ \gamma_c + \alpha_2 A_j + \beta_2 B_k & \text{if therapies assigned concurrently} \end{cases} .$$

That is, the probability of response is assumed to be additive on the logit scale, even though some sort of interaction between the two drugs (as was modeled above using the copula idea) is likely present. The toxicity probabilities, p_{1jk}, are left completely unmodeled, except for the assumption that they are i.i.d. draws from a $Beta(0.1, 0.9)$ distribution *a priori*. The design permits stopping for toxicity, futility, or efficacy; again we defer further details until Sections 4.3 and 4.4. Like other authors in this area, Huang et al. (2007) use simulations to investigate their design's performance across a range of efficacy-toxicity scenarios.

Finally, full-blown decision theoretic approaches can be used. Houede et al. (2010) choose the optimal dose pair of a chemotherapeutic agent and a biologic agent in a phase I/II trial measuring both toxicity and efficacy, where ordinal (rather than merely binary) outcomes are permitted. Joint response probabilities are again obtained via copula modeling, with the marginal outcome probabilities arising from an extension of a model due to Aranda-Ordaz (1983) that permits response probabilities that are not monotone in dose. A particularly novel aspect of this design is that each patient's dose pair (A_j, B_k) is chosen adaptively from a two-dimensional grid by maximizing the posterior expected utility of the patient's outcome. These utilities for each pair are elicited from a panel of physicians using the Delphi method, in the manner of Brook et al. (1986). Because experts are often overconfident in their opinions, even when using a community of experts, elicitation of priors and utilities should be approached with great care; see e.g. the recent text of O'Hagan et al. (2006) for some of the key issues involved. If elicited correctly, the utilities should free us from having to "back out" any aspect of the design from a consideration of its operating characteristics, but the authors still recommend simulations to check those characteristics, an eminently sensible safety feature. See also Section 4.6 for more on decision-theoretic methods.

3.4.4 Dose escalation with two agents

Thall et al. (2003) propose an alternative model-based approach for two-agent dose finding. In spirit the method is similar to the Yin-Yuan combination dose finding described in Section 3.4.1. But instead of the Gumbel model, here we use a 6-parameter bivariate logistic model, and the restriction to adjacent doses is relaxed. Our main motivation to discuss this approach here is the availability of public domain software; see the software notes below.

Consider a phase I oncology trial for the combination of two cytotoxic agents. We assume that each of the two agents has been studied before in single agent trials and that the goal of the new trial is to establish a safe dose combination for the two agents. Let (d_1, d_2) denote the doses of the two cytotoxic agents. Let $\pi^\star$ denote the target toxicity level, and let $d_k^\star$, $k = 1, 2$, denote known single-agent acceptable doses, i.e., doses with mean toxicity equal to $\pi^\star$. In the following discussion we use standardized doses, $x_k = d_k/d_k^\star$, $k = 1, 2$. We do so to avoid scaling problems. Consider a dose combination $\mathbf{x} = (x_1, x_2)$ and let $\pi(\mathbf{x}, \boldsymbol{\theta})$ denote the unknown probability of toxicity at $\mathbf{x}$. Here $\boldsymbol{\theta}$ is a parameter vector that indexes the probability model. We assume

$$\pi(\mathbf{x}, \boldsymbol{\theta}) = \frac{a_1 x_1^{b_1} + a_2 x_2^{b_2} + a_3 \left(x_1^{b_1} x_2^{b_2}\right)^{b_3}}{1 + a_1 x_1^{b_1} + a_2 x_2^{b_2} + a_3 \left(x_1^{b_1} x_2^{b_2}\right)^{b_3}}. \tag{3.8}$$

The model is indexed by $\boldsymbol{\theta} = (a_1, b_1, a_2, b_2, a_3, b_3)$. The model is chosen to allow easy incorporation of information about single-agent toxicities. For $x_2 = 0$ the model reduces to the single agent dose-toxicity curve $\pi((x_1, 0), \boldsymbol{\theta}) \equiv \pi_1(x_1, \boldsymbol{\theta})$ and similarly for π_2. The parameters (a_3, b_3) characterize the two-agent interactions.

Let $\mathbf{Y}_n = (\mathbf{x}_i, y_i; \ i = 1, \ldots, n)$ denote observed indicators for toxicity y_i for n patients treated at dose combinations $\mathbf{x}_i = (x_{i1}, x_{i2})$, $i = 1, \ldots, n$. The outcome is a binary indicator y_i with $y_i = 1$ if patient i experienced a dose-limiting toxicity and $y_i = 0$ otherwise. When the sample size n is understood from the context we will use $\mathbf{Y}$, $\mathbf{x} = (\mathbf{x}_1, \ldots, \mathbf{x}_n)$ and $\mathbf{y} = (\mathbf{y}_1, \ldots, \mathbf{y}_n)$ as short for all data, the vectors of all dose assignments and all responses, respectively. The likelihood function is evaluated as

$$p(\mathbf{y} \mid \boldsymbol{\theta}, \mathbf{x}) = \prod_{i:\, y_i = 1} \pi(\mathbf{x}_i, \boldsymbol{\theta}) \prod_{i:\, y_i = 0} (1 - \pi(\mathbf{x}_i, \boldsymbol{\theta})).$$

Thall et al. (2003) assume independent gamma priors for the parameters,

$$a_j \sim \text{Ga}(\alpha_{1j}, \alpha_{2j}) \text{ and } b_j \sim \text{Ga}(\beta_{1j}, \beta_{2j}),$$

for $j = 1, 2$. Specifically, they adopt informative priors for (a_j, b_j), $j = 1, 2$, corresponding to the single-agent dose-toxicity curves. The hyperparameters $(\alpha_{1j}, \alpha_{2j}, \beta_{1j}, \beta_{2j})$, $j = 1, 2$ are chosen to match the known single-agent toxicity curves as closely as possible. For the interaction parameters we assume independent log normal priors, $\log a_3 \sim N(\mu_{a3}, \sigma_{a3})$ and $\log b_3 \sim N(\mu_{b3}, \sigma_{b3})$. As default choices we propose to use $\mu_{a3} = \mu_{b3} = 0.25$ and $\sigma_{a3}^2 = \sigma_{b3}^2 = 3$. Note that Thall et al. (2003) also use gamma priors for (a_3, b_3), but we found it numerically more stable to work with the normal priors for $(\log a_3, \log b_3)$ instead.

The proposed algorithm proceeds in two stages. First the dose combinations are increased along a pre-determined linear grid D_1 to quickly approximate the desired target toxicity π^*. This pre-determined linear grid is in the bivariate dose space. By default D_1 is defined on a 45 degree line of equal proportions for the two agents. The dose escalation is subject to overdose control. Think of this first stage as a fast climb straight up the expected toxicity surface. In the second stage, we modify the combination of the two doses to explore alternative combinations of the two agents that achieve similar toxicity probabilities. Think of the second stage as moving horizontally along a curve of equal mean toxicity, exploring to either side of the final point on the first stage climb. All moves are based on the currently estimated posterior expected toxicity surface,

$$\bar{\pi}_n(\mathbf{x}) = E[\pi(\mathbf{x}, \boldsymbol{\theta}) \mid \mathbf{Y}_n] = \int \pi(\mathbf{x}, \boldsymbol{\theta}) \, dp(\boldsymbol{\theta} \mid \mathbf{Y}_n) \,.$$

Let $L_2(\pi^\star, \mathbf{Y}_n) = \{\mathbf{x} : \bar{\pi}_n(\mathbf{x}) = \pi^\star\}$ denote the equal (posterior mean) toxicity contour conditional on the current data $\mathbf{Y}_n$.

Let $L_2^{left} = \{\mathbf{x} \in L_2$ and $x_2 > x_1\}$ denote the segment of L_2 above the 45 degree line ($x_1 = x_2$; when D_1 is not defined on the 45 degree line, change L_2^{left} accordingly). Similarly L_2^{right} is the part of L_2 below the 45 degree line. The move in the second stage is restricted on L_2. In alternating cohorts we use L_2^{left} and L_2^{right}. This constraint to alternate moves to either side avoids the algorithm getting trapped. Let L_s^{side} denote the set for the current cohort. To assign the doses in stage 2, we simply randomly select one of the doses in L_2^{side} with equal probability.

Algorithm 3.10 *(Two-agent dose-finding).*

Step 0. Initialization: Define a grid $D_1 = \{\mathbf{x}^{(r)}, \ r = 1, \ldots, R\}$ in the bivariate dose space. By default D_1 is on the 45 degree line.

Initialize the cohort size $K = 3$. Initialize the sample size, $n = 0$, and cohort index, $i = 1$. Fix the treatment dose for the first cohort as $x_1 = x^{(d_0)}$ for some pre-determined d_0.

Fix an assumed true toxicity surface by assuming a parameter vector $\boldsymbol{\theta}_0$ for model (3.8).

Step 1. Stage 1 (initial dose escalation): Escalate on the grid D_1, subject to overdose control.

    Step 1.1. Next cohort: Treat cohort i at dose $\mathbf{x}_i$. Determine the probability of toxicity under the assumed simulation truth, $p = \pi(\mathbf{x}_i, \boldsymbol{\theta}_0)$. Simulate $y_i \sim \text{Bin}(K, p)$ and record the number of observed responses y_i. Increment $n \equiv n + K$.

    Step 1.2. Refining the dose grid: When the first toxicity is observed, i.e. $y_i > 0$, we refine the grid by adding half steps $\frac{1}{2}(\mathbf{x}^{(r)} + \mathbf{x}^{(r+1)})$, $r = 1, \ldots, R - 1$.

    Step 1.3. Posterior updating: Run an MCMC simulation to generate a posterior Monte Carlo sample Θ with $\boldsymbol{\theta} \sim p(\boldsymbol{\theta} \mid \mathbf{Y})$ for all $\boldsymbol{\theta} \in \Theta$, approximately. Using Θ update $\bar{\pi}_n(\mathbf{x}) \equiv \sum_\Theta \pi(\mathbf{x}, \boldsymbol{\theta})$ for all $\mathbf{x} \in D_1$. Increment $n = n + K$.

    Step 1.4. Next dose: Find the dose combination $\mathbf{x}^{(r)} \in D_1$ minimzing $|\bar{\pi}_n - \pi^\star|$, subject to the condition of not skipping any untried dose in D_1 when escalating. Set $x_{i+1} = \mathbf{x}^{(r)}$.

    Step 1.5. Stopping: If $n < n_1$, increment $i = i + 1$ and repeat with Step 1.1. Otherwise continue with step 2.

Step 2. Stage 2 (explore at equal toxicity level): Let $L \equiv L_2^{side}$ denote the current branch of L_2.

Step 2.1. Next dose (uniform assignment): Select $\mathbf{x}_{i+1} \sim \text{Unif}(L)$.

Step 2.2. Next cohort: same as Step 1.1.

Step 2.3. Posterior updating: same as Step 1.3.

Step 2.4. Stopping: If $n < n_1 + n_2$, increment $i \equiv i + 1$ and repeat with step 2.1. Otherwise continue with Step 3.

Step 3. Final recommendation: Let $x_\ell^\star$ denote the optimal dose pair in $L = L_2^{left}$, computed as in Step 2. Similarly, let $x_r^\star$ denote the optimal dose combination in $L = L_2^{right}$, and let $x_m^\star$ denote the optimal dose pair on $L = D_1$.

Report $\{x_\ell^\star, x_m^\star, x_r^\star\}$ as three alternative MTD dose pairs.

■

The MCMC simulation in Steps 1.3 and 2.2. is implemented as a straightforward Metropolis-Hastings algorithm with random walk proposals. In our implementation we used $M = 100$ parallel chains, and 100 iterations each time. The chains were initialized using a normal approximation of the posterior for $\eta = \log \theta$.

Software note: The ToxFinder program offers an implementation of the ideas in this subsection, and can be downloaded from biostatistics.mdanderson.org/ SoftwareDownload/SingleSoftware.aspx?Software_Id=14. In addition, R code for a basic implementation of Algorithm 3.10 is included in the online supplement to this chapter,

www.biostat.umn.edu/~brad/software/BCLM_ch3.html.

Example 3.9 *(Gemcitibine and Cyclophosphamide (CTX) Trial).* We implemented our algorithm for the study that motivated the discussion in Thall et al. (2003) and which therein is described as an example application. The study considers combination chemotherapy with gemcitabine and CTX. The goal of the study is to identify three acceptable dose pairs that can be carried forward in a following phase II trial. We follow Thall et al. (2003), using the same prior means and variances for the first four parameters, namely $E(a_1, b_1, a_2, b_2) = (0.4286, 7.6494, 0.4286, 7.8019)$ with corresponding marginal variances $(0.1054, 5.7145, 0.0791, 3.9933)$. These moments were carefully elicited by Thall et al. (2003). We then found parameters for the scaled gamma priors to match these marginal moments. For the interaction parameters we assumed means $E(a_3, b_3) = (0.25, 0.25)$, and marginal variances $\text{Var}(a_3) = \text{Var}(b_3) = 3$. We then assume independent log normal priors for a_3 and b_3 to match these moments.

The proposed two-agent dose escalation was implemented using maximum sample sizes $n_1 = 20$ and $n_2 = 40$ for stages 1 and 2 and a target toxicity level of $\pi^\star = 0.30$.

Figures 3.18 through 3.20 summarize simulated trial histories under two hypothetical simulation truths. Scenario S2 assumes weak interaction and

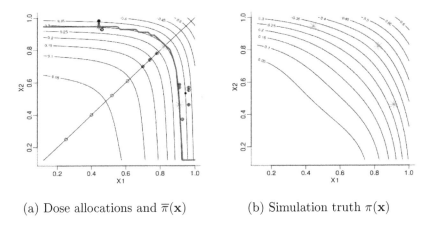

(a) Dose allocations and $\overline{\pi}(\mathbf{x})$ (b) Simulation truth $\pi(\mathbf{x})$

Figure 3.18 *Scenario S2: dose allocations, estimated toxicity surface (conditional on all data) (panel a) and simulation truth (panel b). Empty circles show cohorts with $y_i = 0$, crossed circles show $y_i = 1$, small bullets show $y_i = 2$ and large bullets show $y_i = 3$. The (large) stars show the finally reported three MTD dose pairs. The thick curve in the left panel shows the estimated $\pi^\star$ toxicity curve.*

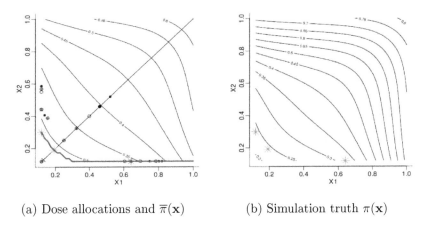

(a) Dose allocations and $\overline{\pi}(\mathbf{x})$ (b) Simulation truth $\pi(\mathbf{x})$

Figure 3.19 *Scenario S4: same as Figure 3.18 for scenario S4.*

moderate toxicity. The second scenario, S4, assumes strong interaction and high toxicity. Figure 3.18 shows the allocated dose combinations as well as the estimated toxicity under S2, while Figure 3.19 shows the same under S4. In both figures we see how the first dose allocations quickly walk up the steep toxicity surface. At the end of Stage 1, the algorithm starts to explore alternative dose combinations off the diagonal that still have the desired target toxicity probability. Note that the dose allocations are always based

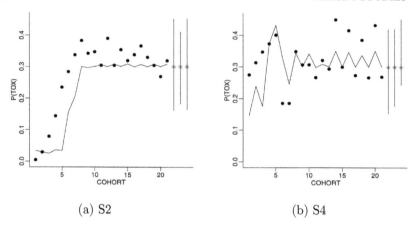

(a) S2   (b) S4

Figure 3.20 *Estimated toxicity probabilities $\bar{\pi}(\mathbf{x}_i)$ (line) and true toxicity prob-abilities $\pi(\mathbf{x}_i)$ (bullets) plotted against cohort i. The last three points show the three reported MTD pairs, together with 95% credible intervals for the true toxi-city $\pi(x^\star)$.*

on currently estimated toxicities. Changes in the posterior estimates lead to some scatter in the assigned dose pairs. The figures also show the esti-mated toxicity surface at the end of the simulated trial and for comparison the assumed simulation truth. The thick lines in the left panels show the estimted sets L_2 at the last step. In both cases, the curves closely track the estimated $\pi^\star = 30\%$ contours for $E(\pi \mid \mathbf{Y})$, except for approximation errors due to the discrete nature of the grid that is used to represent L_2.

Figure 3.20 shows the estimated and true toxicity of the sequence of dose allocations for the same two simulations. We can clearly see the bias in the posterior estimated toxicities that is introduced by the prior model. When the prior assumes higher (lower) toxicities than the simulation truth, the posterior estimates show corresponding positive (negative) biases. ∎

3.5 Appendix: R Macros

The online supplement to this chapter

www.biostat.umn.edu/~brad/software/BCLM_ch3.html

provides the R code that was used to illustrate the examples in this chap-ter. In many cases, the R macros are written to simulate *one* realization of a hypothetical trial using the proposed design. The main function in these examples is named sim.trial(.). To compute operating character-istics one would add an additional loop that repeatedly calls sim.trial. To monitor an ongoing trial one would have to (i) replace the simu-lated data with the actually observed responses, and (ii) strip the top-level loop inside `sim.trial` and use only one iteration. The `CRMinteractive,` `CRMexplore`, and `phaseIsim` programs supporting the work in Section 3.2 are provided on our website in zip files, containing full input, code, and "readme" files.

## CHAPTER 4

Phase II studies

In this chapter we address the design and statistical considerations for the development of "middle phase" clinical trials, especially those associated with phase II cancer trials. Here the focus shifts from toxicity to *efficacy*, and trials are run on much larger groups of patients (say, 40 to 200). We also delve more deeply into the subject of adaptive designs, a subject of greatly increasing interest and utility in middle-phase studies.

After obtaining preliminary information about the safety profile, dose, and administration schedule of a drug in early (phase I) development, the next issue is to examine whether a drug has sufficient efficacy to warrant further development. Phase II studies can be further divided into two parts. The initial assessment of the drug's efficacy is the primary goal for *phase IIA* trials. Typically, phase IIA trials are conducted as single-arm studies to assess the efficacy of new drugs, with the goal of screening out those that are ineffective. Subsequently, *phase IIB* trials are multi-arm studies to compare the efficacy of the new drug versus the standard treatment or other experimental drugs, so that the most promising one can be selected for large scale evaluation in late phase studies. The toxicity profile of the new agents may also be further evaluated in phase II studies.

Phase II studies provide important intermediate steps for a successful drug development. In today's post-genomic and high-throughput era, the number of new candidate agents is growing by leaps and bounds. Since late phase studies are large, time consuming, and expensive, middle phase trials play a critical role in eliminating the "chaff" from our drug collection, so that only the most promising treatments are funneled through to late phase development, thus ensuring a higher overall success rate.

4.1 Standard designs

Traditionally, After the toxicity profile and/or the MTD for a treatment has been investigated, phase II studies are conducted at the MTD or an "optimal biological dose" estimated from phase I to evaluate whether the new agent has sufficient activity and to refine knowledge of its toxicity profile. The primary endpoint of a phase IIA trial is often a binary endpoint of response/no response or success/failure. For cancer trials, the clinical response is defined as complete response (no evidence of disease) or partial response. Partial response is often defined as a 50% or more tumor volume shrinkage based on a two-dimensional measurement, or a 30% or more decrease in the sum of the longest diameters of target lesions based on the one-dimensional RECIST criteria in solid tumors (Therasse et al., 2000, 2006; Eisenhauer et al., 2009). As for phase IIB trials, time-to-event endpoints such as disease-free survival or progression-free survival are often chosen as primary endpoints. Comprehensive overviews on the design and analysis of phase II cancer trials can be found, for example, in papers by Mariani and Marubini (1996), Scher and Heller (2002), and Gray et al. (2006), and Seymour et al. (2010).

4.1.1 Phase IIA designs

To provide an initial efficacy assessment, a phase IIA trial is often designed as a single-arm, open-label study that requires treating 40 to 100 patients in a multistage setting. Multi-stage designs are useful here for early stopping due to lack of efficacy should the interim data indicate that the study drug is inefficacious. In cancer trials, Gehan (1961) proposed the first two-stage design. In the early days of cancer drug development, there were few drugs that had anticancer activity; a drug was considered active if it produced a tumor response rate p of 20% or higher. To test the hypothesis of H_0: $p = 0$ versus H_1: $p = 0.2$, Gehan's design calls for enrolling 14 patients in the first stage. If none of them respond to the treatment, the drug is considered ineffective and the trial is stopped. If at least one tumor response is observed, additional patients (typically 20–40) are enrolled in the second stage such that the response rate can be estimated with a prespecified precision. This design has a Type I error rate of zero (because under the null hypothesis of $p = 0$, no response can occur) and 95% power when $p = 0.2$. The design can also be used to test other alternative response rates under H_1. For example, for $p = 0.1$ or 0.15, the corresponding sample size in the first stage to achieve 95% power will be 29 and 19, respectively. The initial sample size n can be easily calculated by finding the smallest n such that the specified power is greater than or equal to $1 - (1 - p)^n$. The second stage for the sample size can be obtained by finding the total sample size N such that the standard error of the estimated response rate, $\sqrt{p(1 - p)/N}$, is smaller than a certain precision. Here the true parameter p can be estimated by taking, for example, the upper end of a one-sided 75 percent confidence interval, or simply a conservative estimate of $p = 0.5$.

As treatments improve over time, the null response rate corresponding to the response rate of the standard treatment is no longer zero. When the null response is greater than 0, two-stage designs can be constructed to test the hypothesis H_0: $p \leq p_0$ versus H_1: $p \geq p_1$. A primary motivation for a two-stage design is that if the treatment does not work in the first stage, the trial can be stopped early, so that patients are not subjected to a potentially toxic yet ineffective treatment. In addition, resources saved can be devoted to developing other agents.

Among many two-stage designs which control Type I and Type II error rates at α and β, the Simon (1989) optimal design was constructed to minimize the *expected* sample size under the null hypothesis. Alternatively, a *minimax* design can be constructed that minimizes the maximum trial sample size. As in statistical decision theory, minimax designs are rather conservative in that they focus all their attention on the worst-case scenario. For example, when $p_0 = 0.1$ and $p_1 = 0.3$, with $\alpha = \beta = 0.1$, the optimal two-stage design needs to enroll 12 patients in the first stage. If no response or only one response is found, the trial is stopped and the drug is considered ineffective. Otherwise, 23 more patients are enrolled to reach a total of 35 patients. At the end of the trial, if only five or fewer responses are observed, the agent is deemed ineffective. Otherwise (i.e., with 6 or more responses in 35 patients), the agent is considered effective. Under the null hypothesis, there is a 66% chance that the trial will be stopped early. The expected sample size under H_0 is then

$$12 + (35 - 12)(1 - .66) = 19.8 \, ,$$

the first-stage sample size plus the second-stage size times one minus the probability of early stopping.

In comparison, the minimax design enrolls 16 patients in the first stage. If no response or only one response is seen, the trial is stopped early and the drug is considered ineffective. Otherwise, 9 more patients are enrolled in the second stage to reach a total of 25 patients. At the end of the trial, the agent is considered ineffective if four or fewer responses are seen and effective otherwise. The expected sample size is 20.4 and the probability of early stopping is 0.51 under the null hypothesis. In both designs, the trial can be stopped early because of lack of efficacy (i.e., futility), to save patients from receiving ineffective treatments and to save time and resources for developing ineffective treatments. If the treatment works well, there is little reason to stop the trial early in a phase II setting. More patients can benefit from the treatment while the trial continues. Larger sample sizes also increase the precision in estimating the response rate.

A *multi-stage* design with early stopping for futility rules is desirable in phase II settings. Other multi-stage designs can be found in the literature. For example, Fleming (1982) proposed a two-stage design that allows for early stopping due to futility or efficacy. Bryant and Day (1995) developed a two-stage design that allows the investigator to monitor efficacy and toxicity simultaneously. Three-stage designs were proposed by Ensign et al. (1994) and Chen (1997). Three-stage designs improve the efficiency of two-stage designs, but are more complicated to implement and can increase the cost and length of the study. The gain in efficiency of designs with more than three stages often does not justify the additional complexity in conducting them. To derive the sample size and stopping boundaries for a multi-stage design, Schultz et al. (1973) provided a useful recursive formula for computing the tail probabilities to meet the constraints of Type I and Type II error rates.

Software note: A stand-alone program that does Simon two-stage optimal design calculations can be downloaded from `linus.nci.nih.gov/~brb/Opt.htm`. Given a maximum sample size and probabilities of response under the null and alternative hypotheses, the program searches all two-stage designs to find the minimax and optimal designs that satisfy the specified constraints on Type I and II error.

  For those who prefer web-driven calculators (rather than stand-alone programs that need to be installed locally), computations for Simon's two-stage designs are available at `linus.nci.nih.gov/brb/samplesize/otsd.html`. Similarly, calculations for Bryant and Day designs are available online at the website `www.upci.upmc.edu/bf/ClinicalStudyDesign/Phase2BryantDay.cfm`.

  Finally, among many other useful statistical tools, the site `www.crab.org/Statistools.asp`, and the Duke Cancer Center site, `www.cancer.duke.edu/modules/CTDSystems54/index.php?id=3`, provide tools for calculating the performance of general two-stage designs.

4.1.2 Phase IIB designs

After passing the initial efficacy assessment of a new agent in a phase IIA study, the subsequent phase IIB trial is often a randomized, multi-arm study with the goal of identifying the most promising treatment regimen to send to large-scale phase III trials for definitive testing. In addition to testing the response rate, time-to-event endpoints, such as time to disease progression, are often used as the primary endpoint in phase IIB trials. The challenge is to accurately select the most promising regimens among a large number of potentially active regimens for further development.

  Compared to phase III trials, phase IIB trials are by definition smaller and less definitive. They tend to use earlier endpoints, such as disease-free survival, rather than overall survival in order to shorten study duration. They also often have larger Type I and Type II error rates than their phase III counterparts. For example, the acceptable Type I error rate is usually increased from 5% to 10% or even 20%. The maximum Type II error rate still needs to be controlled in the 10 to 20% range. The rationale for this is that, in phase II trials, it is more important to control the Type II error (false-negative) rate than the Type I error (false-positive) rate. By controlling the false-negative rate, active treatments are less likely to be missed. A false-positive result is of less concern in phase II because the final verdict of the effectiveness of a regimen can be provided in another phase II study or a phase III evaluation. A moderate to large expected difference is often assumed for phase II studies as well. Many of the randomized phase II cancer studies apply randomization to achieve patient comparability, while embedding a one-sample phase II design within each treatment arm (Lee and Feng, 2005). Owing to limited sample sizes, such designs typically do not yield sufficient statistical power for a head-to-head comparison between the treatment arms, as is possible in phase III trials.

As an alternative method, Simon, Wittes, and Ellenberg (1985; henceforth abbreviated SWE) proposed a *pick-the-winner* design based on ranking and selection methodology for binary endpoints. Unlike the ordinary hypothesis testing framework which controls both Type I and Type II errors, the ranking and selection procedure controls only Type II errors. Basically, the response rate of each treatment arm is estimated and the arm with the highest response rate is picked as the "winner" for further evaluation. The design is appealing because the required sample size is much smaller than that for a randomized trial under a hypothesis testing framework. For example, N = 146 patients per arm are required for testing the response rates of 10% versus 25% with 90% power and a two-sided 5% Type I error rate. On the other hand, the SWE method requires only N = 21 patients per arm to achieve the same power. The trade-off, however, is that the false-positive rate can range from 20 to over 40%, as reported in simulation studies (e.g. Liu et al., 1999).

The SWE method works best when there is only one true "winner," with all other contenders ranking well behind in efficacy. When there are several comparable, active regimens, the method struggles to accurately differentiate the best one from the other good ones. At the end of the trial, this method always picks the treatment arm with the best observed outcome as the winner, regardless of whether none of the regimens work, some of them work, or all of them work. In addition, another drawback of the SWE method is that it does not provide for early stopping due to futility. Therefore, there is no provision for terminating a non-performing arm early on the basis of interim results. Although the SWE method offers small sample sizes, its ranking and selection methodology does not appear to mesh well with the objectives for phase IIB studies.

Thus, whether based on one-sample or multi-sample hypothesis testing or ranking and selection methods, none of the frequentist methods are fully satisfactory in providing good solutions for phase IIB designs. Although smaller sample sizes are usually found in phase II trials, they should not be thought of as "poor man's phase III trials." Nevertheless, for phase II evaluation, more efficiency is required, and this is where Bayesian methods can often offer a superior approach.

4.1.3 Limitations of traditional frequentist designs

Multi-stage designs achieve better statistical properties than single-stage designs by utilizing information gained in the interim data. By examining the interim data, such designs allow for an earlier decision to stop the trial if convincing evidence to support the null or alternative hypothesis is found. The frequentist analysis of such designs, however, is constrained by the rigid requirement of examining the outcome at the specified sample size at each predetermined stage. The strict sample size guideline in each stage is particularly difficult to adhere to in multi-center trials due to the complexity of coordinating patient accrual and follow-up across multiple sites. Temporarily halting study accrual can also stall the trial's momentum and lower its investigators' enthusiasm for the project. In addition, when actual trial conduct deviates from the original design (e.g., investigators performing interim analyses at unplanned time points), stopping boundaries are left undefined, and the anticipated statistical properties no longer hold. Many authors (Green and Dahlberg, 1992; Herndon, 1998; Chen and Ng, 1998) have recognized these problems and proposed solutions, but none have been completely satisfactory. This lack of design flexibility exposes a fundamental limitation of all such frequentist-based methods, because statistical inferences are made by computing the probability of observing certain data conditioned on a particular design and sampling plan. When there is a disparity between the proposed design and the actual trial conduct (more the norm than an exception in clinical trials), adjustments must be made to all statistical inferences.

All of these reasons support the need for more flexible designs. Bayesian methods offer a different approach for designing and monitoring clinical trials by permitting calculation of the posterior probability of various events given the data. Based on the Likelihood Principle (Subsection 2.2.3), all information pertinent to the parameters is contained in the data and is not constrained by the design. Bayesian methods are particular appealing in clinical trial design because they inherently allow for flexibility in trial conduct and impart the ability to examine interim data, update the posterior probability of parameters, and accordingly make relevant predictions and sensible decisions.

4.2 Predictive probability

In Subsection 2.5.1 we introduced predictive probabilities. In this section we describe their use in the design of phase II clinical trials (e.g., Lee and Liu, 2008). A distinct advantage of this approach is that it mimics the clinical decisionmaking process. Based on the interim data, predictive probability is obtained by calculating the probability of a positive conclusion (rejecting the null hypothesis) should the trial be conducted to the maximum planned sample size. In this framework, the chance that the trial will show a conclusive result at the end of the study, given the current information, is evaluated. The decision to continue or to stop the trial can be made according to the strength of this predictive probability.

4.2.1 Definition and basic calculations for binary data

For a phase IIA trial, suppose our goal is to evaluate the response rate p for a new drug by testing the hypothesis $H_0: p \le p_0$ versus $H_1: p \ge p_1$. Suppose we assume that the prior distribution of the response rate, $\pi(p)$, follows a $Beta(a_0, b_0)$ distribution. As described earlier, the quantity $a_0/(a_0 + b_0)$ gives the prior mean, while the magnitude of $a_0 + b_0$ indicates how informative the prior is. Since the quantities a_0 and b_0 can be considered as the numbers of effective prior responses and non-responses, respectively, $a_0 + b_0$ can be thought of as a measure of prior precision: the larger this sum, the more informative the prior and the stronger the belief it contains.

Suppose we set a maximum number of accrued patients N_{max}, and assume that the number of responses X among the current n patients ($n \le N_{max}$) follows a $Binomial(n, p)$ distribution. By the conjugacy of the beta prior and binomial likelihood, the posterior distribution of the response rate follows another a beta distribution, $p|x \sim Beta(a_0 + x, b_0 + n - x)$. The predictive probability approach looks into the future based on the current observed data to project whether a positive conclusion at the end of study is likely or not, and then makes a sensible decision at the present time accordingly.

Let Y be the number of responses in the potential $m = N_{max} - n$ future patients. Suppose our design is to declare efficacy if the posterior probability of p exceeding some prespecified level p_0 is greater than some threshold θ_T. Marginalizing p out of the binomial likelihood, it is well known that Y follows a *beta-binomial* distribution, $Y \sim Beta\text{-}Binomial(m, a_0 + x, b_0 + n - x)$. When $Y = i$, the posterior distribution of $p|(X = x, Y = i)$ is $Beta(a_0 + x + i, b_0 + N_{max} - x - i)$. The predictive probability (PP) of trial success can then be calculated as follows. Letting $B_i = Pr(p > p_0 \,|\, x, Y = i)$ and $I_i = I(B_i > \theta_T)$, we have

$$
\begin{aligned}
PP &= E\{I[Pr(p > p_0|x, Y) > \theta_T] \,|\, x\} \\
&= \int I[Pr(p > p_0|x, Y) > \theta_T] \, dP(Y|x) \\
&= \sum_{i=0}^{m} Pr(Y = i \,|\, x) \times I(Pr(p > p_0 \,|\, x, Y = i) > \theta_T) \\
&= \sum_{i=0}^{m} Pr(Y = i \,|\, x) \times I(B_i > \theta_T)
\end{aligned}
$$

$$= \sum_{i=0}^{m} Pr(Y = i \mid x) \times I_i .$$

The quantity B_i is the probability that the response rate is larger than p_0 given x responses in n patients in the current data and i responses in m future patients. Comparing B_i to a threshold value θ_T yields an indicator I_i for considering the treatment efficacious at the end of the trial given the current data and the potential outcome of $Y = i$. Example 4.1 below offers a concrete illustration of the calculation of PP using the preceding formulae.

The weighted sum of indicators I_i yields the predictive probability of concluding a positive result by the end of the trial based on the cumulative information in the current stage. A high PP means that the treatment is likely to be efficacious by the end of the study, given the current data, whereas a low PP suggests that the treatment may not have sufficient activity. Therefore, PP can be used to determine whether the trial should be stopped early due to efficacy/futility or continued because the current data are not yet conclusive. We define a rule by introducing two thresholds on PP. The decision rule can be constructed as follows:

Algorithm 4.1 *(Phase IIA basic PP design).*

Step 1: If $PP < \theta_L$, stop the trial and reject the alternative hypothesis;

Step 2: If $PP > \theta_U$, stop the trial and reject the null hypothesis;

Step 3: Otherwise continue to the next stage until reaching N_{max} patients.

■

Typically, we choose θ_L as a small positive number and θ_U as a large positive number, both between 0 and 1 (inclusive). $PP < \theta_L$ indicates that it is unlikely the response rate will be larger than p_0 at the end of the trial given the current information. When this happens, we may as well stop the trial and reject the alternative hypothesis at that point. On the other hand, when $PP > \theta_U$, the current data suggest that, if the same trend continues, we will have a high probability of concluding that the treatment is efficacious at the end of the study. This result, then, provides evidence to stop the trial early due to efficacy. By choosing $\theta_L > 0$ and $\theta_U < 1.0$, the trial can terminate early due to either futility or efficacy. For phase IIA trials, we often prefer to choose $\theta_L > 0$ and $\theta_U = 1.0$ to allow early stopping due to futility, but not due to efficacy.

Example 4.1 *(Calculating phase IIA predictive probabilities).* Suppose an investigator plans to enroll a maximum of $N_{max} = 40$ patients into a phase II study. At a given time, $x = 16$ responses are observed in $n = 23$ patients. What is $P(response\,rate > 60\%)$? Assuming a vague $Beta(0.6, 0.4)$ prior distribution on the response rate p and letting Y be the number of

$Y = i$	$Pr(Y = i\|x)$	$B_i = Pr(p > 0.60 \mid x, Y = i)$	$I(B_i > 0.90)$
0	0.0000	0.0059	0
1	0.0000	0.0138	0
2	0.0001	0.0296	0
3	0.0006	0.0581	0
4	0.0021	0.1049	0
5	0.0058	0.1743	0
6	0.0135	0.2679	0
7	0.0276	0.3822	0
8	0.0497	0.5085	0
9	0.0794	0.6349	0
10	0.1129	0.7489	0
11	0.1426	0.8415	0
12	0.1587	0.9089	1
13	0.1532	0.9528	1
14	0.1246	0.9781	1
15	0.0811	0.9910	1
16	0.0381	0.9968	1
17	0.0099	0.9990	1

Table 4.1 *Bayesian predictive probability calculation for $p_0 = 0.60, \theta_T = 0.90, N_{max} = 40, x = 16, n = 23$, and a $Beta(0.6, 0.4)$ prior distribution on p.*

responses in a future $m = 17$ patients, Y's marginal distribution is *Beta-binomial*$(17, 16.6, 7.4)$. At each possible value of $Y = i$, the conditional posterior of p follows a beta distribution, $p|x, Y = i \sim Beta(16.6 + i, 24.4 - i)$. In this example, we set $\theta_T = 0.90$.

As can be seen from Table 4.1, when Y lies in $[0, 11]$, the resulting $P(response\ rate > 0.60)$ ranges from 0.0059 to 0.8415. Hence, we would conclude H_0 for $Y \leq 11$. On the other hand, when Y lies in $[12, 17]$, the resulting $P(response\ rate > 0.60)$ ranges from 0.9089 to 0.9990. In these cases we would instead decide in favor of H_1. The predictive probability is then the weighted average (weighted by the probability of the realization of each Y) of the indicator of a positive trial should the current trend continue and the trial be conducted until the end of the study. The calculation yields $PP = 0.5656$. If we were to choose $\theta_L = 0.10$, the trial would not be stopped due to futility because PP is greater than θ_L. Similarly, if we were to choose $\theta_U = 0.95$, the trial would not be stopped due to efficacy either. Thus based on the interim data, we should continue the study because the evidence is not yet sufficient to draw a definitive conclusion in either direction. ∎

4.2.2 Derivation of the predictive process design

In this subsection we illustrate how to design a trial using the PP approach by searching for N_{max}, θ_L, θ_T, and θ_U values that satisfy a particular set of Type I and Type II error rate constraints. Given p_0, p_1, the prior distribution on the response rate $\pi(p)$, and the cohort size for interim monitoring, we search the aforementioned design parameters to yield a design having satisfactory operating characteristics. As mentioned earlier, we choose $\theta_U = 1.0$ because if the treatment is working, there is little reason to stop the trial early; enrolling more patients to the active treatment is good. Treating more patients until the maximum sample size is reached (usually, less than 100) can also increase the precision in estimating the response rate. Given N_{max}, the question is, "Are there values of θ_L and θ_T that yield desirable design properties"? Our goal is to identify the combinations of θ_L and θ_T to yield the desired power within the error constraints. There may exist ranges of θ_L and θ_T that satisfy the constraints. By varying N_{max} from small to large, the design with the smallest N_{max} that controls both the Type I and Type II error rates (α and β, respectively) at the nominal level is the one we choose. This idea is similar to finding the minimax design (where we minimized the maximum sample size).

The framework of this PP method allows the investigator to monitor the trial either continuously or by any cohort size. To implement Algorithm 4.1, we recommend computing PP and making interim decisions only after the first 10 patients have been treated and evaluated for their response status. Although the choice of treating a minimum of 10 patients is somewhat arbitrary, a minimum number of patients is required to provide information sufficient to obtain a good estimate of the treatment efficacy, and avoid making premature decisions based on spurious results from a small number of patients. After 10 patients, we calculate PP continuously (i.e., with cohort size of 1) to monitor the treatment efficacy. A sufficiently low PP (e.g., PP $\leq \theta_L$) suggests that the trial could be stopped early due to futility (lack of efficacy). Note that PP can be computed for any cohort size and at any interim time. A trial can be stopped anytime due to excessive toxicity, however.

Example 4.2 *(Lung cancer trial).* The primary objective of this study is to assess the efficacy of a particular combination therapy as front-line treatment in patients with advanced non-small cell lung cancer. The study involves a new epidermal growth factor receptor tyrosin kinase inhibitor. The primary endpoint is the clinical response rate (i.e., the rate of complete response and partial response combined) for the new regimen. The current standard treatment yields a response rate of approximately 20% (p_0). The target response rate of the new regimen is 40% (p_1). With the constraint of both Type I and Type II error rates ≤ 0.1, Simon's optimal two-stage design yields $n_1=17$, $r_1=3$, $N_{max}=37$, $r=10$, $PET(p_0)=0.55$ and

$E(N\,|\,p_0)$=26.02 with α=0.095 and β=0.097, where $PET(p_0)$ and $E(N|p_0)$ denote the probability of early termination and the expected sample size under the null hypothesis, respectively. Here, n_1 is the sample size for the first stage; if there are r_1 or fewer responses, the trial will be stopped early and the treatment is considered ineffective. Otherwise, a total of N_{max} patients will be enrolled. If there are a total of r responders or less, the treatment is declared ineffective. On the other hand, if there are at least $r+1$ responders, the null hypothesis is rejected and the treatment is considered effective. The corresponding minimax design yields n_1=19, r_1=3, N_{max}=36, r=10, $PET(p_0)$ =0.46, and $E(N\,|\,p_0)$=28.26 with α=0.086 and β=0.098.

Switching to the PP approach, we assume a vague $Beta(0.2, 0.8)$ prior distribution for the response rate p. The trial is monitored continuously after evaluating the responses of the first 10 patients. For each N_{max} between 25 and 50, we search the θ_L and θ_T space to generate designs that have both Type I and Type II error rates under 0.10. Table 4.2 lists some of the results in order of increasing maximum sample size N_{max}. Among all the designs, the design with $N_{max} = 36$ (third line of the second portion of the table) is the design with the smallest N_{max} that has both Type I and Type II error rates less than 0.1. Note that for $N_{max} = 35$, Type I and Type II error rates cannot both be controlled at rates less than 0.1. For example, the first line with $N_{max} = 35$ shows that when Type I error is constrained to be under 0.1, Type I error is greater than 0.1. Likewise, the second line shows that when Type I error is controlled, Type II error is not. Because there is no solution for this (and smaller) sample sizes that meets both the specified Type I and Type II error constraints, the parameters θ_L, θ_T, the rejection boundary r, the probability of early stopping, and the expected sample size under the null hypothesis are not provided for these cases.

Based on this setting, θ_L and θ_T are determined to be 0.001 and any value in [0.852, 0.922], respectively. The corresponding rejection regions (in number of responses / n) are 0/10, 1/17, 2/21, 3/24, 4/27, 5/29, 6/31, 7/33, 8/34, 9/35, and 10/36. The trial will be stopped and the treatment determined to be ineffective at the first moment when the number of responses falls into the rejection region. Based on these boundaries, if the true response rate is 20%, the probability of accepting the treatment is 0.088. On the other hand, if the true response rate is 40%, the probability of accepting the treatment is 0.906. The probability of stopping the trial early is 0.86 and the expected sample size is 27.67 when the true response rate is 20%. Compared to Simon's minimax two-stage design, the PP design monitors the data more frequently, yet also has a larger probability of early termination and a smaller expected sample size in the null case. Both designs have the same maximum sample size with controlled Type I and Type II error rates.

Figure 4.1 shows the stopping regions for Simon's minimax design (de-

Simon's Minimax/Optimal Two-Stage designs:

	r_1/n_1	r/N_{max}	$PET(p_0)$	$E(N|p_0)$	α	β
Minimax	3/19	10/36	0.46	28.26	0.086	0.098
Optimal	3/17	10/37	0.55	26.02	0.095	0.097

Predictive Probability-based designs:

θ_L	θ_T	r/N_{max}	$PET(p_0)$	$E(N|p_0)$	α	β
		NA/35			0.126	0.093
		NA/35			0.074	0.116
0.001	[0.852,0.922]	10/36	0.86	27.67	0.088	0.094
0.011	[0.830,0.908]	10/37	0.85	25.13	0.099	0.084
0.001	[0.876,0.935]	11/39	0.88	29.24	0.073	0.092
0.001	[0.857,0.923]	11/40	0.86	30.23	0.086	0.075
0.003	[0.837,0.910]	11/41	0.85	30.27	0.100	0.062
0.043	[0.816,0.895]	11/42	0.86	23.56	0.099	0.083
0.001	[0.880,0.935]	12/43	0.88	32.13	0.072	0.074
0.001	[0.862,0.924]	12/44	0.87	33.71	0.085	0.059
0.001	[0.844,0.912]	12/45	0.85	34.69	0.098	0.048
0.032	[0.824,0.898]	12/46	0.86	26.22	0.098	0.068
0.001	[0.884,0.936]	13/47	0.89	35.25	0.071	0.058
0.001	[0.868,0.925]	13/48	0.87	36.43	0.083	0.047
0.001	[0.850,0.914]	13/49	0.86	37.86	0.095	0.038
0.020	[0.832,0.901]	13/50	0.86	30.60	0.100	0.046

Table 4.2 *Operating characteristics of Simon's two-stage designs and the PP design with Type I and Type II error rates 0.10, a Beta(0.2, 0.8) prior for p, $p_0 = 0.2$, and $p_1 = 0.4$. The intervals in the second column indicate any θ_T in the given closed interval (endpoints included) will deliver the operating characteristics shown.*

noted as "M"), the optimal two-stage design (denoted as "O"), and the predictive probability design (denoted as "PP"). The "regions" for both two-stage designs are at two discrete points (corresponding to the first and second stages of the design), while the stepwise stopping boundaries for the PP design allows continuous monitoring of the trial. Under the PP approach, the trial can be stopped when there are no responses in the first 10-16 patients, 1 response in the first 17-20 patients, 2 responses in the first 21-23 patients, and so on. Thus the PP design allows more flexible and frequent monitoring. In addition, compared to the two-stage designs,

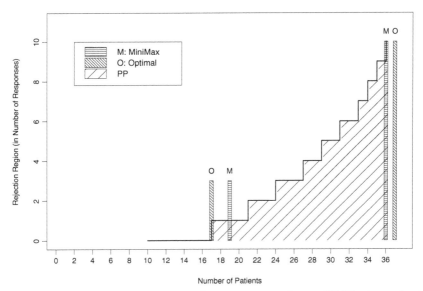

Figure 4.1 *Stopping regions for the Simon minimax design ("M"), the optimal design ("O"), and the predictive probability design ("PP").*

it is harder to stop a trial under the PP design at 17 or 19 patients. For example, with 0, 1, 2, or 3 responses in 17 patients, the trial will be stopped under the two-stage optimal design, but the PP design only stops the trials with 0 or 1 responses at this point. It is often undesirable to stop the trial too early in phase II development. The PP design allows the trial to be stopped at any time if the accumulating evidence does not support the new treatment's efficacy over the standard therapy.■

Software note: As usual, software to carry out PP calculations like those above is available online. After specifying a relatively small sample size and the design parameters p_0, p_1, α, and β, the software we used performs a two-dimensional search over θ_T and θ_L to find a design satisfying the desired constraints on α and β. If both the α and β constraints are met then we have a solution; we can even reduce the sample size and try again. If however there is no solution, the current sample size is not big enough, and so the software increases the sample size by 1 and tries again. The desktop version of this software, **Phase II PP Design**, is available on the web at the M.D. Anderson software download website, **biostatistics.mdanderson.org/SoftwareDownload**.

4.3 Sequential stopping

One of the advantages of a Bayesian approach to inference is the increased flexibility to include sequential stopping compared to the more restrictive requirements under a classical approach. Noninformative stopping rules are irrelevant for Bayesian inference. In other words, posterior inference remains unchanged no matter why the trial was stopped. By contrast, the classical p-value depends crucially on the design of the experiment, of which the stopping mechanism is a key component. The only condition placed on the Bayesian is that the stopping rule be noninformative. Technically this means that the stopping rule and the parameters need to be independent *a priori*. See, however, the discussion near the end of Subsection 2.5.4 concerning frequentist stopping bias. Several designs make use of this feature of Bayesian inference to introduce early stopping for futility and/or for efficacy.

4.3.1 Binary stopping for futility and efficacy

Thall and Simon (1994) and Thall, Simon, and Estey (1995) introduce a class of phase II Bayesian clinical trial designs that include stopping rules based on decision boundaries for clinically meaningful events. To illustrate, let $y_i \in \{0, 1\}$ denote an indicator for response for the i-th patient. Let θ_E and θ_S denote the probability of response under the experimental therapy (E) and standard of care (S), respectively. As mentioned earlier, many phase IIA studies do not include randomization to control. In such cases we assume that either θ_S is known, or at least that an informative prior distribution $p(\theta_S)$ is available. Let $\mathbf{y} = (y_1, \ldots, y_n)$ denote all data up to patient n. We can meaningfully evaluate posterior probabilities of the form

$$\pi_n = p(\theta_E > \theta_S + \delta \mid \mathbf{y}). \tag{4.1}$$

The probability π_n is the posterior probability that the response probability under the experimental therapy dominates that under the standard of care by at least δ. The offset δ is fixed by the investigator, and should reflect the minimum clinically meaningful improvement. It also depends on the nature of the response, the disease and the range of θ_S. The probability π_n is updated after each patient (or patient cohort), and is subsequently used to define sequential stopping rules reminiscent of Algorithm 4.1 of the form

$$
\text{decision} = \begin{cases}
\text{stop and declare } E \text{ promising} & \text{if } \pi_n > U_n \\
\text{continue enrolling patients} & \text{if } L_n < \pi_n < U_n \\
\text{stop and declare } E \text{ not promising} & \text{if } \pi_n < L_n
\end{cases}.
$$

$$\tag{4.2}$$

The decision boundaries $\{(L_n, U_n), \; n = 1, 2, \ldots\}$ are parameters of the design. For example, one could use $L_n \equiv 0.05$ and $U_n \equiv 0.95$ for all n. The considerations that enter the choice of these boundaries are similar to those for choosing stopping boundaries for frequentist group sequential designs (e.g., Jennison and Turnbull, 2000, Sec. 2.3).

In practice, one starts with a reasonable first choice, evaluates frequentist operating characteristics (see Section 2.5.4), and iteratively adjusts the decision boundaries until desired operating characteristics are achieved. For example, we might start with $L_n = 1\%$ and $U_n = 80\%$. Next we compute operating characteristics. We might consider two scenarios: a null scenario $S0$ with $\theta_E = \theta_S$, and an alternative scenario $S1$ with $\theta_E > \theta_S + \delta$ as the simulation truth. Type I error is then the probability with respect to repeat experimentation under $S0$ of ending the trial with the (wrong) conclusion that E is promising, while power is the probability, with respect to repeated simulation of possible trial histories under $S1$, that the trial ends with the (correct) conclusion that E is promising. Assume we find that the Type I error implied by rule (4.2) is 8%, a bit larger than desired. We would next try an increased lower bound L_n to reduce the Type I error. Now we might find an acceptable Type I error under $S0$, but a power of only 70% under $S1$. To increase power we might now try to reduce the upper bound, say to $U_n = 75\%$. A sequence of such iterative corrections will eventually lead to a set of bounds that achieve desirable operating characteristics.

4.3.2 Binary stopping for futility, efficacy, and toxicity

Thall et al. (1995) extend the design from a single outcome to multiple outcomes, including, for example, an efficacy and a toxicity outcome. This allows us to consider the phase II analog of Section 3.3, where we described phase I-II dose-finding trials that traded off efficacy and toxicity following the approach of Thall and Cook (2004). In our present context, let CR denote an efficacy event (e.g., complete response) and TOX a toxicity event. Thall et al. (1995) describe an example with $K = 4$ elementary events $\{A_1 = (CR, TOX), A_2 = (noCR, TOX), A_3 = (CR, noTOX), A_4 = (noCR, noTOX)\}$. Efficacy is $CR = A_1 \cup A_3$, while toxicity is $TOX = A_1 \cup A_2$, etc. The design again involves stopping boundaries as in (4.2), but now using posterior probabilities of CR and TOX.

Let $(p_T(A_1), p_T(A_2), p_T(A_3), p_T(A_4))$ denote the (unknown) probabilities of the four elementary events A_1, A_2, A_3, and A_4 under treatment T, where $T \in \{E, S\}$ (experimental or standard therapy). Suppose we assume a Dirichlet prior for these probabilities. Under standard therapy, we assume a $priori$ that $(p_{S1}, \ldots, p_{S4}) \sim Dir(\theta_{S1}, \ldots, \theta_{S4})$. Similarly, under experimental therapy we assume $(p_{E1}, \ldots, p_{E4}) \sim Dir(\theta_{E1}, \ldots, \theta_{E4})$. The parameters θ_S and θ_E are fixed. Let y_i^n denote the number of patients among the first n who report event A_i and let $y^n = (y_1^n, \ldots, y_4^n)$. The conjugate Dirichlet prior allows for easy posterior updating, since

$$p_E(p_1, \ldots, p_4 \mid y^n) = Dir(\theta_{E1}^n, \ldots, \theta_{E4}^n) ,$$

where $\theta_{Ei}^n = \theta_{Ei} + y_i^n$. Let $\eta_S(CR) = \sum_{A_i \in CR} p_{Si}$ denote the probability of complete remission under standard therapy, and similarly for $\eta_E(CR)$, $\eta_S(TOX)$ and $\eta_E(TOX)$. The posterior $p(\eta_E(CR) \mid y^n)$ then emerges as a beta distribution, $\text{Be}(\theta_{E1}^n + \theta_{E3}^n, \theta_{E2}^n + \theta_{E4}^n)$. Here we used the fact that the beta is the special case of a Dirichlet distribution having just two probabilities. Similarly, $p_E(\eta_E(TOX) \mid y^n) = \text{Be}(\theta_{E1}^n + \theta_{E2}^n, \theta_{E3}^n + \theta_{E4}^n)$. The distributions for $\eta_S(\cdot)$ remain unchanged throughout as $p(\eta_S(TOX)) = \text{Be}(\theta_{S1} + \theta_{S2}, \theta_{S3} + \theta_{S4})$, and similarly for $\eta_S(CR)$.

As before, thresholds on posterior probabilities determine sequential stopping. We track the two posterior probabilities

$$\pi_n(CR) = Pr(\eta_E(CR) > \eta_S(CR) + \delta_{CR} \mid y^n) \qquad (4.3)$$
$$\text{and } \pi_n(TOX) = Pr(\eta_E(TOX) > \eta_S(TOX) + \delta_{TOX} \mid y^n) .$$

After each patient cohort, the posterior probabilities $\pi_n(\cdot)$ are updated and compared against thresholds (in this sequence):

$$\text{decision} = \begin{cases} \text{stop, declare } E \text{ not promising} & \text{if } \pi_n(CR) < L_n(CR) \\ \text{stop, declare } E \text{ too toxic} & \text{if } \pi_n(TOX) > U_n(TOX) \\ \text{stop, declare } E \text{ promising} & \text{if } \pi_n(CR) > U_n(CR) \\ \text{continue enrolling patients} & \text{otherwise} \end{cases}$$

$$(4.4)$$

The evaluation of $\pi_n(CR)$ requires integration with respect to the two independent beta-distributed random variables $\eta_E(CR)$ and $\eta_S(CR)$, and similarly for $\pi_n(TOX)$.

Software note: Designs of this type are implemented in public domain software `MultcLean` that is available from `http://biostatistics.mdanderson.org/SoftwareDownload/`. A basic implementation using R functions is shown in this chapter's online supplement.

The following algorithm explains in detail all the steps involved in the implementation of the approach described above. This algorithm pertains to a single-arm trial with all patients assigned to the experimental therapy. Thus the parameters θ_S never change; only the prior on θ_E is updated.

Algorithm 4.2 *(Phase II stopping for futility, efficacy, and toxicity).*

Step 0. Initialization: Initialize $\theta_E^0 = \theta_E$ (posterior parameters = prior parameters). Set $n = 0$ (number of patients), $n_1 = 0$ (number of patients with observed response), $t = 0$ (calendar time in months), $y_j^n = 0$, $j = 1, \ldots, 4$ (number of patients with event A_i), and $k = 4$ (cohort size). If using this algorithm as part of a simulation of operating characteristics, fix an assumed scenario (simulation truth) which we notate as $p_{Ej}^o \equiv Pr(A_j)$

Step 1. Posterior updating: Update the posterior parameters $\theta_{Ej}^n = \theta_{Ej} + y_j^n$.

Step 2. Posterior probabilities: Evaluate $\pi_n(CR)$ and $\pi_n(TOX)$ using Monte Carlo simulation as follows:

Step 2.1. Simulate probabilities under S: For $m = 1, \ldots, M$, simulate $\eta_S^m(CR) \sim \text{Be}(\theta_{S1} + \theta_{S3}, \theta_{S2} + \theta_{S4})$ and $\eta_S^m(TOX) \sim \text{Be}(\theta_{S1} + \theta_{S2}, \theta_{S3} + \theta_{S4})$.

Step 2.2. Estimate π_E: $\pi_E(CR) \approx \frac{1}{M} \sum Pr(\eta_E(CR) > \eta_S^m(CR) + \delta_{CR} \mid y^n)$ and $\pi_E(TOX) \approx \frac{1}{M} \sum Pr(\eta_E(TOX) > \eta_S^m(TOX) + \delta_{TOX} \mid y^n)$. The probabilities in the sums are probabilities under the Beta distributions given earlier.

Step 3. Stopping: If $\pi_E(CR) < L_n(CR)$, stop for lack of efficacy. If $\pi_E(TOX) > U_n(TOX)$, stop for excessive toxicity. If $\pi_n(CR) > U_n(CR)$ then stop for efficacy. If $n_1 > n_{\max}$, stop for maximum enrollment. Otherwise continue to Step 4.

Step 4. Next cohort: If $n < n_{\max}$ then recruit a new cohort, $i = n + 1, \ldots, n + k$, using $Pr(x_i = j) = p_{Ej}^o$ and recruitment time $t_{i0} = t$. Update $n \equiv n + k$, $t = t + 1$, y_i^n and $n_1 = \sum_{i=1}^n I(t \geq t_{0i} + 3)$. Repeat from Step 1.

∎

Example 4.3 *(A BMT trial).* We implement the algorithm for an example reported in Thall et al. (1995, Section 3.1). These authors considered a trial with patients who received bone marrow transplant (BMT) from partially matched donors. The study was a phase II trial of a post-transplant prophylaxis for graft versus host disease (GVHD). Patients were monitored for 100 days post transplant. If no GVHD occurs within 100 days, the treatment is considered successful. A major complication here is transplant rejection (TR). They implement Algorithm 4.2 using $CR = \{\text{no GVHD within 100 days}\}$, and $TOX = \{\text{TR within 100 days}\}$, again resulting in $K = 4$ elementary events. Let G and T indicate the events of observing GVHD and TR within 100 days and let $\bar{G}$ and $\bar{T}$ denote the complementary events. The elementary events are thus $\{\bar{G}\bar{T}, \bar{G}T, G\bar{T}, GT\}$. We use the Dirichlet prior from Thall et al. (1995), $p(p_{E1}, \ldots, p_{E4}) = Dir(\theta_{E1}, \ldots, \theta_{E4})$ with $\theta_E \propto (2.037, 6.111, 30.555, 2.037)$ and $\sum \theta_{Ej} = 4$. The other design parameters are $\delta_{CR} = 20\%$, $\delta_{TOX} = 5\%$, and $n_{\max} = 75$. The probability bounds are $L_{CR} = 2\%$ and $U_{TOX} = 80\%$ (both constant over n). No upper threshold U_{CR} is used, i.e., we do not consider early stopping for efficacy.

The simulation output is summarized in Figure 4.2. The figure shows efficacy and toxicity probabilities under the assumed simulation truth. The two horizontal lines show the lower bound L_{CR} (at 2%) and the upper bound U_{TOX} (at 80%). Crossing these bounds triggers the stopping decisions described in (4.4). At time $l = 0$ months we start with $\pi_n(TOX)$ and $\pi_n(CR)$ for $n = 0$ computed under the prior model. As new data is

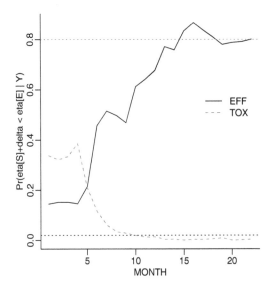

Figure 4.2 *Toxicity intervals: Posterior estimated probabilities of complete re-mission,* $E(\pi_n(CR) \mid data)$, *and toxicity,* $E(\pi_n(TOX) \mid data)$, *plotted against month; see (4.3).*

accrued, the posterior distributions are updated and the posterior means for $\eta_E(CR)$ and $\eta_E(TOX)$ quickly move down and up, respectively. Note the 100 day ($\approx$ 3 month) delay in the change of both posterior means. ∎

4.3.3 Monitoring event times

The stopping rules discussed in the previous section are based on a binary response variable. The nature of a response of this sort varies across studies. For example, a typical response might be an indicator for patient survival beyond seven months. Response variables based on a dichotomized contin-uous outcome involve a loss of information compared to the original data. Their main advantage is increased robustness; it is easy to be very general about a probability model for a binary outcome. By contrast, inference is often very sensitive with respect to the choice of a specific parametric form for the distribution of a continuous outcome. On the other hand, the likelihood function for the continuous outcome is more informative (i.e., more peaked) and allows more decisive inference with fewer observations. In other words, we achieve faster learning with the same number of pa-tients. Also, in some studies it is scientifically inappropriate to reduce the outcome to a dichotomized binary variable. Another limitation of binary outcomes is their inherent delays. For example, we might have to wait up

to 100 days after treatment to record a response when the binary outcome
is defined as transplant rejection within 100 days, as in Example 4.3.

Thall, Wooten, and Tannir (2005) propose study designs that allow early
stopping for futility and/or efficacy based on a time-to-event outcome. Assume that an event time T_i is recorded for each patient; say, time to disease
progression (TTP). We assume a parametric model for the sampling distribution; say, an exponential distribution. Let μ_S denote the mean event
time under the standard of care, and let μ_E denote the unknown mean
event time under the experimental therapy. Rather than reducing T_i to a
binary outcome (such as $TTP > 7$), Thall et al. (2005) replace the posterior probabilities π_n in (4.1) with corresponding probabilities on the μ
scale, e.g.

$$\pi_n = p(\mu_E > \mu_S + \delta \mid \mathbf{y}) .$$

On the basis of π_n they define stopping rules similar to (4.2); for example, stop for futility when $\pi_n < L_n$, stop for efficacy when $\pi_n > U_n$, and
continue enrollment otherwise. As before, the tuning parameters δ and
$\{(L_n, U_n),\ n = 1, 2, \ldots\}$ are fixed to achieve desired operating characteristics.

Software note: A public domain software implementation of this approach is
   available from
   http://biostatistics.mdanderson.org/SoftwareDownload/.

Thall et al. (2005) also discuss extensions to multiple event times, such as
time to disease progression, severe adverse event, and death.

4.4 Adaptive randomization and dose allocation

In this section we consider a randomized phase IIB multi-arm clinical trial.
The multiple arms could be different treatments (possibly including a control arm), different doses or schedules of the same agent, or any combination
of such comparisons. There are many good reasons to introduce randomization in the assignment of patients to the competing arms; see e.g. Subsection 2.2.6 for a discussion. But most of the arguments for randomization
do not require randomization with equal probabilities to all arms. *Adaptive dose allocation* is an attractive device to maintain the advantages of
randomization while introducing increased assignment of patients to more
promising treatments.

4.4.1 Principles of adaptive randomization

Adaptive dose allocation as we discuss it here still includes randomization.
It is distinct from deterministic adaptive dose assignment, such as play-the-
winner rules. Berry and Eick (1995) give a comparative discussion of play-
the-winner versus various randomization rules, including equal randomization, adaptive randomization, and a decision-theoretic solution. Here we

focus on outcome-adaptive designs, as opposed to covariate-adaptive designs that seek to balance covariates across treatments.

The idea of adaptive allocation goes back at least to Thompson (1933) and, more recently, to Louis (1975, 1977). A recent review appears in Thall and Wathen (2007), whose approach we discuss in more detail below because it emphasizes practical applicability and because an implementation in public domain software is available. Assume there are two arms, A_1 and A_2. Let $p_{1<2}$ denote the posterior probability that arm A_2 dominates arm A_1. For example, assume that the outcome is a binary efficacy response, and let θ_1 and θ_2 denote the probability of response under each treatment arm. Let $\mathbf{y}$ generically denote the currently available data. Then $p_{1<2} = p(\theta_1 < \theta_2 \mid \mathbf{y})$. Thall and Wathen (2007) propose to randomize to treatments A_1 and A_2 with probabilities proportional to $r_2(\mathbf{y}) = \{p_{1<2}(\mathbf{y})\}^c$ and $r_1(\mathbf{y}) = \{1 - p_{1<2}(\mathbf{y})\}^c$. In general, for more than two arms, use

$$r_j(\mathbf{y}) \propto \{p(\theta_j = \max_k \theta_k \mid \mathbf{y})\}^c. \tag{4.5}$$

Thall and Wathen (2007) propose using $c = n/2N$, where N is the maximum number of patients and n is the number of currently enrolled patients. This recommendation is based on empirical evidence under typical scenarios. Wathen and Cook (2006) summarize extensive simulations and give specific recommendations for the implementation of Bayesian adaptive randomization. Thall and Wathen (2005) apply the approach to a study where the probability model for an ordinal outcome includes a covariate. The outcome is trinary (response, stable, failure), while the covariates are two binary patient-specific baseline values. The definition of (4.5) remains unchanged; only the relevant probability model with respect to which the posterior probabilities are evaluated changes. Cheung et al. (2006) applies the method with r_j based on posterior probabilities of survival beyond day 50 under three competing treatment regimens.

Software note: The Adaptive Randomization (AR) package, a Windows application for designing and simulating outcome-adaptive randomized trials with up to 10 arms, is another of those freely available from the M.D. Anderson software website, biostatistics.mdanderson.org/SoftwareDownload. Outcomes may be either binary or time-to-event (TITE). Adaptively randomized trial designs are popular at M.D. Anderson and other institutions because such designs place more patients on the more effective treatments while also preserving the benefits of randomization. Between 2005 and 2009, there were 583 registered downloads of Adaptive Randomization.

We now describe the capabilities of the AR package in some detail, but only for the binary response case; the program's handling of the TITE case is somewhat restrictive at present, permitting only an exponential survival model with a conjugate inverse gamma prior. By contrast, the binary response cases assumes a beta prior for the probability of response

θ_k in Arm k, still conjugate but plenty general for most applications. AR seeks to unbalance the randomization probabilities using (4.5) to favor the treatment experiencing better interim results. The program comes with an easy-to-read user's guide, available online; here we summarize the main points.

In a binary response setting, our goal may be to find the k corresponding to the largest θ_k (if the endpoint is efficacy), or the smallest θ_k (if the endpoint is toxicity). In either case, we begin by specifying the $Beta(\alpha_k, \beta_k)$ prior distributions for the θ_k in one of three ways: either by choosing the (α_k, β_k) pairs directly, or indirectly by specifying either two quantiles for the distribution or the mean and the variance, since either permits AR to "back out" the (α_k, β_k). Then assuming independent binary responses in group k of which x_k are positive and $n_k - x_k$ are negative, the posterior for θ_k emerges immediately as the familiar $Beta(x_k + \alpha_k,\ n_k - x_k + \beta_k)$ distribution. This beta posterior is then used to define a variety of stopping rules, as follows.

Algorithm 4.3 *(Phase IIB AR design)*

Step 1. Early loser: If the probability that treatment arm k is the best falls below some prespecified probability p_L, i.e., if

$$P(\theta_k > \theta_{j \neq k} | Data) < p_L ,$$

then arm k is declared a loser and is suspended. Normally one takes p_L fairly small; say 0.10 or less. We note that the software does permit an arm to return to active status later in the trial if the other arms grow worse and arm k becomes competitive again.

Step 2. Early winner: If the probability that treatment arm k is the best exceeds some prespecified probability p_U, i.e., if

$$P(\theta_k > \theta_{j \neq k} | Data) > p_U ,$$

then arm k is declared the winner and the trial is stopped early. Normally one takes p_U fairly large; in a two-arm trial we would take $p_U = 1 - p_L$, or else only one among this rule and the previous rule would be active.

Step 3. Final winner: If, *after all patients have been evaluated*, the probability that treatment arm k is the best exceeds some prespecified probability p_U^*, i.e., if

$$P(\theta_k > \theta_{j \neq k} | Data) > p_U^* ,$$

then arm k is declared the winner. If however *no* treatment arm can meet this criterion, AR does not make a final selection. One typically sets $p_U^* < p_U$ (say, between 0.70 and 0.90) to increase the chance of obtaining a final winner.

Step 4. Futility: If the probability that treatment arm k is better than some prespecified minimally tolerable response rate θ_{min} falls below some prespecified probability p_L^*, i.e., if

$$P(\theta_k > \theta_{min}|Data) < p_L^* ,$$

then arm k is declared futile and will not accrue more patients. (This rule applies only when the goal is to find the largest θ_k, i.e., efficacy trials.) We take p_L^* quite small, typically 0.10 or less. Once an arm is declared futile, it cannot be re-activated.

∎

As each new patient enters the trial, the randomization probability for each arm is updated using (4.5) and the available outcome data from all currently enrolled patients. Thus for a trial with m arms, the probability of arm k being assigned next is

$$\frac{P(\theta_k = \max_j \theta_j|Data)^c}{\sum_{i=1}^{m} P(\theta_k = \max_j \theta_j|Data)^c} ,$$

where $c \geq 0$ (and clearly $c = 0$ corresponds to equal randomization). As mentioned above, we might take c to be some significant fraction of the maximum sample size. This is a rather conservative approach, allowing a substantial amount of information to be gained about both treatment arms before significant adapting occurs. The AR user manual recommends values of c near 1, and perhaps no bigger than 2, depending on accrual rates relative to observation time. That is, larger c may be appropriate for trials with slow relative accrual. The user can also specify a minimum randomization probability (say, 0.10), as well as an initial number of patients to randomize fairly, before adaptive randomization begins. Both of these are safeguards against excessively adapting away from a treatment arm. A minimum number of trial patients (say, 10) can also be specified.

The software then permits the establishment of various "scenarios" that describe certain true states of nature (e.g., a null case where the arms actually all have the same effectiveness). Data are then simulated from each scenario, with patients randomized according to the rules established. Repeating this process some large number of times (say, 100 for a quick investigation, and 1000 or 10,000 for final reporting), the design's operating characteristics (i.e., empirical probabilities of selection, early selection, early stopping, and the number of patients randomized for each arm) and average trial length can be evaluated. Various designs can then be compared across scenarios in terms of their performance. We illustrate the mechanics of doing this by means of the following example:

Example 4.4 *(Sensitizer trial).* We illustrate the use of the AR package with a University of Minnesota trial designed to assess the efficacy of a "sensitizer," intended to be given concurrently with a certain chemotherapeutic

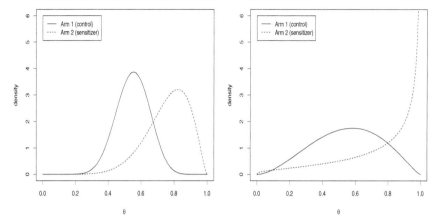

Figure 4.3 *Prior distributions for θ: left, standard priors; right, conservative priors. Both Arm 1 priors have mean 0.55 and both Arm 2 priors have mean 0.75; conservative priors have standard deviations equal to twice those of the standard priors.*

agent to enhance its effectiveness. A previous statistical consultant retained by the investigator had concluded that 49 patients would be required to implement a one-arm phase II investigation of the sensitizer's effectiveness as measured by complete remission (CR) at 28 days post-treatment using a Simon two-stage design. The investigator, however, would prefer to run a two-arm comparison of the drug-plus-sensitizer versus the drug alone, and fears the sample size required would likely be near 100, which is too large to be practical with her expected patient accrual rate (about 30 per year). She does have some prior information she is willing to use, and is hoping that using a Bayesian adaptive design will also save enough patients that she can reasonably expect success with, say, 60 total patients.

We use the AR software to design such a trial. Choosing the binary endpoint option (CR/no CR), we set the maximum patient accrual to 60, and the minimum randomization probability to 0.10, and specify that the first 14 patients should be randomized fairly (7 to each arm) before adaptive randomization begins. We then set the crucial tuning parameter $c = 1$; recall larger values of c correspond to potentially greater deviation from equal randomization (after the first 14 patients).

Turning to the prior distributions, the investigator wishes to specify response rates of .55 in the control arm and .75 in the sensitizer arm. Assuming standard deviations of 0.10 and 0.13 in the two arms, respectively, determines the two beta distributions shown in the left panel of Figure 4.3. The right panel of this figure shows two "conservative" versions of these

Scenario 1
Average Trial Length: 22.5 months

Arm	True Pr (success)	Pr (select)	Pr(select early)	Pr(stop early)	# Patients (2.5%, 97.5%)
Arm1	0.55	0.01	0	0.11	19.6 (5, 38)
Arm2	0.55	0.16	0.11	0	35.6 (8, 53)

Scenario 2
Average Trial Length: 16.4 months

Arm	True Pr (success)	Pr (select)	Pr(select early)	Pr(stop early)	# Patients (2.5%, 97.5%)
Arm1	0.55	0	0	0.55	10.1 (4, 22)
Arm2	0.7	0.74	0.55	0	30.8 (4, 51)

Scenario 3
Average Trial Length: 10.8 months

Arm	True Pr (success)	Pr (select)	Pr(select early)	Pr(stop early)	# Patients (2.5%, 97.5%)
Arm1	0.55	0	0	0.89	7.01 (4, 16)
Arm2	0.8	0.96	0.89	0	20.1 (4, 51)

Table 4.3 *Operating characteristics, sensitizer trial design using the standard prior and standard stopping rule.*

two priors, obtained simply by doubling their standard deviations (to 0.20 and 0.26, respectively).

For our stopping rules, we begin with a "standard" rule that sets the early loser selection probability $p_L = 0.025$, the early winner selection probability $p_U = 0.975$, the final winner selection probability $p_U^* = 0.90$, and the futility parameters $\theta_{min} = 0.50$ and $p_L^* = 0.05$. We also consider a more "liberal" stopping rule that instead uses $p_L = 0.05$ and $p_U = 0.95$, making early losing and winning somewhat easier to achieve. We then run AR, comparing results from three different scenarios:

- Scenario 1: true response rates of .55 in both groups (the "null" scenario),
- Scenario 2: true response rates of .55 control, .70 sensitizer (the "most likely" scenario), and
- Scenario 3: true response rates of .55 control, .80 sensitizer (the "optimistic" scenario).

Tables 4.3–4.5 give the simulated operating characteristics for three dif-

Scenario 1
Average Trial Length: 21.0 months

Arm	True Pr (success)	Pr (select)	Pr(select early)	Pr(stop early)	# Patients (2.5%, 97.5%)
Arm1	0.55	0.19	0.05	0.15	26.2 (5, 45)
Arm2	0.55	0.16	0.13	0.09	25.4 (4, 47)

Scenario 2
Average Trial Length: 18.1 months

Arm	True Pr (success)	Pr (select)	Pr(select early)	Pr(stop early)	# Patients (2.5%, 97.5%)
Arm1	0.55	0.04	0.02	0.39	15.2 (4, 44)
Arm2	0.7	0.52	0.39	0.02	29.4 (4, 49)

Scenario 3
Average Trial Length: 14.3 months

Arm	True Pr (success)	Pr (select)	Pr(select early)	Pr(stop early)	# Patients (2.5%, 97.5%)
Arm1	0.55	0	0	0.63	10.6 (2, 26)
Arm2	0.8	0.8	0.63	0	25.6 (3, 50)

Table 4.4 *Operating characteristics, sensitizer trial design using the conservative prior and standard stopping rule.*

ferent designs. All of our results are based on just 100 simulated trials each — probably too small to be considered reliable for practical use, but large enough for us to illustrate the differences across designs and scenarios. First, Table 4.3 shows the results from the design using the standard prior and standard stopping rule. This design has pretty good Type I error (17% total selection probability in the "null" scenario), good power (74%) in the "most likely" scenario, and outstanding power (96%) in the "optimistic" scenario. But the total sample sizes are fairly high (10.1 + 30.8 ≈ 41 in the most likely scenario), and the average trial lengths are fairly long (16.4 months in the most likely scenario, under our assumed accrual rate of 2.5 patients per month, or 30 per year).

By contrast, Table 4.4 shows the results from the design using the conservative prior with the standard stopping rule. As expected, this design is more conservative, borrowing far less strength from the investigator's clinical opinion and thus forcing the data to largely stand on their own. As

Scenario 1
Average Trial Length: 18.2 months

Arm	True Pr (success)	Pr (select)	Pr(select early)	Pr(stop early)	# Patients (2.5%, 97.5%)
Arm1	0.55	0	0	0.33	18.1 (2, 39)
Arm2	0.55	0.37	0.33	0	26.4 (3, 49)

Scenario 2
Average Trial Length: 11.3 months

Arm	True Pr (success)	Pr (select)	Pr(select early)	Pr(stop early)	# Patients (2.5%, 97.5%)
Arm1	0.55	0	0	0.73	9.56 (2, 26)
Arm2	0.7	0.82	0.73	0	19.1 (2, 48)

Scenario 3
Average Trial Length: 8.15 months

Arm	True Pr (success)	Pr (select)	Pr(select early)	Pr(stop early)	# Patients (2.5%, 97.5%)
Arm1	0.55	0	0	0.92	7.2 (1, 27)
Arm2	0.8	0.93	0.92	0	13.5 (2, 46)

Table 4.5 *Operating characteristics, sensitizer trial design using the standard prior and liberal stopping rule.*

a result, Type I errors are a bit higher, and power a bit lower. Still, the investigator might adopt this design since thanks to adaptivity it continues to save patient resources: it uses just 36 on average in the optimistic case, and 44 in the most likely case (recall the Simon two-stage design required 49 patients in the *one-arm* case).

Finally, Table 4.5 shows the results from the design that returns to the standard prior, but now couples it with the more liberal stopping rule. Again as expected, this design has somewhat higher Type I error (37%, all of it due to incorrect selections of the sensitizer arm) than the baseline design in Table 4.3. But this design also finishes much more quickly, taking just 11.3 months and using only 29 patients on average (instead of 16.4 and 41 for the baseline design) in the most likely scenario.

In summary, all three designs have strengths and weaknesses. And this analysis was certainly not intended to be exhaustive: the investigator (or her statistician) would likely wish to consider even more designs. For example, if we sought to reduce Type I error, we might consider a more conservative stopping rule that sets $p_L = 0.01$ and $p_U = 0.99$. ∎

4.4.2 Dose ranging and optimal biologic dosing

Dose ranging studies are phase II trials that seek to find the dose with highest efficacy within a range of safe doses. Many traditional designs assume that the probability of toxicity increases monotonically with dose. However, the increased use of molecularly targeted therapies requires alternative statistical approaches that target an optimal biological dose (OBD) *without* assuming a monotone dose-response relationship. The OBD is the dose with maximum therapeutic effect.

One of the few such approaches is that of Bekele and Shen (2005), who define dose-finding based on *jointly* modeling toxicity and biomarker response. The marginal model for toxicity is a probit model with monotone dose-specific means, while the marginal model for biomarker response is a dynamic *state space model* (defined below). The two marginal models are linked by introducing correlation of dose-specific parameters for toxicity and biomarker response.

Similar state space models for flexible dose-response curves are also used in Müller et al. (2006) and in Smith et al. (2006). Let $f(d)$ denote the mean response at dose d. Before we describe details of the model, we outline some important features. Let D_j, $j = 1, \ldots, J$, denote the range of allowable doses, and $\theta_j \equiv f(D_j)$ the vector of mean responses at the allowable doses. The underlying idea is to formalize a model which locally (i.e., for d close to D_j) fits a straight line for the response y,

$$y = \theta_j + (d - D_j)\delta_j ,$$

having level θ_j and slope δ_j. When moving from dose D_{j-1} to D_j, the parameters $\alpha_j = (\theta_j, \delta_j)$ change by adjusting the level to $\theta_j = \theta_{j-1} + \delta_{j-1}$ adding a (small) so-called *evolution noise* e_j.

Let Y_{jk}, $k = 1, \ldots, \nu_j$, denote the k-th response observed at dose D_j, i.e., $\mathbf{Y}_j = \{Y_{jk}, \ k = 1, \ldots, \nu_j\}$ is the vector of responses y_i of all patients with assigned dose $d_i = D_j$. Note the notational convention of using upper case symbols for quantities D_j and Y_{jk} indexed by doses, and lower case y_i and d_i for quantities indexed by patients. Also, we will use $\mathbf{Y}^{(j)} = (\mathbf{Y}_1, \ldots, \mathbf{Y}_j)'$ for all responses up to and including dose D_j, and $\mathbf{y}^{(n)} = (y_1, \ldots, y_n)'$ for all data up to and including the n-th patient. The resulting model is

$$Y_{jk} = \theta_j + \epsilon_{jk}, \quad j = 1, \ldots, n, \ k = 1, \ldots, \nu_j$$

and

$$(\theta_j, \, \delta_j) = (\theta_{j-1} + \delta_{j-1}, \, \delta_{j-1}) + e_j , \tag{4.6}$$

with independent errors $\epsilon_j \sim N(0, V\sigma^2)$ and $e_j \sim N_2(w, W\sigma^2)$. The first equation describes the distribution of Y_{jk} conditional on the state parameters $\alpha_j = (\theta_j, \delta_j)$ and is referred to as the *observation* equation; the second equation formalizes the change of α_j between doses and is referred to as the *evolution* (or *state*) equation. For a given specification of (V, W) and priors $p(\alpha_0) = N(m_0, C_0)$ and $p(\sigma^{-2}) = Gamma(v_0/2, S_0/2)$ with given moments m_0, C_0 and S_0, and degrees of freedom v_0, there exists a straightforward recursive algorithm to compute posterior distributions $p(\alpha_j | Y_1, \ldots, Y_j)$ and any other desired posterior inference. The algorithm, known as *Forward Filtering Backward Sampling* (FFBS), is described in Frühwirth-Schnatter (1994).

Software note: Smith et al. (2006) and Smith and Richardson (2007) include WinBUGS code to implement the FFBS for a normal dynamic linear model. We outline an FFBS algorithm for our setting below, with an R implementation again given in this chapter's software page,

$$\text{www.biostat.umn.edu/~brad/software/BCLM\_ch4.html}$$

The approach from Müller et al. (2006) is described by the following algorithm, which implements the simulation of one possible trial history under an assumed scenario $\theta^o = (\theta_1^o, \ldots, \theta_J^o)$. In addition to the model for the unknown mean response curve, implementation of trial simulation requires the specification of a dose allocation rule and stopping rules.

Dose allocation: Let $D^\star = D^\star(\theta)$ denote the (unknown) ED95 dose defined by $\theta_{j^\star} = \min \theta_j + 0.95(\max \theta_j - \min \theta_j)$. Usually equality cannot be achieved; the ED95 is then defined as the dose with mean response closest to the target. Let $\mathbf{r} = (r_1, \ldots, r_J)$ denote the probability of allocating the next patient to dose j, $j = 1, \ldots, J$. We use $r_j \propto \sqrt{Pr(D^\star = j \mid \mathbf{y}^{(n)})}$, subject to $r_1 \geq 10\%$ allocation to placebo. The allocation probability r_j is a variation of the adaptive allocation rule (4.5) discussed in Subsection 4.4.1.

Sequential stopping: Let Δ denote the smallest mean response that would be considered a success. We follow the example from Krams et al. (2005) who apply the proposed design to a stroke trial. The outcome is an improvement in stroke score, with an improvement of at least 3 points being considered a success. Let $s_j = Pr(\theta_j > 3 \mid \mathbf{y}^{(n)})$. Following Krams et al. (2005) we define the following stopping rules: (i) Stop for futility when $\max_j s_j < 0.05$, and (ii) stop for efficacy when $s_{\hat{D}^\star} > 0.95$, where $\hat{D}^\star$ is the currently estimated ED95.

Algorithm 4.4 *(Optimal Biologic Dose).*

Step 0. Initialization: Use $r_j = 1/J$. Initialize sample size $n = 0$, and maximum sample size $n_{\max}$ (say, to 100).

Step 1. Next patient cohort: Select doses d_i, $i = n+1, \ldots, n+k$ using the current allocation probabilities r_j. Generate (simulated) responses $y_i \sim N(\theta_j^o, \sigma^2)$. Increment $n \equiv n + k$.

Step 2. Posterior updating: Use FFBS (see Algorithm 4.5) to summarize $p(\theta \mid \mathbf{y}^{(n)})$. Record $s_j = Pr(\theta_j > 3 \mid \mathbf{y}^{(n)})$ and $\hat{D}^\star = D_{j^\star}$ where $j^\star = \arg\max_j \{Pr(D_j = D^\star \mid \mathbf{y}^{(n)})\}$.

Step 3. Stopping: If $\max_j s_j < 0.05$ stop for futility. If $s_{\hat{D}^\star} > 0.95$ stop for efficacy and report $\hat{D}^\star$ as the recommended dose. If $n > n_{\max}$ stop for maximum sample size. Otherwise continue with step 1. Note that the stopping criterion includes stopping for both efficacy and futility.

∎

Step 2 requires an implementation of the FFBS algorithm. This chapter's software page,

www.biostat.umn.edu/~brad/software/BCLM_ch4.html

includes R macros for a basic FFBS implementation. The algorithm is exact, and consists of two finite iterations. In the first loop we evaluate $p(\alpha_j \mid \mathbf{Y}^{(j)})$, $j = 1, \ldots, J$. In the second loop we evaluate $p(\alpha_j \mid \alpha_{j+1,\ldots,J}, \mathbf{Y}^{(J)})$ and $\bar{\mu}_j \equiv E(\theta_j \mid \mathbf{Y}^{(J)})$, $j = 1, \ldots, J$. All distributions are normal, and fully characterized by the first two moments. In the following description $p(\alpha_j \mid \mathbf{Y}^{(j-1)}) = N(r_j, R_j)$, $p(\alpha_j \mid \mathbf{Y}^{(j)}) = N(m_j, C_j)$ and $p(\alpha_j \mid \alpha_{j+1}, \mathbf{Y}^{(J)}) = N(\mu_j(\alpha_{j+1}), \Sigma_j)$ define three sequences of posterior distributions. The three sets of posteriors condition upon the data up to the $(j-1)$st dose, up to the jth dose, and on all data (and α_{j+1}), respectively. A prior $p(\alpha_0) = N(m_0, C_0)$ defines a starting condition for the following iteration.

Algorithm 4.5 *(FFBS)*.

Step 0. Initialize: We formalize prior information by including additional fake observations $y_j^o \sim N(\theta_j, \sigma^2/n_j^o)$. Using fractional values for n_j^o allows us to specify arbitrarily accurate prior equivalent sample sizes.

Step 1. Forward filtering: For $j = 1, \ldots, J$ carry out the following update. Let

$$y_j = \frac{\nu_j \sum_k Y_{jk} + n_j^o y_j^o}{\nu_j + n_j^o}$$

and $n_j = \nu_j + n_j^o$ denote the sample mean and sample size of all observations (including the prior equivalent data) at dose j. Update the posterior moments as $R_j = GC_{j-1}G' + \tau I$, $r_j = Gm_{j-1}$ and $C_j^{-1} = R_j^{-1} + Z'Zn_j/\sigma^2$, $m_j = C_j(R_j^{-1}r_j + n_j/\sigma^2 Z'y_j)$.

Step 2. Backward smoothing: Set $\Sigma_J = C_J$ and $\mu_J = m_J$. For $j = J-1, \ldots, 1$, evaluate $\Sigma_j^{-1} = C_j^{-1} + GG'/\tau^2$ and $\mu_j = \Sigma_j\left(C_j^{-1}m_j + G'\mu_{j+1}\right)$.

Step 3. Posterior simulation: For the evaluation of the posterior distribution of the unknown ED95, $D^\star$ it is useful to include (exact) posterior simulation. We generate a set of M posterior draws $\theta^m \sim p(\theta_1, \ldots, \theta_J \mid D_J)$, $m = 1, \ldots, M$. To do this, we start with the highest dose and work our way down. That is, start with $\theta_J^m \sim N(\mu_J, \Sigma_J)$, and then for

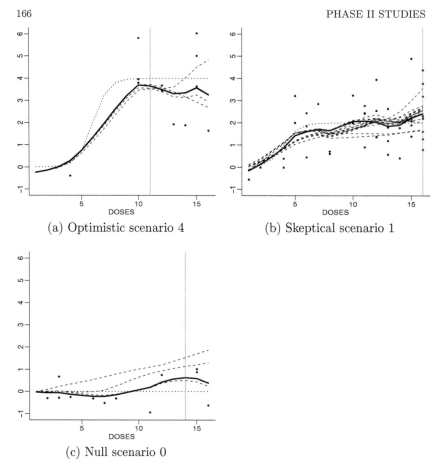

(a) Optimistic scenario 4   (b) Skeptical scenario 1

(c) Null scenario 0

Figure 4.4 *The three plots summarize the simulation of one possible trial history under three alternative curves as simulation truth (dotted curves in panels a, b, and c). The figures show the posterior estimated curves after each cohort (thin dashed) and after stopping (thick solid), the data (dots), and the estimated ED95 at the end of the trial (vertical line).*

$j = J - 1, \ldots, 1$, evaluate $\mu_j^m = \Sigma_j (C_j^{-1} m_j + 1/\tau^2 G' \theta_{j+1}^m)$ and generate $\theta_j^m \sim N(\mu_j^m, \Sigma_j)$.

■

Example 4.5 *(Stroke trial).* We implemented Algorithm 4.5 for the stroke study in Berry et al. (2001), where again the response y_i is improvement in stroke score over a 90-day period. We assume a range of $J = 16$ possible doses, $j = 1, \ldots, J$, including placebo as $D_1 = 0$. The maximum number of patients was set to $n_{\max} = 100$. We use three alternative scenarios of assumed true response profiles as simulation truth. The scenarios presented here correspond to an optimistic assumption of a significant treatment effect at higher doses (scenario 4), a skeptical scenario with a moderate treatment effect only (scenario 1) and a null scenario assuming no treatment effect (scenario 0). The three scenarios are shown in Figure 4.4. The figure shows the simulated responses under one simulated realization of the entire trial. The data are shown as dots. Also shown are the posterior mean response curve $E(\theta_1, \ldots, \theta_J \mid \mathbf{y}^{(n)})$ (thick line), the simulation truth (dotted line), and random draws from $p(\theta_1, \ldots, \theta_J \mid \mathbf{y}^{(n)})$ (dashed lines). The latter illustrate posterior uncertainty.

Under all three scenarios the sequential stopping rule leads to early termination. Under scenario 4, the simulation stopped early for efficacy after $n = 12$ patients. Under scenarios 1 and 0, the simulation stopped early for futility after $n = 46$ and after $n = 12$ patients, respectively. ∎

4.4.3 Adaptive randomization in dose finding

The adaptive randomization ideas of Subsection 4.4.1 can be applied much more broadly than just adaptively randomizing to two treatments. Blending in the ideas of the previous subsection, an adaptive randomization can also be to one of K competing *dose levels*, bringing us into the area of *adaptive dose allocation*. Here we offer a simple example based on an setting already seen in Chapter 3.

Example 4.6 *(Stroke trial revisited)*. The stroke trial of Example 4.5 included adaptive dose allocation. A variation of the allocation probabilities (4.5) was used. We defined

$$r_j(\mathbf{y}) \propto \sqrt{Pr(D^\star = D_j \mid \mathbf{y})} \, .$$

Recall that $D^\star$ denoted the (unknown) ED95 dose. Under the model used in Example 4.5, the posterior distribution of $D^\star$ is only available via simulation. The underlying model is not critical. For example, under an alternative implementation with, say, a shifted and scaled logistic dose/response curve, the posterior probabilities for $D^\star$ would also be easily available by posterior simulation. In either case, for each dose D_j one would evaluate the posterior probability $Pr(D^\star = D_j \mid \mathbf{y})$. Using the allocation probabilities r_j, we favor allocation of the next patient cohort at doses that are likely to be the desired ED95 dose. The adaptive allocation rule $r_j(\mathbf{y})$ formalizes Step 2 in Algorithm 4.4.

For the implementation described in Example 4.5, Figure 4.5 shows the sequence of dose allocations over time for one realization of the trial. Notice how the allocation probabilities differ under the three considered scenarios. Recall that the three scenarios were an optimistic scenario assuming a maximum benefit over placebo of up to 4 points (Scenario 4), a sceptic scenario with only a moderate 2-point advantage over placebo (Scenario

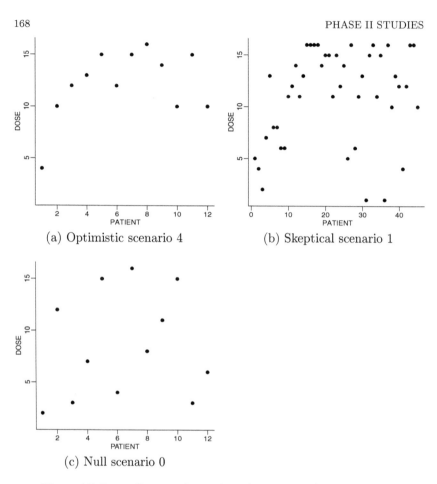

(a) Optimistic scenario 4   (b) Skeptical scenario 1

(c) Null scenario 0

Figure 4.5 *Dose allocation (vertical axis) by patient (horizontal axis).*

1) and a null scenario with a horizontal line at 0 points advantage over placebo (Scenario 0). The algorithm correctly zooms in on the range of interesting doses. For a practical implementation of adaptive dose allocation it is important that the adaptation not be too greedy. In this example this is achieved by enforcing a minimum allocation probability at placebo, and by using a square root transformation. ∎

4.4.4 Outcome adaptive randomization with delayed survival response

Many clinical studies involve responses that are observed with a substantial delay between assignment of a treatment and the recording of the outcome. A typical example is tumor response in phase II trials, as in Example 4.2. For solid tumors, response might be defined in terms of tumor size after a fixed number of days. Another example is the phase II trial discussed in Example 4.3. There the outcome was defined as occurrence of graft versus host disease (GVHD) within 100 days. In either case the investigator would have to wait for the response of the currently recruited patients before being able to make a decision about sequential stopping or treatment allocation for the next patient.

The Bayesian paradigm provides a principled approach to address such complications. If a decision is desired before all responses from the previous patient (or patient cohort) are available, the investigator can proceed on the basis of the partial information. Inference is based on the posterior distribution conditional on all data available at the time of making the decision. Subsection 4.3.3 discussed a trial design based on event times, while the TITE-CRM design discussed in Subsection 3.2.3 used partial information for a binary tumor response. The TITE-CRM assumed that the response is an indicator for an event time occuring within a specified period.

Some designs go a step further by introducing available early responses. Let S denote an early response (for example, complete response based on tumor size) and let T denote the desired final response (for example progression-free survival, PFS). Modeling the joint distribution of S and T, we can use available data on S to update posterior inference on parameters related to T. This allows the construction of more efficient clinical trial designs.

Recall that in Example 4.5 we discussed a stroke trial. The outcome here was improvement by day 90 in stroke score over baseline. However, in stroke patients most of the improvement occurs over the first few weeks, making it particularly attractive to use early responses to improve the trial design. Let T denote the final day 90 response and let S_t denote the improvement by week t, $t = 1, \ldots, 12$. In the implementation of this trial, Berry et al. (2001) used a joint probability model for T and $(S_1, \ldots, S_{12})$ to address some of the challenges related to the delayed 90-day response.

Another good example of this strategy is the design proposed in Huang et al. (2009). These authors propose a study design that uses progression-free survival (henceforth simply "survival") for adaptive treatment allocation. They consider a phase IIb trial with two treatment arms, A and B. They argue that one of the reasons for the high failure rate of phase III therapeutic trials is the use of tumor shrinkage, rather than the ultimately important survival outcome, as a primary endpoint in phase IIb trials. The main reason why investigators nevertheless continue to use tumor shrinkage are the practical complications arising from the substantial lag between treatment assignment and reporting of a delayed survival response.

Huang et al. (2009) propose a design that combines the relative advantages of both the easily observed tumor response and the ultimately relevant survival endpoint. The key feature of the design is a joint probability model for tumor response (S) and survival (T). Let $x_i \in \{A, B\}$ denote the treatment assignment for the i-th patient, and let (S_i, T_i, δ_i) denote the outcome for the i-th patient, with S_i denoting tumor response (i.e., tumor shrinkage), T_i denoting the survival time, and $\delta_i \in \{0, 1\}$ a binary indicator with $\delta_i = 1$ when T_i is observed and $\delta_i = 0$ when only a censored time $t_i \leq T_i$ is recorded. In other words, at calendar time t the recorded response for a patient who was recruited at (calendar) time t_i^0 is $t_i = \min(T_i, t - t_i^0)$, with δ_i indicating whether t_i is an observed survival time. The authors assume that tumor response is reported as a categorical outcome with 4 possibilities, $S_i \in \{1, 2, 3, 4\}$, referring to resistance to treatment or death $(S_i = 1)$, stable disease $(S_i = 2)$, partial remission $(S_i = 3)$, and complete remission (CR; $S_i = 4$). The joint probability model for (S_i, T_i) is

$$P(S_i = j \mid x_i = x) = p_{xj} \text{ and } P(T_i \mid S_i = j, x_i = x) = \text{Exp}(\lambda_{xj}), \quad (4.7)$$

where $\text{Exp}(\lambda)$ indicates an exponential distribution with mean $\mu = 1/\lambda$. The model is completed with a prior

$$(p_{x1}, \dots, p_{x4}) \sim \text{Dir}(\gamma_{x1}, \dots, \gamma_{x4}), \text{ and } \mu_{xj} \equiv \frac{1}{\lambda_{xj}} \sim IG(\alpha_{xj}, \beta_{xj}) \quad (4.8)$$

independently for $x \in \{A, B\}$. Here $\text{Dir}(a_1, \dots, a_4)$ denotes a Dirichlet distribution with parameters $(a_1, \dots, a_4)$ and $IG(a, b)$ is an inverse gamma distribution with mean $b/(a - 1)$. The model is chosen to allow closed-form posterior inference. Let $n_{xj} = \sum_{i=1}^{n} I(S_i = j \text{ and } x_i = x)$ denote the number of patients with response j under treatment x, let t denote the current calendar time, let $\gamma'_{xj} = \gamma_{xj} + n_{xj}$, and let

$$\alpha'_{xj} = \alpha_{xj} + \sum_{i:\, S_i = j,\, x_i = x} \delta_i \text{ and } \beta'_{xj} = \beta_{xj} + \sum_{i:\, S_i = j,\, x_i = x} t_i \quad (4.9)$$

with $t_i = \min\{T_i, t - t_i^0\}$ denoting the observed survival time T_i if $\delta_i = 1$, and the censoring time $t - t_i^0$ if $\delta_i = 0$. Letting Y generically denote the observed data, we have

$$p(p_{x1}, \dots, p_{x4} \mid Y) = \text{Dir}(\gamma'_{x1}, \dots, \gamma'_{x4}) \text{ and } p(\mu_{xj} \mid Y) = IG(\alpha'_{xj}, \beta'_{xj}).$$
$$(4.10)$$

Huang et al. (2009) propose a trial design that includes continuous updating of the posterior distributions (4.10), adaptive allocation based on current posterior inference and early stopping for futility and for superiority. For adaptive allocation they consider the posterior probability

$$p = P(\mu_A > \mu_B \mid Y),$$

with $\mu_x = \sum p_{xj}\mu_{xj}$ for $x \in \{A, B\}$ indicating the mean PFS on treatment arm x. By allocating patients to arm A with probability p, the design increases the probability that patients receive the best treatment. The same posterior probability is used to define early stopping for futility when $p <$

p_L and for superiority when $p > p_U$, using, for example, $p_L = 0.025$ and $p_U = 1 - p_L$. The proposed design is summarized in the following algorithm.

Algorithm 4.6 *(Adaptive allocation with survival response).*

Step 0. Initialization: Initialize sample size and calendar time $n = 0$ and $t = 0$. Initialize $p = 0.5$.

Step 1. Next cohort: Recruit the next cohort of patients, $i = n+1, \ldots, n+ k$, and then:

- Allocate treatments A and B with probabilities p and $q = 1 - p$, respectively, by generating x_i with $P(x_i = A) = p$ and $P(x_i = B) = q$.
- Increment calendar time by one week, $t = t + 1$.
- Simulate tumor responses, $S_{i,k}$, $k = 1, \ldots, 4$ for the newly recruited patients.
- Generate simulation truth for the (future) progression free survival times T_i for the newly recruited patients, and record recruitment time (calendar time), $t_i^0 = t$.
- Increment $n \equiv n + k$.

Step 2. Posterior updating: Update the posterior parameters $\alpha'_{xj}, \beta'_{xj}$ and γ'_{xj} defined in (4.9). Compute and record $p = P(\theta_A > \theta_B \mid Y)$, with $\theta_x = \sum_j p_{xj} \mu_{xj}$, $x \in \{A, B\}$.

Step 3. Stopping: If $p < p_L$ then stop for futility. If $p > p_U$ stop for efficacy.

If $t > t_{max}$ stop for having reached the maximum horizon.

Otherwise continue with step 1.

∎

Note that this algorithm describes the simulation of one trial realization. For the evaluation of operating characteristics, we would use repeated simulation under an assumed simulation truth, generating the tumor responses from (4.7). By contrast, for use in an actual implementation of the trial design, to evaluate the stopping criterion and the treatment allocation for the respective next patient, we would start with Step 2 and use the actual data in place of any simulated responses.

Software note: A basic R implementation of this algorithm is included in the online supplement to this chapter,

www.biostat.umn.edu/~brad/software/BCLM_ch4.html .

The R code carries out simulation of one hypothetical realization of a trial following the proposed algorithm. The code includes a loop over patient cohorts. Within the loop we carry out posterior updating before recruiting the respective next cohort. One of the posterior summaries is the probability of superiority for treatment arm A, $p = P(\mu_A > \mu_B \mid y)$. We use

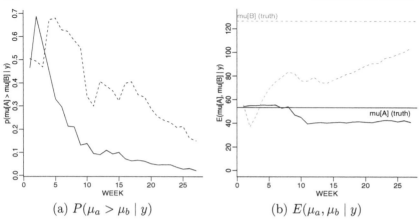

(a) $P(\mu_a > \mu_b \mid y)$ (b) $E(\mu_a, \mu_b \mid y)$

Figure 4.6 *Adaptive leukemia trial with survival response. Posterior probability of superiority by week (a) and posterior mean survival time by week (b). In panel (a) the solid line shows the $P(\mu_a > \mu_b \mid y)$ under the proposed model (4.7) and (4.8). The dashed line shows the same probability under a corresponding model without regression on early responses.*

independent Monte Carlo simulation to numerically evaluate p and use p to carry out the stopping decision.

Example 4.7 *(Adaptive leukemia trial with survival response).* Huang et al. (2009) discuss an application of the proposed design to a phase II trial for acute myelogenous leukemia. One of their scenarios (Scenario 3 in the paper) assumes a simulation truth with higher response rates and longer response durations (i.e., PFS) under treatment B. The simulation truth is model (4.7) with $p_A = (0.2, 0.4, 0.1, 0.3)$, $p_B = (0.1, 0.1, 0.2, 0.6)$, $\mu_A = (4, 30, 75, 110)$ and $\mu_B = (6, 45, 112, 165)$. The implied true marginal mean PFS is 53 weeks under treatment A and 126 weeks under treatment B.

We implemented Algorithm 4.6 for this application. We assumed a maximum number of $n = 120$ patients, accruing one patient per week. After enrolling the last patient we allow the trial to continue for up to 40 weeks, recording survival times for the already enrolled patients. However, under the stopping rule in Algorithm 4.6 the protocol almost always stops early. Huang et al. (2009) report an average number of $n = 62$ patients. Figure 4.6 summarizes one simulated trial realization. The solid curve in panel (a) plots the posterior probability $p = P(\mu_A > \mu_B \mid y)$ as a function of the sample size. When p crosses the threshold $p < p_L = 0.025$, the trial stops for futility around $t = 27$ weeks.

For comparison we also evaluated posterior inference under an alternative probability model without regression on early responses S_i. The alternative model assumes $P(T_i \mid S_i = j) = \text{Exp}(\lambda_x)$ with a conjugate inverse gamma prior $\mu_x \sim IG(\alpha_x, \beta_x)$ for $\mu_x = 1/\lambda_x$. Huang et al. (2009) refer to the alternative model as the "common model." We fix the prior with $\alpha_x = 2$ and $\beta_x = 60$, $x \in \{A, B\}$. The dashed curve in Figure 4.6(a) shows the sequence of posterior probabilities $p = P(\mu_A > \mu_B \mid y)$ under the common model. Eventually the probabilities under the two models converge. However, notice the substantial differences around Week 15. The posterior probabilities p (correctly) decrease more steeply when we include regression on early responses. ∎

4.5 Hierarchical models for phase II designs

Hierarchical models are one of the big successes stories of Bayesian biostatistics. Hierarchical models are used to formalize borrowing strength across related subpopulations; for example, different trials of the same treatment in slightly different populations, or different treatments of the same disease. An important feature is that this sharing of information is done in a coherent fashion. The use of an underlying encompassing probability model across related submodels ensures coherent behavior. In Section 2.4 we reviewed the basic setup of hierarchical models and showed an example from the realm of metaanalysis, including WinBUGS and BRugs code. In this section we elaborate on the use of hierarchical models in phase II clinical trial design.

Thall et al. (2003) develop a phase II design for related trials. Their motivating application is a phase II trial for 12 different sarcomas. On the one hand it would be inappropriate to pool all patients across the 12 disease subtypes. On the other hand, one would certainly want to use information from other subtypes when making a judgment about any of the subpopulations. A practical limitation is the very slow accrual. Only very small sample sizes (6 or fewer) are expected for some subtypes, making it impossible to run separate trials. Besides practical concerns, there are important ethical considerations that require investigators to pool across closely related subpopulations.

Let $j = 1, \ldots, J$ index J related subpopulations (for example, the $J = 12$ sarcomas). Let y_j generically denote the data for the j-th subpopulation. Within each subpopulation we assume a submodel $P(y_j \mid \theta_j)$. The submodels are combined into a joint encompassing hierarchical model by assuming $\theta_j \sim P(\theta_j \mid \phi)$. The following algorithm outlines the specific steps of a phase II trial across subpopulations. Let n_j denote the number of patients enrolled in population j. We assume that the submodel in population j is binomial sampling, $y_j \sim \text{Bin}(n_j, \pi_j)$. The binomial success probabilities are transformed to $\theta_j = \log(\pi_j/(1 - \pi_j))$ and given a common hyperprior with moments $\boldsymbol{\eta} = (\mu, \Sigma)$. In summary,

$$y_j \mid \theta_j \sim \text{Bin}(n_j, \pi_j(\theta_j)) \text{ and } \theta_j \sim N(\mu, \Sigma) . \tag{4.11}$$

The model is completed with a hyperprior on $\boldsymbol{\eta} = (\mu, \Sigma)$. We assume $\Sigma = \tau I$, where

$$\mu \sim N(m_\mu, s_\mu) \text{ and } \tau \sim Gamma(a_0, b_0) .$$

The following algorithm outlines the simulation of a hypothetical trial using the design proposed in Thall et al. (2003). Let $\mathbf{y}^{(t)}$ denote all data up to and including month t. Thall et al. (2003) propose a design that involves continuous updating of

$$p_{30,j} = P(\pi_j > 30\% \mid \mathbf{y}^{(t)}).$$

Accrual for subpopulation j is stopped if $p_{30,j} < 0.05$ at any time. We assume known accrual rates. Let k_j denote the number of recruited patients in subpopulation j in a given month. We assume $P(k_j = k) = a_{jk}$ is known, with an upper bound $k_j \leq K$. We assume a simulation truth π_j^o.

Algorithm 4.7 *(Phase II design for related subpopulations).*

Step 0. Initialize: Initialize $n_j = 0$, $j = 1, \ldots, J$, $t = 0$, and the prior moments (m_0, s_0).

Step 1. Simulate patient cohort: Generate a random cohort size k_j, where $P(k_j = k) = a_{jk}$, $j = 1, \ldots, J$, $k = 0, \ldots, K$. Simulate responses $x_j \sim \text{Bin}(k_j, \pi_j^o)$, update $n_j \equiv n_j + k_j$, and augment y_j with the new responses x_j to $y_j \equiv y_j + x_j$. Increment $t = t + 1$.

Step 2. Update posterior inference: Evaluate posterior probabilities $p_{30,j} = P(\pi_j > 30\% \mid \mathbf{y}^{(t)})$ and posterior moments $E(\pi_j \mid \mathbf{y}^{(t)})$. The computation of these posterior summaries requires several posterior integrations. (A possible implementation is outlined in Algorithm 4.8.)

Step 3. Drop trials: Identify all subpopulations with $p_{30,j} < 0.05$ and exclude them from further recruitment.

Step 4. Stopping: If all subpopulations are dropped, then stop the trial for lack of efficacy in all subpopulations. If the maximum enrollment is reached, $n = \sum n_j > n_{\max}$, stop for maximum enrollment. Otherwise repeat with Step 1.

∎

The evaluation of $p_{30,j}$ in Step 2 requires the evaluation of the marginal posterior distribution for π_j, i.e., marginalization with respect to π_h, $h \neq j$ and μ, τ. Such posterior integrations can be routinely carried out using MCMC posterior simulation when they are required once. The challenge here is that these posterior probabilities are required for all J subpopulations, for each period t of the trial, and for massive repeat simulation during the evaluation of operating characteristics. We therefore use a fast approximation based on adaptive bivariate quadrature for the integration over $(\mu, \log \tau)$ and then exploiting the conditional (posterior) independence of π_j, $j = 1, \ldots, J$, given (μ, τ). The latter reduces the integration with respect to the J-dimensional parameter vector $(\pi_1, \ldots, \pi_J)$ to J univariate integrations. We use adaptive quadrature for each of these univariate integrations. We use the R package adapt for the bivariate adaptive quadrature, and the R function integrate for the univariate adaptive quadrature.

Software note: The R package adapt (Lumley and Maecher, 2007) is available in CRAN at http://cran.r-project.org/src/contrib/Archive/adapt/.

Let $\mathbf{m}_t = E(\mu, \log(\tau) \mid \mathbf{y}^{(t)})$, $s^2_{\mu t} = \text{Var}(\mu \mid \mathbf{y}^{(t)})$, $s^2_{\tau t} = \text{Var}(\tau \mid \mathbf{y}^{(t)})$ and $\mathbf{s}_t = (s_{\mu t}, s_{\tau t})$ denote marginal means, variances and standard deviations for (μ, τ). The following algorithm implements posterior integration to evaluate $p_{30,j}$ and $E(\pi_j \mid \mathbf{y}^{(t)})$.

Algorithm 4.8 *(Numerical posterior integration for $p_{30,j}$).*

Step 1. Marginal posterior for $\mu, \log \tau$: Find the (marginal) posterior distribution $P(\mu, \log \tau \mid \mathbf{y}^{(t)})$ for any $(\mu, \log \tau)$; we use (univariate) numerical integration with respect to π_j, $j = 1, \ldots, J$. Let (y_j, n_j) denote the number of successes and number of patients in subpopulation j, and let $\sigma = exp(-.5 \log \tau)$. The marginal likelihood is given by

$$P(y_j \mid \mu, \tau) = \int \text{Bin}(y_j; \, n_j, \pi_j) \, N(\theta_j; \, \mu, \sigma) \, d\theta_j \, ,$$

with $\pi_j = 1/(1 + \exp(-\theta_j))$. We evaluate the integral by numerical quadrature using the R function integrate(). The desired posterior is then determined by

$$P(\mu, \tau \mid \mathbf{y}^{(t)}) \propto p(\mu) \, p(\tau) \prod_{j=1}^{J} p(y_j \mid \mu, \tau) \qquad (4.12)$$

Step 2. $p_{30,j}$, integration with respect to $\mu, \log \tau$: The posterior probability $p_{30,j}$ is obtained by another numerical integration. Letting $\theta_{30} = \log(0.3/0.7)$, we have

$$P(\pi_j > 0.30 \mid \mu, \tau, \mathbf{y}^{(t)}) = \int_{\theta_{30}}^{\infty} \frac{\text{Bin}(y_j; \, n_j, \pi_j) \, N(\theta_j; \, \mu, \sigma)}{p(y_j \mid \mu, \tau)} \, d\theta_j$$

Recall that $\theta_j = \log(\pi_j/(1 - \pi_j))$. The marginal probability $p_{30,j} = \int P(\pi_j > 0.30 \mid \mu, \tau, \mathbf{y}^{(t)}) \, dp(\mu, \tau \mid \mathbf{y}^{(t)})$ is found by bivariate adaptive quadrature, using (4.12) and the R package adapt.

Step 3. $E(\pi_j \mid \mathbf{y}^{(t)})$: The marginal expectations are found similarly, using

$$E(\pi_j \mid \mu, \tau, \mathbf{y}^{(t)}) = \int \pi_j \frac{\text{Bin}(y_j; \, n_j, \pi_j) \, N(\theta_j; \, \mu, \sigma)}{p(y_j \mid \mu, \tau)} \, d\theta_j$$

■

Example 4.8 *(Imatinib in sarcoma).* We implement the proposed design for the example discussed in Thall et al. (2003). They consider a phase II trial of imatinib in sarcoma. Sarcoma is a very heterogeneous disease. In this particular trial patients with $J = 10$ different subtypes of sarcoma are enrolled. The observed outcome is success defined as a reduction in tumor volume. Let π_j denote the unknown success probability for sarcoma type j. We define a hierarchical model as in (4.11) with a binomial sampling model, a normal prior on the logit scale, and a conjugate hyperprior. Following Thall et al. (2003) we set the hyperprior distributions as $\mu \sim N(-1.386, 10)$ with the mean chosen to match a logit of 0.20, and $\tau \sim \text{Ga}(2, 20)$ with $E(\tau) = 0.10$.

Figure 4.7 summarizes a trial simulation under the assumed truth $\pi = (3, 1, 1, 1, 1, 3, 1, 1, 1, 1)/10$. Assumed accrual rates are $E(k_j) = 5.5$ for $j = 1, \ldots, 5$ and $E(k_j) = 2$ for $j = 6, \ldots, 10$. Thus the total sample size is around $n_j = 44$ for the first 5 subtypes and $n_j = 16$ for the last 5, rarer subtypes.

Panel (a) shows the posterior means $E(\pi_j \mid \mathbf{y}^{(t)})$ plotted against t. The two bullets at 0.1 and 0.3 indicate the simulation truths. Note the separation into two clearly distinguished groups according to the simulation truth. Note how posterior inference for the rare subtypes borrows strength from the more prevalent subtypes. Posterior inference for all subtypes quickly moves away from the prior distribution centered around $\pi_j = 0.20$. Panel (b) plots the posterior probabilities $p_{30,j}$ against t. The horizontal dashed line indicates the cutoff at $\epsilon = 0.05$. When a posterior probability $p_{30,j}$ drops below the cutoff the corresponding subtype is closed for recruitment, although data from the already accrued patients continues to be used in posterior computations. ∎

4.6 Decision theoretic designs

4.6.1 Utility functions and their specification

Clinical trial design is naturally described as a decision problem (Berry and Ho, 1988). Studies are usually carried out with a well-defined primary objective. Describing that objective as choosing an action d to maximize some utility function specifies a formal decision problem. As already outlined in Subsection 1.4.1, a utility function is the opposite of a loss function: it describes the amount we "gain" (in some suitable units, such as dollars, patient lives, QALYs, and so on) when we choose action d. The utility function typically involves unknown quantities, including future data y and unknown parameters θ. For example, in a phase II study d could be a sequential stopping decision, y could be the observed outcomes and θ could be unknown true success probabilities for a list of possible dose levels. The utility function $u(d, \theta, y)$ could be a combination of the number of successfully treated patients, sampling cost for the recruited patients, and a large

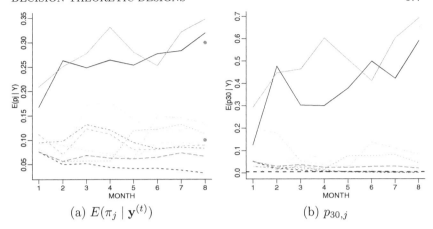

(a) $E(\pi_j \mid \mathbf{y}^{(t)})$ (b) $p_{30,j}$

Figure 4.7 *Hierarchical model. Panel (a) shows the posterior estimated success probabilities for $J = 10$ sarcoma subtypes, plotted against month $t = 1, \ldots, 6$. The points at $t = 6$ indicate the simulation truth. Panel (b) shows the posterior estimated probabilities $p_{30,j}$.*

reward if a subsequent phase III trial concludes with a significant result. Under the expected utility maximization paradigm, the optimal decision is determined by maximizing the utility $u(\cdot)$, conditional on all data that is available at the time of decisionmaking, and marginalizing with respect to all future data y and all unknown parameters θ.

In Subsection 2.5.5 we discussed a particular fully Bayesian method for incorporation of trial costs via decision theoretic methods. In practice, however, decision theoretic clinical trial design remains relatively uncommon. The main reasons for this lack of applications are fundamental concerns with the decision theoretic setup, and practical difficulties in the implementation. Perhaps the most relevant concern is the difficulty of specifying a good utility function. To start, *whose* utility is relevant? Assume we are willing to settle this question by choosing the investigator's utility. Part of the investigator's utility function is the need to satisfy regulatory requirements. This naturally adds additional perspectives into the problem. For example, the utility in a phase II trial might include a large reward for a significant outcome in the following confirmatory trial. Another problem is that the choice of a utility function and a probability model implicitly specifies the optimal rule for the trial design. The implicit nature of this specification is sometimes awkward, as it might lead to counterintuitive rules. For example, consider a dose finding trial to find the optimal dose of a drug. Assume that the outcome is desirable and the underlying probability model assumes a nonlinear regression of outcome on dose with a monotone increasing mean function. Let LD95 denote the dose that achieves 95% of the maximum possible benefit over placebo. Assume that the utility function is posterior precision of the mean response at the LD95. The optimal rule might allocate all patients at placebo and maximum dose only. This is because the mean response at the LD95 is a deterministic function of mean response at placebo and maximum dose. Of course no investigator would want to use this rule. Another generic problem is the use of randomization. For many good reasons randomization is desirable for trials that involve multiple treatment arms. Yet, under a strict decision theoretic framework there is an optimal treatment assignment for each patient, and thus no good reason for randomization. The issue can be finessed, but the basic problem remains that randomization is not natural under a decision theoretic paradigm.

The other big impediment to wider use of decision theoretic rules is the often computationally intensive nature of the solution. For example, consider the adaptive dose allocation problem. The problem is a sequential decision problem. The expected utility calculation for the dose assignment for the i-th cohort requires that we know the optimal dose allocation for the $(i + 1)$-st cohort, etc. In general such sequential decision problems are computationally intractable.

However, several strategies exist to mitigate these problems and make decision theoretic designs feasible. One difficulty in the choice of utility functions is the specification of tradeoff parameters for competing goals, for example sampling cost, successful treatment of patients in the trial, and treatment success for future patients. In general, utility functions often involve some parameters that are difficult to fix. A common strategy is to fix these parameters by considering (frequentist) operating characteristics of the implied designs and then choose the utility parameters to achieve desired operating characteristics. For example, consider a decision $d = (t_1, \ldots, t_n, t_{n+1})$ that includes treatment allocation $t_i(y_1, \ldots, y_{i-1})$, $i = 1, \ldots, n$ for n patients in a clinical trial, and upon conclusion of the trial a treatment recommendation $t_{n+1}(y_1, \ldots, y_n)$ for a generic $(n + 1)$-st future patient. Assume y_i is a binary indicator for treatment success. The utility function could then be $u(y, d, \theta) = \sum_{i=1}^{n} y_i + \lambda p(y_{n+1} = 1)$. Consider a grid on λ and for each value of λ, compute operating characteristics, such as Type I error probabilities and power under assumed true scenarios. We might then fix λ to best match desired operating characteristics.

Another important strategy is the use of decision boundaries to simplify sequential decision problems; we will discuss an example in the next subsection. Finally, we note that randomization is often introduced by randomizing among a set of near-optimal decisions and similar compromises.

4.6.2 Screening designs for drug development

Rossell et al. (2007) propose a Bayesian decision theoretic solution to the drug screening problem. Consider a setup where new treatment options for a well-defined patient population arise in each period. We index treatments in the order of appearance, $i = 1, 2, \ldots$. At any given time, a number of experimental treatments n_t are being considered. Let A_t denote the set of indices of treatments that are being studied at time t. For each treatment $i \in A_t$ we observe responses y_{ti}, and have to decide for which treatments we should stop recruitment (stopping, $d_{ti} = 0$), and for which we should continue accrual (continuation, $d_{ti} = 1$). Upon stopping we make a terminal decision of whether the treatment should be abandoned ($a_i = 0$) or recommended for a confirmatory phase III study ($a_i = 1$). Discontinued treatments ($d_{ti} = 0$) are removed from the active set A_t, and new treatments are added to form the new set A_{t+1}. We assume a finite horizon T. In the last period, T, continuation is not possible and $d_{Ti} = 0$ for all treatments under study.

Rossell et al. (2007) assume a binomial sampling model for y_{ti}. Let N_{ti} denote the accrual for treatment i in period t, and let θ_i denote an unknown success probability for treatment i, so that

$$y_{ti} \sim \text{Bin}(N_{ti}, \theta_i)$$

for all $i \in A_t$. The model is completed with a prior $\theta_i \sim \text{Be}(u, v)$ and independent hyperpriors $u \sim \text{Ga}(a_u, b_u)\, v \sim \text{Ga}(a_v, b_v)$, subject to $u + v \leq 10$.

Before we continue the discussion of the decision theoretic setup, we state the final algorithm. Let (m_{ti}, s_{ti}) denote the posterior mean $E(\theta_i \mid y)$ and standard deviation $SD(\theta_i \mid y)$ conditional on all data up to time t. We construct decision boundaries for $(\log s_{ti}, m_{ti})$. The decision boundaries form a cone in the $(\log s_t i, m_t i)$ plane; see Figure 4.8. The sequential stopping condition d_{it} is determined by these boundaries. While inside the cone, continue $d_{it} = 0$. Once we cross the boundaries, stop, $d_{it} = 1$.

We now discuss one possible construction of these decision boundaries. An alternative approach is outlined in Example 4.9. The construction will involve the consideration of a follow-up confirmatory phase III trial for selected treatments ($a_i = 1$). Let $\tau = \min\{t : d_{ti} = 0\}$ denote the time of stopping accrual for treatment i. We assume that the confirmatory trial is set up as a two-arm randomized trial with the same binary success outcome. Let θ_0 denote the assumed known success probability under standard of care. We assume that a simple z-test is used to test $H_0 : \theta_i = \theta_0$ versus the alternative $H_a : \theta_i = m_{ti}$ for a given significance level α_3 and power $1 - \beta_3$, where the "3" subscripts here refer to the phase III study. The required sample size for the follow-up confirmatory trial is

$$n_3(m_{\tau i} = m, s_{\tau i} = s)$$
$$= 2 \left(\frac{z_{\beta_3}\sqrt{m(1-m)+\theta_0(1-\theta_0)}+z_{\alpha_3}\sqrt{2\overline{m}(1-\overline{m})}}{m-\theta_0} \right)^2.$$

Here $\overline{m} = (m_{\tau i} + \theta_0)/2$ and z_p is the standard normal $(1-p)$ quantile. Let B denote the event that the z-statistic falls in the rejection region. We have

$$p(B \mid y) = P(\hat{\theta}_i - \hat{\theta}_0 > z_{\alpha_3/2}\sqrt{2\overline{m}(1-\overline{m})/n_3} \mid y)$$

where $y = (y_1, \ldots, y_\tau)$ and $\hat{\theta}_i$ and $\hat{\theta}_0$ are the proportions of successes under treatment and control in the z-test. The probability $p(B \mid y)$ can be approximated based on a normal approximation of the posterior predictive distribution for $\hat{\theta}_i - \hat{\theta}_0$ (Rossell et al., 2007, Section 2.2).

Algorithm 4.9 *(Decision-theoretic screening design).*

Step 0. Decision boundaries in $(\log s_{ti}, m)$: Consider two half lines in the $(\log s, m)$ plane that form a cone intersecting at $(\log s_0, b_0)$ and passing through $(\log s_1, b_1)$ and $(\log s_1, b_2)$, respectively (see Figure 4.8 for an illustration). Here s_0 and s_1 are fixed. For example, fix s_0 to be a minimum standard deviation and s_1 to approximately match the marginal prior standard deviation. The parameters (b_0, b_1, b_2) will be determined below. The two half lines are decision boundaries that determine d_{ti}:

$$d_{ti} = \begin{cases} 1 & \text{if } (\log(s_{ti}), m_{ti}) \text{ lies between the two lines} \\ 0 & \text{otherwise} \end{cases}$$

Step 1. Utility parameters. Fix c_1 and c_2 to reflect the relative cost of recruiting one patient and the reward that is realized if a following confirmatory trial ends with a significant result (e.g., $c_1 = 1$ and $c_2 = 10,000$). Define a utility function

$$u(b,y) = -c_1 \sum_t \sum_{i \in A_t} N_{ti}$$
$$+ \sum_{i:a_i=1} \left[-c_1 n_3 + c_2 P(B \mid y_1, \ldots, y_{\tau_i}) E(\hat{\theta}_i - \hat{\theta}_0 \mid B, y_1, \ldots, y_{\tau_i}) \right].$$
$$(4.13)$$

For given data y and decision boundaries b, the realized utility $u(b,y)$ can be evaluated.

Step 2. Forward simulation: Simulate many possible trial realizations, without stopping, i.e., using $d_{ti} = 1$ for $t = 1, \ldots, T-1$, and save the realized trajectories $\{\log(s_{ti}, m_{ti})\}$.

Step 3. Optimal decision boundaries: For a grid of (b_0, b_1, b_2) values, evaluate the average realized utility $u(b,y)$, averaging over all simulations saved in Step 3. Denote the average as $U(b)$. The optimal decision boundary $b^\star$ is the one with maximum $U(b)$.

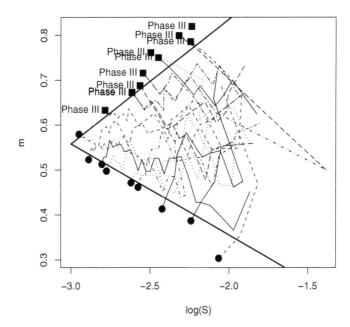

Figure 4.8 *Decision boundaries in the* $(\log s, m)$ *plane. The two half lines are the decision boundaries intersecting at* $(\log s_0, b_0)$. *The trajectories show some forward simulations* $(\log s_{ti}, m_{ti})$, *together with the final decision* a_i *when the trajectories cross the decision boundaries* $(d_{ti} = 0)$.

Step 4. Trial conduct: Use the optimal decision boundary $b^\star$ to decide continuation versus stopping for all treatments $i \in A_t$ at each time $t = 1, \ldots, T$.

■

The algorithm is justified as an approximation of the optimal sequential stopping rule under the utility function $u(\cdot)$. The nature of the approximation is that we only allow sequential stopping rules that depend on the full data indirectly through the summaries (m_{ti}, s_{ti}).

Software note: Designs of this type are implemented in an R package written by David Rossell called *sesdesphII*. The package is available at
                    http://rosselldavid.googlepages.com/software   .
The program requires only specification of the hyperparameters u, v, s_0, s_1 and the grids on b_0, b_1, and b_2.

Example 4.9 *(Clinical immunology).* We summarize an application to designing a screening study for vaccines discussed in Rossell et al. (2007). The

α_{max}	β_{max}	b_0^*	b_1^*	b_2^*	$\overline{N}$	α	β
0.05	0.05	0.45	0.64	0.24	31.78	0.04	0.04
0.05	0.10	0.53	0.67	0.37	15.77	0.05	0.10
0.05	0.15	0.57	0.64	0.52	9.96	0.05	0.14
0.10	0.05	0.49	0.51	0.26	17.17	0.09	0.03
0.10	0.10	0.43	0.46	0.37	7.16	0.10	0.10
0.10	0.15	0.38	0.43	0.37	7.05	0.09	0.10
0.15	0.05	0.43	0.46	0.22	13.13	0.15	0.02
0.15	0.10	0.34	0.41	0.31	6.19	0.12	0.09
0.15	0.15	0.34	0.41	0.31	6.19	0.12	0.09

Table 4.6 *Summary statistics for clinical immunology example.*

utility function is a variation of the one in (4.13), using the average number of patients needed to recommend one treatment. Letting $M = \sum_{i=1}^{n_T} a_i$ denote the number of treatments that are recommended for phase III, the utility chosen is $u(b, y) = 1/M \sum_{t=t_{0i}}^{t_{1i}} \sum_{i=1}^{n_T} N_{ti}$. We assume that the success probability for the standard of care is $\theta_0 = 0.5$, and use a Beta prior $\theta_i \sim Be(0.3188, 0.5327)$, chosen to match the moments observed in historical data, $E(\theta_i) = 0.3743$ and $Var(\theta_i) = 0.1265$.

We evaluate designs with $M = 1000$ simulations on a grid with 20 equally spaced values of b_0 in $[0.3, 0.7]$, b_1 in $[0.3, 0.8]$, and b_2 in $[0.2, 0.6]$, and use cohorts of $N = 2$ patients. After each batch, the posterior moments are evaluated and the decision to stop is taken as in Step 0 above. For the terminal decision we use a fixed rule. Upon stopping the enrollment, a treatment is recommended when stopping was indicated by crossing the upper boundary, whereas a treatment is abandoned if stopping was indicated by crossing the lower boundary. We then select b to maximize $U(b)$, the Monte Carlo sample average utility in the forward simulation. The maximization is restricted to designs b that satisfy constraints on Type I error α and power $1 - \beta$. Here α is the fraction of treatments with (simulation) truth $\theta_i < \theta_0$ and $a_i = 1$, and β is the fraction of treatments with $\theta_i > \theta_0$ and $a_i = 0$. The maximization over $U(b)$ is restricted to designs b with $\alpha \leq \alpha_{max}$ and $\beta \leq \beta_{max}$.

Table 4.6 summarizes results for several choices of α_{max} and β_{max}. The column $\overline{N} \equiv U(b)$ reports the average number of patients necessary to recommend one treatment. ∎

4.7 Case studies in phase II adaptive design

In this section we present two recent high-profile trials that employ innovative trial designs using the approaches introduced earlier in this chapter. Both trials are good examples of the benefits that can be achieved through a Bayesian adaptive approach. While we are not yet able to reveal final results in either case, we do discuss the conditions that encourage the adoption of an adaptive Bayesian viewpoint, as well as corresponding implementational details.

4.7.1 The BATTLE trial

The use of adaptive designs has gained much attention lately thanks to its potential for improving study efficiency by reducing sample size, resulting in higher statistical power in identifying efficacious drugs or important biomarkers associated with the drug efficacy, and treating more patients with more effective treatments during the trial. As mentioned earlier, both the Center for Drug Evaluation and Research (CDER) and the Center for Biologics Evaluation and Research (CBER) at the U.S. FDA have issued guidance documents for the use of adaptive methods in clinical trials (see the Preface of this book for the websites of these two documents).

In this section, we illustrate an adaptive design case study, the *Biomarker-integrated Approaches of Targeted Therapy for Lung Cancer Elimination* (BATTLE) trial (Zhou et al., 2008). The goal of this trial is to evaluate the efficacy of four targeted treatments in patients with advanced non-small cell lung cancer. The four treatments to be compared are erlotinib (TX 1), sorafenib (TX 2), vandetanib (TX 3), and the combination of erlotinib and bexarotene (TX 4). To enroll in the study, all patients are required to have biopsies to measure a tumor's biomarker profile. Based on this profile, patients are assigned to one of the five marker groups: EGFR mutation/amplification (MG 1), K-ras and/or B-raf mutation (MG 2), VEGF and/or VEGFR expression (MG 3), RXR and/or cyclin D1 expression (MG 4), or no marker group (MG 5) if all markers are negative or there are insufficient tissues for marker analysis. It is assumed that each treatment may be more efficacious in patients having a biomarker profile that matches the agent's mechanism of action. Therefore, the specific goal of this trial is to test the efficacy of these targeted agents, and identify the corresponding predictive biomarkers. In addition, the trialists aim to take advantage of the information learned from the interim data, so as to treat more patients with better therapies during the trial. The primary endpoint is the 8-week disease control rate (DCR), which is defined as the proportion of patients without disease progression 8 weeks after randomization. We apply a Bayesian hierarchical model to characterize the DCR, and use response adaptive randomization (RAR) to assign more patients into more effective treatments based on the accumulating trial data.

Hierarchical probit model

The Bayesian probit model (Albert and Chib, 1993) is used to define the DCR for each treatment (TX) by marker group (MG). A probit link function is chosen to model the binary disease control status. A latent continuous variable is introduced to model the hierarchical relationship of the response data in treatment by marker groups. Let j denote the treatment, k the marker group, and i the index for the patient running from 1 to n_{jk}, where n_{jk} is the total number of patients in TX j and MG k. Let y_{ijk} be the binary disease control random variable (progression-free at 8 weeks), which takes the value 0 if the patient experiences progression or dies within eight weeks of the TX, and 1 otherwise. A latent continuous variable z_{ijk} is then introduced to model the DCR; let

$$y_{ijk} = \begin{cases} 0 & \text{if } z_{ijk} \leq 0 \\ 1 & \text{if } z_{ijk} > 0 \end{cases} \tag{4.14}$$

The DCR for TX j and MG k is the probability that the latent variable is greater than 0, defined as $\gamma_{jk} = P(y_{ijk} = 1) = P(z_{ijk} > 0)$. For each subgroup, we assume that z_{ijk} follows a normal distribution with mean μ_{jk}. Note that because only the sign of z_{ijk} matters for determining y_{ijk}, the model can be identified only up to a multiplicative constant on z_{ijk}. To ensure identifiability, we thus set the variance of z_{ijk} to 1 (Albert and Chib, 1993; Johnson and Albert, 2000). For a given marker group, a $N(\phi_j, \sigma^2)$ hyperprior is imposed on the location parameters μ_{jk} of the latent variables. The parameter ϕ_j is also assumed normal with mean 0 and variance τ^2, which allows for the exchange of information across different treatments. This hierarchical model allows borrowing information across different marker groups (k) within a treatment (j). The full hierarchical model is thus

$$\begin{aligned} z_{ijk} &\sim N(\mu_{jk}, 1), \text{ for all } i, j, \text{ and } k \\ \mu_{jk} &\sim N(\phi_j, \sigma^2), \text{ for all } j \text{ and } k \\ \text{and } \phi_j &\sim N(0, \tau^2), \text{ for all } j \, . \end{aligned} \tag{4.15}$$

The parameters σ^2 and τ^2 control the extent of the borrowing across marker groups within each treatment and across all treatments, respectively. Our default configuration is to use a vague specification, namely $\sigma^2 = \tau^2 = 10^6$. The posterior distributions can be routinely computed via Gibbs sampling from the full conditional distributions given below.

Denote L_{ijk} as the likelihood for patient i in marker group k receiving TX j. Assuming independence across patients, the overall likelihood is the product $L = \prod_j \prod_k \prod_{i=1}^{n_{jk}} L_{ijk}$, where L_{ijk} is

$$\left(Pr(z_{ijk} \geq 0|\mu_{jk}, \phi_j, \sigma^2, \tau^2)\right)^{I(y_{ijk}=1)} \left(Pr(z_{ijk} < 0|\mu_{jk}, \phi_j, \sigma^2, \tau^2)\right)^{I(y_{ijk}=0)}$$
$$= \left\{\int_0^\infty f(z_{ijk}|\mu_{jk}, 1)\right\}^{I(y_{ijk}=1)} \left\{\int_{-\infty}^0 f(z_{ijk}|\mu_{jk}, 1)\right\}^{I(y_{ijk}=0)}.$$

The full conditional distributions for the μ_{jk} and ϕ_k are normal thanks to our use of conjugate priors. The latent variables z_{ijk} follow *truncated* normal distributions. The distributions required for the Gibbs sampler are thus

$$z_{ijk} \mid y_{ijk}, \mu_{jk} \propto \begin{cases} N(\mu_{jk}, 1)I(-\infty, 0) & \text{if } y_{ijk} = 0 \\ N(\mu_{jk}, 1)I(0, \infty) & \text{if } y_{ijk} = 1 \end{cases}$$
$$\mu_{jk} \mid z_{ijk}, \phi_j \propto N(\sum_{i=1}^{n_{jk}} z_{ijk} + \phi_j/\sigma^2, \; 1/(n_{jk} + 1/\sigma^2))$$
$$\text{and } \phi_j \mid \mu_{jk} \propto N(\sum_{k=1}^5 \mu_{jk}, \; 1/(5 + 1/\tau^2)).$$

Note that a truncated normal can be straightforwardly sampled by simple rejection, or via a more efficient one-for-one sampling algorithm using only the normal cdf and inverse cdf; see Carlin and Louis (2009, p.362)

Adaptive randomization

A response adaptive randomization (AR) is proposed for the BATTLE trial. Because patients with certain biomarker profiles may respond differently to different treatments, the biomarker profile must be taken into consideration when assigning patients into various treatments. For example, if patients with EGFR mutation are more likely to respond to erlotinib than other treatments, it is desirable to assign more such patients to erlotinib. Because the true DCR for each of the treatment (TX) by marker group (MG) combinations is unknown when the trial begins, we apply equal randomization (ER) in the first part of the trial until at least one patient with a known disease control status is enrolled in each TX by MG. Subsequent to this, patients are adaptively randomized. Under the Bayesian probit model described above, all accumulative data are used in computing the posterior DCR, and thus in determining the randomization ratio. The randomization rate is computed based on the estimated posterior mean of the DCR of each TX in each MG.

The randomization ratio for a patient in MG k to receive TX j is taken as proportional to the estimated mean DCR in that subgroup. That is,

$$\hat{\gamma}_{jk} / \sum_{w \in \Omega} \hat{\gamma}_{wk}, \tag{4.16}$$

where $\hat{\gamma}$ corresponds to the posterior mean of the DCR, and Ω indicates the subset of all eligible and non-suspended treatments for that patient at the time of randomization. Note that another commonly used alternative is to randomize patient in MG k to TX j with probability $Pr(\gamma_{jk} > \gamma_{j'k}, j \in$

$\{1, 2, 3, 4\}, j' \neq j$). To ensure a certain minimal probability of randomization for each non-suspended treatment, if the estimated DCR is less than 10%, 10% is used as the randomization percentage for this treatment. AR is carried out until the last patient is enrolled, unless all four treatments have been suspended due to futility. R code was developed to facilitate the visualization of the dynamic nature of AR.

Interim and final decision rules

We also add an early futility stopping rule to the trial design. If the current data indicate that a treatment is unlikely to be beneficial to patients in certain marker groups, randomization to that treatment is suspended. Specifically, denote the target DCR by θ_1 and the critical probability for early stopping (i.e., suspension of randomization due to futility) by δ_L. The trial will be suspended for TX j and MG k if the probability that the estimated DCR is at least θ_1 is less than or equal to δ_L, i.e.,

$$Pr(\gamma_{jk} \geq \theta_1 | Data) \leq \delta_L . \tag{4.17}$$

We choose $\theta_1 = 0.5$ and $\delta_L = 0.1$. The stopping rule will be applied after AR begins.

Next, let θ_0 and δ_U be the DCR for standard treatment and the critical probability for declaring an effective treatment, respectively. The treatment will be considered a success at the end of a trial if the probability that the estimated DCR being at least θ_0 is greater than δ_U, i.e.,

$$Pr(\gamma_{jk} \geq \theta_0 | Data) > \delta_U . \tag{4.18}$$

In this study, we set $\theta_0 = 0.3$ and $\delta_U = 0.8$.

Finally, note that the trial design has no early stopping rule for effective treatments. If a treatment shows early signs of efficacy, more patients will continue to be enrolled to that treatment under the AR scheme, and the declaration of efficacy will occur at the end of the trial.

Operating characteristics

As usual, we evaluate the operating characteristics of the proposed trial design through simulation. In this phase II trial with four treatments, five marker groups, and a limited sample size of 200 evaluable patients, our target is to achieve a 20% false positive rate (i.e., when we conclude a non-effective treatment to be effective), and 80% power (i.e., concluding the effective treatments effective). A higher false positive rate than 0.10 (commonly accepted in phase II trials) is allowed so that we will not miss any potentially effective treatments. Once effective treatments are identified, they will be confirmed by larger studies in the future.

We conduct simulations with 1,000 generated datasets. We assume that for MG 1, the true DCR for Treatment 1 is 80%, but only 30% for all

			Marker Group		
TX	1	2	3	4	5
	true disease control rate / observed disease control rate				
1	0.80/0.77	0.30/0.22	0.30/0.24	0.30/0.22	0.30/0.20
2	0.30/0.21	0.60/0.54	0.30/0.24	0.30/0.24	0.30/0.18
3	0.30/0.22	0.30/0.22	0.60/0.57	0.30/0.23	0.30/0.19
4	0.30/0.22	0.30/0.23	0.30/0.24	0.60/0.55	0.30/0.19
	average sample size (column percentage)				
1	13.0 (43.2)	7.6 (19.1)	10.8 (17.9)	9.0 (18.1)	4.6 (22.9)
2	5.4 (17.9)	15.4 (38.8)	11.1 (18.4)	9.3 (18.7)	4.3 (21.4)
3	5.7 (18.9)	7.7 (19.4)	25.9 (43.0)	9.3 (18.7)	4.4 (21.9)
4	5.7 (18.9)	7.6 (19.1)	10.9 (18.1)	20.7 (41.6)	4.5 (22.4)
none	0.3 (1.0)	1.4 (3.5)	1.7 (2.8)	1.5 (3.0)	2.2 (10.9)
total	30.1	39.7	60.3	49.8	20.1
	P(declaring an effective TX) / P(suspending an ineffective TX)				
1	0.95/0.04	0.14/0.56	0.14/0.63	0.12/0.61	0.14/0.57
2	0.13/0.56	0.82/0.12	0.14/0.61	0.14/0.58	0.14/0.61
3	0.17/0.54	0.15/0.58	0.90/0.07	0.14/0.60	0.13/0.57
4	0.14/0.53	0.14/0.56	0.14/0.62	0.86/0.09	0.15/0.57

Table 4.7 *Operating characteristics for the BATTLE trial with one effective treatment for Marker Groups 1-4 and no effective treatment for Marker Group 5.*

other treatments. We assume that for MG 2, the true DCR for Treatment 2 is 60%, with 30% for all other treatments. Similarly, we assume MG 3 and MG 4 have only one effective treatment, but that there is no effective treatment in MG 5.

Table 4.7 shows that the crude observed (sample mean) DCRs underestimate the true rates due to the AR. The model-based (posterior mean) DCR estimates (not shown) also underestimate these true rates, but by uniformly smaller margins.

With AR and an early stopping rule, more patients are randomized into more effective treatments. The percentage of patients receiving effective treatments are 43.2% for MG 1, 38.8% for MG 2, 43.0% for MG 3, and 41.6% for MG 4, compared to just 25% under ER. For patients in MG 5, since there is no effective treatment, percentages of patients randomized into Treatments 1-4 are about the same, with a 10.9% chance that no treatments are assigned to patients because all four treatments are inefficacious. These patients may of course receive other treatments off-protocol. The total number of patients in each MG is estimated from prior data.

The probabilities of declaring effective treatments are also shown. When the treatments are efficacious, the powers are 95%, 82%, 90%, and 86% for TX1/MG1, TX2/MG2, TX3/MG3, and TX4/MG4, respectively. The false positive rates for declaring ineffective treatments effective (not shown in the table) range between 0.12 to 0.17. The probabilities of suspending treatments are also listed. When the treatments are effective, the probabilities of suspension are no larger than 0.12 (occurs in TX2/MG2). Conversely, for ineffective treatments, the probabilities of suspension all exceed 0.53 (occurs in TX4/MG1).

Scenarios with different informative priors obtained by varying σ^2 and τ^2 were also evaluated. Basically, when the treatment effect is more homogeneous across treatments or MGs, more borrowing yields better results with respect to less biased estimates of DCR and more accurate declarations of effective treatments. On the other hand, when the treatment effects are heterogeneous, too much borrowing can lead to a higher chance of false positive conclusions. The amount of borrowing should be carefully calibrated to ensure good control of false positive rates.

Discussion

In this case study, we illustrated an RAR design under the framework of a hierarchical Bayes model. Based on simulation studies, we have shown that with a total of 200 evaluable patients, the trial design has desirable operating characteristics that select clinically effective agents with a high probability and ineffective agents with a low probability, treat more patients with effective agents according to their tumor biomarker profiles, and suspend ineffective agents from enrollment with a high probability by applying an early stopping rule. The Bayesian AR design is a smart, novel, and ethical design. In conjunction with an early stopping rule, it can be applied to efficiently identify effective agents and eliminate ineffective ones. By aligning effective treatments with patients' biomarker profiles, more patients are treated with effective therapies, and hence, more patients could reach disease control status. AR design with early stopping is ideally suitable for the development of targeted therapy. The proposed trial design continues to "learn" by updating the posterior distribution and improves the estimates as the trial progresses. It is a "smart" design that matches patients with the drugs best suited for them. This trial design presents a step towards personalized medicine.

However, the success of the response adaptive randomization trial depends on several key factors. First, the time for a patient's biomarker assessment needs to be relatively short (e.g., in a few days) because the patient's treatment assignment depends on the determination of the marker profile. Second, the time for outcome assessment must be relatively short as well, so that the decision based on up-to-date data can provide appropriate guidance for subsequent treatment assignments. Third, the trial accrual cannot be too fast. If a trial has a fast accrual rate, many patients may have been enrolled into the trial before the outcome data becomes available to provide useful information for the adaptive randomization. Therefore, quick and easily assessable endpoints and slow to moderate accrual rates (relative to the outcome assessment time) are most suitable for RAR designs. Lastly, for AR to work, we must have good markers and good treatments.

4.7.2 The I-SPY 2 trial

I-SPY 2 (Barker et al., 2009) is an adaptive phase II clinical trial of neoadjuvant treatments for women with locally advanced breast cancer; the reader may see http://vimeo.com/10266694 for the launch of this trial with a press conference at the National Press Club. The name of the trial derives from the phrase, "Investigation of Serial studies to Predict Your Therapeutic Response with Imaging And moLecular analysis"; see ispy2.org. The trial caught the attention of mainstream media, including the *Wall Street Journal* (see the writeup of April 19, 2010) and NBC's News 4 (WRC-TV, Washington DC). Speakers at the press conference included Senator Arlen Specter (D-PA) and Congresswoman Jackie Speier (D-CA).

There are good reasons for the hype. The trial is revolutionary, albeit not for the mathematics; the underlying methods and models are sophisticated, but not mathematically difficult. The revolutionary aspect is that, similar to BATTLE, the trial seeks to identify effective drugs and drug combinations for specific subtypes of the disease. Subtypes are characterized by combinations of biomarkers, including binary indicators for hormone receptor status, HER2 status (+/-) and MammaPrint status. The latter is recorded as a binary indicator for low versus high MammaPrint risk score (Mook et al., 2007). Combinations and unions of combinations of these markers define ten possible subpopulations (using practical relevance and clinical judgment to narrow down from 255 combinatorially possible subpopulations). The primary endpoint is pathologic complete response at 6 months (pCR).

Learning occurs as the trial proceeds, and data from all patients is used to inform inference about any drug and any subpopulation. Also the word "Your" in the name of the trial suggests another revolutionary aspect. Using adaptive treatment allocation, patients in each subpopulation are assigned the treatments that are considered most promising for them. Many of the elements of this trial are similar to the methods described earlier in this chapter.

Sequential stopping

The protocol includes the evaluation of predictive probabilities as described in Section 4.2. The trial uses a variation of Algorithm 4.2 to decide about dropping or graduating drugs from the trial. Drugs are dropped when there is little hope of future success, and graduated and recommended for further development when results are promising. Specifically, for each drug we compute posterior predictive probabilities of success in a hypothetical future phase III trial. The future phase III trial is set up to compare the drug under consideration versus control in a phase III trial with fixed sample size. If the posterior predictive probability of success in this future trial falls below a lower threshold for all possible subgroups, then the drug is dropped from consideration ("defeat"). If on the other hand, the posterior predictive probability of success in the future phase III trial is beyond an upper threshold for some subpopulation, then the drug graduates from the phase II trial and is recommended for a follow-up phase III study ("victory"). The use of success in a hypothetical future phase III study as a criterion for selecting drugs in a phase II screening design is similar to the drug screening trial discussed in Subsection 4.6.2.

Subpopulations

The outcome of I-SPY 2 is a stream of drugs that are recommended for further development. One of the critical features of I-SPY 2 is that each recommendation includes an identification of an appropriate subpopulation, characterized by the recorded biomarkers. Such recommendations are facilitated by the use of a hierarchical model across all possible subpopulations. The model is similar to the models described in Section 4.5.

   The clinical relevance of this feature cannot be overstated. Despite widely reported promise of biomarkers for informing all aspects of drug development, the practical implementation of developing and validating biomarkers has proven extremely challenging. The hierarchical model together with other features of I-SPY 2 promises to break this "biomarker barrier."

Adaptive allocation

Patients are allocated to the competing treatment arms using adaptive randomization. In Section 4.4 we described the general paradigm. Let $\pi(z, t)$ denote the probability of pCR for a patient characterized by biomarkers z under treatment t. I-SPY 2 uses adaptive allocation probabilities proportional to

$$P(\pi(z, t) > \pi(z, t'),\ t' \neq t \mid data),$$

i.e., the posterior probability of treatment t being optimal for subgroup z. As usual the randomization is restricted to some minimum allocation probability for all active treatment arms.

Delayed responses

A potential limitation of I-SPY 2 is the delayed nature of the primary
endpoint pCR at 6 months. The need to wait 6 months for the outcome
would limit the benefits of the adaptive features in the trial design. I-SPY 2
overcomes this limitation by using longitudinal magnetic resonance imaging
(MRI) measurements. Correlating the MRI measurements with the final
response allows the investigators to impute the missing final response for
patients who were recruited within the last 6 months. One of the important
features of the trial is that this imputation is done with full consideration
of the related uncertainties. Rather than relying on a plug-in estimate,
posterior inference in I-SPY 2 repeatedly imputes the missing outcomes,
thereby correctly adjusting for the uncertainty.

In summary, I-SPY 2 applies an innovative Bayesian design to screen
novel phase II drugs for women with locally advanced breast cancer. The
design allows for rapid identification of effective drugs *and* biomarkers that
characterize the breast cancer subtypes that are most susceptible to the
respective drug.

4.8 Appendix: R Macros

The online supplement to this chapter

> www.biostat.umn.edu/~brad/software/BCLM_ch4.html

provides the R code that was used to illustrate the examples of this section.
In the typical case, as in the previous chapter, the R macros are written to
simulate one realization of a hypothetical trial using the proposed design.
The main function in these examples is named sim.trial(.). To compute
operating characteristics one would add an additional loop that repeatedly
calls sim.trial. To monitor an ongoing trial one would instead replace the
simulated data with the actually observed responses, and strip the top-level
loop inside sim.trial, using only one iteration.

## CHAPTER 5

Phase III studies

In this chapter, we turn to Bayesian design and analysis of phase III studies. These are typically randomized controlled multicenter trials on large patient groups (300-3,000 or more, depending upon the disease/medical condition studied) aimed at being the definitive assessment of how effective the drug is, in comparison with current "gold standard" treatment. Such trials are often called *confirmatory trials*.

The approach of the chapter is to focus on what is different for a Bayesian statistician in a confirmatory trial. The development here is not meant as a general reference for designing or analyzing confirmatory trials, but rather as a description and exemplification of the features and challenges for a Bayesian. Especially early in the chapter, we rely heavily on demonstrating these features and challenges through a running "example trial" that we construct for pedagogical purposes. This chapter is not meant as a precise recipe for doing every possible Bayesian confirmatory trial. In fact, we believe such an attempt would be counterproductive, both to the Bayesian approach and to science in general. After all, an important aspect of the Bayesian approach is its flexibility and synthetic nature. The ability to create a unique design specific to the challenges of each problem, guided by Bayesian principles and philosophy, is one of the strengths of the approach. Any attempt to describe in overly "cookbook-y" steps how this should be done is likely to stifle its effectiveness.

5.1 Introduction to confirmatory studies

There are multiple issues that arise in many applications we have seen. We highlight these and discuss how we deal with and solve these issues in practice. The regulatory industry is ever changing and so these issues may become increasingly or decreasingly relevant through time, but despite this it is unlikely that they will lose relevance any time soon. The issues that are highlighted in the chapter are not specific to any particular therapeutic area, regulatory agency, or type of medical therapy. Section 5.8 offers a full case study of a confirmatory trial involving a medical device.

Confirmatory studies raise different statistical challenges. The most im-

portant statistical aspect is that the confirmatory study is typically over-
seen and judged by a regulatory agency. This creates predetermined statistical thresholds or "hurdles" that must be met in order for the regulatory
agency to approve the medical therapy for public use. Earlier phase studies typically have learning goals, such as finding the largest safe dose or
the minimum effective dose. These trials' goals are clearly articulated, but
their definitions of statistically important effects are not regulated by agencies. These "learning" studies typically allow better decisions to be made
in later phases of medical therapy development. The desired result of a
confirmatory trial is the approval of a therapy for public use.

The industry standard has been to design a fixed sample size trial with
a defined analysis on a defined endpoint. The statistical hurdle is to get a
statistically significant result at a specified Type I error level, typically the
0.05 level (could be one- or two-sided). At the conclusion of the study the
data are unblinded and analyzed according to the pre-planned endpoint
and analysis for statistical significance at the agreed upon level. The power
of the design is relevant in the acceptance of the design by regulatory
agents, but at the analysis stage, at the completion of the study, the power
is irrelevant. The critical aspect is significance at the specified level, which
makes the Type I error of the design the most important regulatory hurdle.
The exact Type I error of an adaptive Bayesian design can be extremely
difficult, if not impossible, to calculate. The many different adaptive aspects
of the design can have implications to the Type I error which individually
are hard to capture. Thus the standard way to measure the Type I error
of the adaptive features is through simulations. In this chapter simulations
are described and presented.

As discussed in Section 1.3, there are many different adaptive features
that have and can be employed in confirmatory trials. The first and most
common is to adapt the sample size. Despite the early phase trials, the effect
of a treatment, and especially relative to a blinded control, is still uncertain
at the outset of phase III. The ability to adapt the sample size to the results
of the trial creates an appropriate sample size, resulting in a more efficient
trial. This adaptation of sample size includes the appropriate sample size to
determine success of the treatment, but also the ability to determine when
the treatment is unlikely to show trial success and, thus, stop the trial for
futility. Second, some trials may start with multiple treatment arms with
the desire that one of the arms may be dropped during the trial. A decision
may be made between two active treatment arms, whether it be different
schedules, doses, regimen, or device styles, as to which is more appropriate
to carry forward in the confirmation of the therapy. Finally, a trial may
start with multiple doses of an experimental agent, where the first stage of
the trial determines the dose arm to move forward to a second stage that
undertakes a more traditional comparison to a control arm. This type of
confirmatory trial is referred to as a *seamless phase II/III* trial.

All adaptive designs discussed in this book are *prospectively* adaptive designs. By this we mean the design is completely specified before the start of the trial. The results of the trial may change the trial's features, but these changes are by design, not ad hoc retrospective changes. We do not consider having a committee of three people choosing a dose to move to the second stage of the design to be a prospective adaptive design. The methodology of selecting the dose moving forward is uncertain. Such a design cannot be simulated and the operating characteristics are unknown. There are certainly times in which such a design may be reasonable, but it is not part of our investigation – especially in confirmatory trials. As described, a regulatory agency is typically the consumer of the results of a confirmatory trial and the ability to completely define a design, and to understand the behavior of the design with its operating characteristics is critical to the acceptance of adaptive designs.

5.2 Bayesian adaptive confirmatory trials

In this section we describe common issues that arise in a Bayesian confirmatory design. These typically involve the adaptive features of the design and their affects on the Type I error. The selection of priors for confirmatory trials is rarely an issue, as non- or minimally informative priors are typically chosen. We return to the prior distributions and their effects in Section 5.5.

To demonstrate the idea of a confirmatory trial we develop a very simple example trial, and subsequently build upon it to add adaptive aspects. The example is simple to allow the adaptive aspects and the effects of these adaptive features to be clear. We carry the following example through much of this chapter.

Example 5.1 *(Basic confirmatory trial)*. Suppose we have a one-armed trial in which each subject is considered a success or failure. The information on whether a subject is a success or failure is observed immediately. This may be the case in a pain study where the endpoint is "two hours pain free" (in the world of clinical trials this is essentially immediate). Let the probability a subject is a success be p. Each observation is assumed independent. Therefore, for n observations the number of successes is

$$X \mid p \sim \text{Binomial}(n, p)$$

Assume the regulatory agency agrees that to demonstrate statistical success of the medical therapy the trial must show $p > 0.5$. In a hypothesis testing framework,

$$H_0 : p \leq 0.5$$

$$H_A : p > 0.5.$$

A fixed sample size trial at the one-sided 0.05-level, with $n = 100$, would result in a successful trial if $X \geq 59$. The probability of $X \geq 59$, assuming $p = 0.5$ is 0.0443. A cutoff for success of $X \geq 58$ would result in a one-sided Type I error of 0.066. For this example we assume the regulatory restriction is a one-sided Type I error of 0.05. Thus the trial would be considered successful if $X \geq 59$. Observing 58 successes would be considered a failed study. In reality this is not always the case as secondary endpoints and additional information may mean that regulators allow the therapy to be marketed. For our purposes, we focus on achieving statistical significance with the primary endpoint.

Suppose instead that a Bayesian approach is now used for the primary analysis. The primary analysis is to conclude statistical success if the posterior probability of H_A is greater than 95%. For a Bayesian analysis we assume a prior distribution of

$$p \sim \text{Beta}(1, 1) \equiv \text{Unif}(0, 1) \,,$$

resulting in the posterior distribution

$$p \mid X \sim \text{Beta}(1 + X, 1 + N - X) \,.$$

The posterior probabilities of superiority, $Pr(p > 0.5 | X)$ for $X = 57, 58, 59$, and 60 are 0.918, 0.945, 0.964, and 0.977, respectively. Therefore, the rule that statistical success is a posterior probability of superiority of at least 0.95 corresponds to a rule that 59 or more successes implies statistical success. ∎

Consistent with regulatory experience, this Bayesian rule above would be completely acceptable for the primary analysis. In this case the Type I error for this Bayesian rule is 0.044, identical to the traditional frequentist rule, as the rule is effectively the same. Regulatory agencies typically do not have "rules" around the level of posterior probability that needs to be achieved, but rather that the Bayesian rules have acceptable frequentist properties. Therefore, in order to adjust Bayesian analyses for acceptable frequentist characteristics the "hurdle," in this case a posterior probability of 0.95, can be adjusted to have adequate Type I error characteristics. This idea is demonstrated below. We also note that adjusting the Bayesian analysis to fit frequentist properties has consequences for the use of prior distributions and the Bayesian paradigm (see Section 5.5).

5.2.1 Adaptive sample size using posterior probabilities

To enhance the fixed Bayesian design of Example 5.1 we create a Bayesian adaptive design. Prospectively, we add the following interim analysis rules to the design. If at $n = 50$ or $n = 75$ there is at least a 0.95 posterior probability of superiority, then statistical success will be claimed. This rule corresponds to claiming success if $X_{50} \geq 31$ or $X_{75} \geq 45$; this is in addition to the claim of success if $X_{100} \geq 59$. At any of these thresholds the posterior probability of superiority is at least 0.95. From a frequentist perspective, the Type I error of this design is 0.0958. The design is simple enough that exact calculation of the Type I error is possible in this case (assuming $p = 0.5$):

$$1 - \sum_{i=0}^{30} \sum_{j=i}^{\min(25+i,44)} \sum_{k=j}^{\min(25+j,58)} \Pr(X_1 = i) \Pr(X_2 = j - i) \Pr(X_3 = k - j),$$

where X_1, X_2, and X_3 are independent binomial random variables with sample sizes $50, 25$, and 25, respectively, and a probability of success p. An implementation of the above in R is simple enough that we provide it here, as well as on the book's website:

R code
```
simulateP <- 0.5
answer <- 0
for (i in 0:30){
    for (j in i:min(44,25+i)){
        for (k in j:min(58,25+j)){
            pri <- dbinom(i,50,simulateP)
            prj <- dbinom(j-i,25,simulateP)
            prk <- dbinom(k-j,25,simulateP)
            answer <- answer + pri*prj*prk
        }
    }
}

> 1-answer
[1] 0.09578662
```

While this calculation is straightforward, we also provide a simulation of the design. In almost every Bayesian adaptive trial there is some form of simulation, and this simple example offers a good opportunity for illustration.

Example 5.2 *(Basic confirmatory trial, continued)*. The following R code (again provided both here and online) provides an example function, adapt1, which simulates the above design. The result of the function is the probability of statistical success (win), the mean and standard deviation of the resulting sample size, and the probability of each possible sample size. The output of this function for one million simulated trial runs is presented below. The resulting probability of statistical success, 0.09577, is based on $1,000,000$ simulated trials assuming that the true probability of success is 0.5. Recall that the theoretical value was calculated above at 0.09579.

R code
```
adapt1 <- function(simulateP,nsims,postcut,hypothesisP,nCuts){
    win <- logical(nsims)
    ss <- numeric(nsims)
```

```
    nInts <- nCuts
    for (i in 2:length(nCuts)){
       nInts[i] <- nCuts[i] - nCuts[i-1]
    }

    for (i in 1:nsims){
       x <- rbinom(length(nCuts),nInts,simulateP)
       x <- c(x[1],x[1]+x[2],x[1]+x[2]+x[3])
       ProbSup <- 1 - pbeta(hypothesisP,1+x,1+nCuts-x)

  # Probability of Success
       win[i] <- any(ProbSup > postcut )
  # Sample size
       ss[i] <- min(nCuts[ProbSup > postcut],max(nCuts))
    }
    out <- c(length(win[win])/nsims,mean(ss),
                     sqrt(var(ss)),table(ss)/nsims)
    names(out) <- c('Pr(win)','MeanSS','SD SS',as.character(nCuts))
    out
}


## Input these values for the Type I error of Example 5.2.1:
> nsims <- 1000000
> postcut <- 0.95
> hypothesisP <- 0.5
> simulateP <- 0.5
> nCuts <- c(50,75,100)
> out <- adapt1(simulateP,nsims,postcut,hypothesisP,nCuts)

> out
  Pr(win)    MeanSS      SD SS         50         75        100
 0.095770 96.455625 12.247579   0.059165   0.023445   0.917390
```

The Type I error of this design would likely be judged too high by regulatory agencies. A standard remedy for this is to raise the threshold of posterior probability until the Type I error is less than the "required level," which we are assuming is 0.05 in this setting. Table 5.1 provides the Type I error probability for various posterior thresholds, P_{cut}.

The posterior probability threshold creates a Bayesian rule for defining a statistical success. This Bayesian threshold creates the three success thresholds (at the looks of 50, 75, and 100) that define success. This situation creates an integer value problem and so the Type I error probabilities shown in Table 5.2 have discrete drops. The posterior probability threshold of $P_{cut} = 0.976$ creates a trial in which the Type I error probability, 0.0423, has been "controlled" at the one-sided 0.05 level. This posterior probability threshold implies that the values of 33, 47, and 60 successes are needed to claim success at each of the three looks ($n = 50, 75, 100$). Table 5.2 shows

P_{cut}	Type I error
0.95	0.0958
0.96	0.0692
0.97	0.0591
0.9725	0.0591
0.975	0.0532
0.976	0.0423
0.9775	0.0347
0.98	0.0347
0.99	0.0195

Table 5.1 *The Type I error for different posterior probability levels of success* (P_{cut}) *for Example 5.2.1.*

p	Pr(Win)	Mean SS	SD SS	Pr(50)	Pr(75)	Pr(100)
0.50	0.0421	98.9	6.9	0.017	0.011	0.972
0.55	0.217	94.7	14.2	0.077	0.058	0.864
0.60	0.578	84.1	21.0	0.237	0.162	0.601
0.65	0.889	69.0	21.1	0.504	0.229	0.266
0.70	0.989	57.0	14.2	0.780	0.160	0.060
0.75	0.999	51.5	6.53	0.944	0.051	0.005

Table 5.2 *Operating characteristics of the adaptive design with early stopping for success for Example 5.2.1.*

the operating characteristics of this adaptive Bayesian design for assumed probabilities that are larger than $p = 0.5$, and thus represent power calculations. These simulations (using the R function adapt1) are based on $100,000$ simulations for each case. ∎

The operating characteristics of the design demonstrate the Type I error control of the design in the previous example having Type I error of 0.0421. The power of the design for a hypothesized value of 0.65 is 0.889. Under this hypothesized value the mean sample size is 69, with a 0.504 probability of stopping for success at the 50-subject interim analysis. The larger the assumed probability of success the smaller the mean sample size. Under the hypothesis that the probability of success is 0.65 the average sample size of the adaptive trial would be 69. If a fixed trial of 69 subjects were conducted the power under the alternative hypothesis of 0.65 would be 0.802. Thus the fixed trial and the adaptive trial have the identical mean sample size,

69, yet the adaptive design has a power of 0.889 relative to 0.802 for the fixed design.

These are common operating characteristics that are created in order to justify a Bayesian design to a regulatory agency. The critical aspect of these is the Type I error of the design; the power of the design is typically not a major concern. Of course, if the design has very poor power then the regulatory agency would likely deem it unethical to conduct such a study, as it would be of little scientific credibility. In our experience, there is rarely an interaction in which 80% or 90% power – or any other level – is a regulatory restriction.

Of course, the power of a design is certainly an issue for the trial's *sponsor*. The amount of risk and the cost benefit of different sample sizes and adaptive features is of paramount concern. The power presented above is a "frequentist" calculation and is done by conditioning on a specific value. As discussed in Section 2.5, a Bayesian form of the power of this design can be found by integrating over a company-specific prior distribution. Suppose the sponsor had early phase data on the medical therapy in which there were 7 successes in 10 subjects. Using the subjective company-specific prior distribution (in this case, a Beta(7, 3)) would result in a predictive probability of success of 0.807, with a mean sample size of 62.1 (standard deviation of 20.7). The probability of stopping at the first look (50 subjects) is 0.734 and 0.049 at the second (75 subjects). These may be contrasted with the frequentist operating characteristics achieved when conditioning on the value of $p = 0.7$, which is the mean of the Beta(7,3) prior distribution.

Frequentists refer to the need for a "penalty" when performing interim analyses. This is a reference to the idea seen here that by increasing the number of opportunities for success, the Type I error is increased. Therefore a penalty (in the form of requiring a more stringent stopping threshold) must be paid at each analysis. In this example such a penalty has been implemented by increasing the threshold for the probability of success from 0.95 at the final look to 0.976 at each of the three looks. Therefore if the trial gets to the final analysis, the probability of success must be greater than 0.976, rather than 0.95. We find the term "penalty" here to be unnecessarily pejorative; in fact, the Bayesian adaptive design has merely redistributed the Type I error across several analyses to produce a design that is more powerful (as seen by the 0.889 > 0.802). The paradigm conflict inherent in tweaking Bayesian designs using frequentist criteria is discussed further in Section 5.5.

5.2.2 Futility analyses using predictive probabilities

Thus far our trial adaptation has been based only on success. Just as important is stopping for failure, or what is often termed futility. At each of the interim analysis points, 50 and 75, we could stop the trial when the likelihood of trial success is small. Stopping for success is based on reaching a threshold of posterior probability, which is the agreed upon regulatory hurdle for statistical success.

Stopping for futility based on posterior probabilities at the current look is awkward. If the posterior probability of superiority is 0.05, 0.50, or 0.75 at the interim analysis this provides little relevant information about whether the trial is ultimately going to be successful. We utilize predictive probabilities to address the likelihood that the final statistical hurdle will be met. Predictive probabilities are incredibly important tools in Bayesian adaptive designs. The following subsection introduces futility analysis using predictive probabilities.

Example 5.3 *(Basic confirmatory trial, re-continued).* Continuing on with our running example, suppose our goal is to create rules for stopping the trial for futility at the 50- and 75-subject look, or at any other time point of interest. In order to stop at the 50-subject look we are interested in the probability that the trial will be successful if it continues accruing subjects. For example, at the 50-subject look, suppose there are 25 successes. The posterior probability of superiority is 0.50. This quantity provides little information about the likelihood that the trial will result in statistical success. A big difference between earlier phase trials and confirmatory trials are the strict hurdles for success. The structure of confirmatory trials is that the hurdle for statistical success, whether based on a p-value or Bayesian posterior probability, is the most important metric and provides a clear measure of success.

Conditional on observing 25 successes and 25 failures at the 50-subject look, the current posterior distribution for p is a Beta($\alpha = 26, \beta = 26$). The predictive distribution for the next n subjects is a *beta-binomial* distribution, having a probability density function for generic α and β of

$$f(x) = \frac{\Gamma(\alpha + \beta)\Gamma(n + 1)\Gamma(x + \alpha)\Gamma(n - x + \alpha)}{\Gamma(\alpha)\Gamma(\beta)\Gamma(x + 1)\Gamma(n - x + 1)\Gamma(n + \alpha + \beta)} .$$

Figure 5.1 shows this predictive distribution of the next 25 and the next 50 observations, based on the currently observed values of 25 successes in 50 subjects and the Beta(1,1) prior distribution. The trial is defined so that statistical success occurs if 47 of the first 75 or 60 of the 100 total subjects are successes. These regions are shown on the predictive distributions using thicker line segments. The predictive probability of success at the $n = 75$ look is 0.00078, and is 0.0256 for the final analysis at $n = 100$.

As part of our adaptive design, we can create stopping rules for futility based on these predictive probabilities of success – typically the predictive probability of success at the final analysis. In this simple design, calculating the predictive probability of success at any time was not difficult, but in more complicated designs it can be quite difficult (because of the additional adaptive aspects which may themselves require predictive probabilities).

Predictive Distribution for Success at n=75

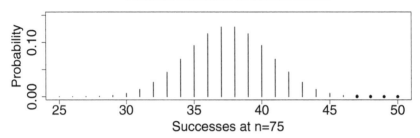

Predictive Distribution for Success at n=100

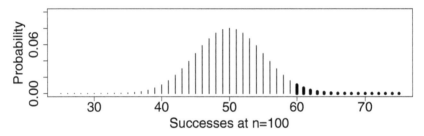

Figure 5.1 *The predictive distribution of the number of successes at the 75 and 100 subject looks for the trial in Subsection 5.2.2.*

Suppose we enhance the design by adding in a futility rule that if the probability of success at the final analysis is less than 0.05 then the trial will stop for futility. In such a design, the result of 25 successes and 25 failures at the 50-subject look would result in stopping the trial for futility. Despite the posterior probability of superiority still being moderate, the probability that the trial will ultimately result in a statistical success is remote. ■

Adding futility rules to a design does not increase the probability of a Type I error, it usually decreases it. Table 5.3 presents the operating characteristics of the adaptive design with an added rule that if at the 50- or 75-subject looks there is less than a 0.05 predictive probability of success, then the trial stops for futility. The table presents the probability of stopping for each look for success (upper number of the pair provided) and for futility (lower number). The futility rule has little impact on the probability of concluding success or failure; rather, it simply makes the same decision sooner. The mean sample sizes in the statistically easier scenarios are small, with mean sample sizes of 64.3 and 51.5 in the two extreme scenarios. In the more statistically challenging cases, such as $p = 0.55$ and $p = 0.60$, the mean sample sizes are the largest, with means of 74.1 and 76.1, respectively. In the case where $p = 0.60$ the power is 0.569,

p	Pr(Win)	Mean SS	SD SS	Pr(50)	Pr(75)	Pr(100)
0.50	0.0407	64.3	18.2	0.016	0.011	0.014
				0.555	0.275	0.129
0.55	0.215	74.1	20.7	0.078	0.059	0.078
				0.283	0.253	0.248
0.60	0.569	76.1	21.1	0.238	0.161	0.170
				0.099	0.122	0.210
0.65	0.882	67.3	20.1	0.506	0.227	0.148
				0.021	0.028	0.069
0.70	0.987	56.8	13.9	0.782	0.158	0.048
				0.003	0.003	0.008
0.75	0.999	51.5	6.4	0.945	0.050	0.005
				0.000	0.000	0.000

Table 5.3 *Operating characteristics of the adaptive design in Subsection 5.2.2 with early stopping for success and futility. The two numbers in each of the last three rows represent the probability of stopping for success (top) and futility (bottom).*

which compares to 0.578 without the futility rule. In the columns (50 and 75) where early futility is demonstrated (with probability 0.099 and 0.122, respectively), these are not necessarily "errors." They are indeed incorrect conclusions from the study, but they are almost always the same decision that would have been made had the study continued to the full sample size. These are circumstances where the early poor performance (due to randomness) caused the trial to stop earlier because the final conclusion of "fail" was inevitable.

Stopping a trial for futility does not imply that the evidence is conclusive, that the medical therapy is detrimental, or that it is conclusively inferior. It is only conclusive that the statistical hurdle is very unlikely to be met. If there are 41 successes and 34 failures at the 75-subject look then the futility rule stops the trial. (If the maximum sample size were larger, this futility rule would be different; if the maximum were 150 then 38 or fewer successes among the first 75 would lead to stopping for futility.) The predictive probability rule is driven by the current trial and the conclusions drawn in the current trial — not by some measure of learning or inference.

5.2.3 Handling delayed outcomes

One of the ways in which Example 5.3 is simple is its notion that the information on *all* of the subjects is known immediately. During an interim analysis point (say, at the 50-subject look), it is assumed that the information on all 50 subjects is known. But in many trials, the time to information for these subjects is such that there is a lag between the number of subjects in the trial and the information known at the time of the analysis. In this section we discuss adaptive sample sizes in the case where the analyses taking place have incomplete information on the subjects in the trial.

Suppose in Example 5.3 that each subject is labeled a success or failure based on a delayed outcome, such as a one-month visit for success. We assume for now that this measure of success is a medical test that is conducted one month after treatment, such that there is no information gained earlier than one month. We discuss in Subsection 5.4 the ubiquitous problem of handling longer-term outcomes when there is, possibly, information gained earlier than the final endpoint.

We extend Example 5.3 in the following way. Assume that the result for each subject is observed one month after treatment. The accrual rate of subjects then becomes an important part of the design itself. If accrual is slow relative to the one-month outcome (say, 1 subject per month) then this lag-time in outcome is essentially irrelevant, as information on almost all subjects is known at the time of an interim analysis. If there are 100 subjects accrued in a month then this lag-time in outcome would make adaptation worthless, as no information would be gained soon enough for any informed adaptations to a 100-subject trial. For this example we assume an accrual rate of 20 subjects per month. Then at any particular look at the data, there will be a lag of 20 subjects with no information. We still wish to look when 50 and 75 subjects have been enrolled, for the possibility of a smaller sample size. These looks at the data are statistically different than those in the previous trials of this chapter, in which we assumed complete information was available at each look. If the trial is stopped at the 50-subject look for (expected) success based on the 30 subjects with complete information, it may be that the data on the remaining 20 that will be collected will be negative and thus the result of the 50-subject trial will be failure.

Consistent with the Bayesian approach we employ predictive probabilities to determine when stopping is appropriate; that is, the likelihood of success for the trial is high when the "lag" of 20 subjects is observed. We consider the following design:

Algorithm 5.1 *(Adaptive design with delayed outcomes).*

Step 1: When 50 subjects are enrolled, a predictive probability of trial success for the current 50 is calculated; if greater than 0.90, the trial is stopped for expected success. If the predictive probability of trial success for the maximum number of subjects, 100, is 0.05 or less, the trial is stopped for futility.

Step 2: When 75 subjects are enrolled, a predictive probability of trial success for the current 75 is calculated; if greater than 0.90, the trial is stopped for expected success. If the predictive probability of trial success for the maximum number of subjects, 100, is 0.05 or less, the trial is stopped for futility.

Step 3: The final analysis is conducted when the trial is complete; that is, when all subjects have complete information. The prior distribution assumed for p at this point is a Beta(1,1). If the posterior probability of superiority at the final analysis is at least P_{cut}, then statistical success is claimed.

■

Example 5.4 *(Basic confirmatory trial with delayed outcomes).* Recall from Table 5.1 that when there was complete information on each subject, the threshold, P_{cut}, was set to 0.976. In this analysis the same number of interim looks are employed, but these interim looks are different. The action that is taken by these looks is to stop accrual, but there is still a reasonable amount of data that must be collected. Therefore these looks have a different implication for the Type I error. This is a common phenomenon with the advent of new adaptive designs, where the adaptive actions taken have unclear and unknown effects on the Type I error.

In this example we determine the effect by simulation. By simulating this design under the null hypothesis that $p = 0.5$, we find the effect that all the adaptive features combined have on the Type I error and then adjust the statistical hurdle P_{cut} appropriately to control the Type I error. Table 5.4 shows the Type I error for this design for different values of P_{cut} based on 100,000 simulated trials.

A very important part of adaptive designs such as this is the accrual rate. We have made the assumption in each of these simulations that the accrual rate is 20 per month. If the accrual were 100 per month then the trial would go to the maximum of 100 each time and the appropriate threshold would be $P_{cut} = 0.95$. If accrual were slow enough that all subjects' data were known then the interim analyses would be perfect information looks, as in the previous example, thus the appropriate cutoff would be $P_{cut} = 0.96$. We typically provide a range of accrual rates within the realm of possible values. Table 5.4 shows the probability of a Type I error for accrual rates of 10, 20, and 30 per month. Based on this range of accrual rates the threshold of $P_{cut} = 0.96$ is selected for the trial.

The operating characteristics for this trial, based on an accrual rate of 20 per month, are shown in Table 5.5. Relative to the values for all p, the chance of early stopping at the 50-subject look is reduced relative to Table 5.3, due to the loss of information. R code to evaluate the operating

P_{cut}	10/month	Pr(Win) 20/month	30/month
0.95	0.0551	0.0521	0.0495
0.955	0.0518	0.0471	0.0453
0.96	0.0489	0.0454	0.0452
0.97	0.0372	0.0321	0.0311
0.976	0.0316	0.0288	0.0280
0.98	0.0217	0.0195	0.0184
0.99	0.0114	0.0110	0.0104

Table 5.4 *The Type I error from different posterior probability levels of success and different monthly accrual rates in Subsection 5.2.3.*

p	Pr(Win)	Mean SS	SD SS	Pr(50)	Pr(75)	Pr(100)
0.50	0.0454	76.3	20.2	0.005 0.296	0.008 0.337	0.032 0.322
0.55	0.235	85.1	18.9	0.025 0.141	0.047 0.214	0.163 0.409
0.60	0.602	86.7	18.3	0.086 0.056	0.158 0.088	0.358 0.254
0.65	0.891	79.5	19.7	0.218 0.019	0.322 0.023	0.352 0.066
0.70	0.986	68.5	18.4	0.430 0.005	0.387 0.003	0.169 0.005
0.75	0.999	59.1	13.8	0.673 0.001	0.288 0.000	0.037 0.000

Table 5.5 *Operating characteristics of the adaptive design in Subsection 5.2.3 with a lag-time in information. The two numbers in each of the last three rows represent the probability of stopping for and achieving success (top) and failure (bottom).*

characteristics of this design is described in the appendix to this chapter, and provided on the book's website.

The adaptive looks in this trial are different from traditional group sequential methods because these looks do not result in a claim of success. The looks set the appropriate sample size based on the accruing information. The selection of the cutoffs for stopping for the appropriate sample size are typically sponsor- or designer-specified, based on the various costs and utilities of the outcomes.

There are really two different uses of "priors" in Algorithm 5.1. The first is for the final analysis at the conclusion of the study, where a Beta(1,1) prior is selected. We refer to this prior distribution as the *regulatory prior*; it is analogous to a skeptical *analysis prior* in Section 2.5. This is the prior that is important to regulatory agents and which dictates what prior is used for the final primary analysis. In Section 5.5 we discuss further the idea of using subjective priors for the regulatory prior. Barring extenuating circumstances, such as relevant historical or clinical information, the regulatory prior is flat or non-informative. The regulatory prior is rarely controversial or in dispute.

The second use of a prior distribution here is the prior that is used in the calculation of the predictive distribution. There is no reason, either foundationally Bayesian or regulatory, that these two distributions must be the same. Indeed, their roles are quite different in the trial. The regulatory prior is clear, but the prior used for the predictive distribution carries the risk of the sponsor in selecting the appropriate sample size. In many applications this prior distribution is based on either historical or sponsor-related information, similar to the *design prior* in Section 2.5. This is not unlike a fixed sample size in a classically designed trial that is typically based on the sponsor's beliefs about the relative efficacy. In an adaptive trial like this, the sponsor information is updated based on accruing information and the ability to select a more appropriate sample size. ∎

In some circumstances, selection of a noninformative prior for the purposes of sample size selection can lead to poor performance. For example, the "bathtub-shaped" Beta(0.01,0.01) prior is considered non-informative, and is arguably less informative than our standard Beta(1,1). If a predictive distribution is created from a Beta(0.01,0.01) prior when there are either no successes or no failures, this will result in a predictive distribution that is incredibly heavily centered on future results being all failures or all successes, respectively. This predictive distribution can lead to hasty decisions regarding expected success or futility. Therefore, careful consideration should be given to the prior distribution used in the sample size selection. When the trial is complete, the regulatory prior is used in the final analysis, and the prior distribution used in the design stage is no longer relevant.

p	Pr(Win)	Mean SS	SD SS	Pr(50)	Pr(75)	Pr(100)
0.50	0.0485	81.3	19.3	0.011 0.194	0.006 0.333	0.032 0.424
0.55	0.241	87.7	18.2	0.048 0.093	0.035 0.174	0.158 0.492
0.60	0.606	85.6	20.1	0.150 0.050	0.115 0.062	0.342 0.281
0.65	0.886	76.2	21.9	0.332 0.028	0.217 0.015	0.337 0.070
0.70	0.980	64.3	18.9	0.577 0.012	0.247 0.002	0.157 0.006
0.75	0.997	55.7	12.3	0.802 0.002	0.162 0.000	0.034 0.000

Table 5.6 *Operating characteristics of the adaptive design with a lag-time in information, $Beta(8,2)$ design prior. The two numbers in each of the last three rows represent the probability of stopping for and achieving success (top) and failure (bottom).*

Table 5.6 presents the operating characteristics for the previous example when the prior distribution used for the sample size selection is a $Beta(8,2)$, rather than the $Beta(1,1)$; the regulatory prior remains a $Beta(1,1)$. In this example the same cutoff value of 0.96 is used, resulting in a Type I error of no more than 0.05. The effect of the $Beta(8,2)$ design prior is that the trial stops sooner for expected success, but takes longer to stop for futility. There is little overall impact to the power or Type I error, but the total sample size is affected.

5.3 Arm dropping

There are many different adaptive features that can happen within a confirmatory trial. The ability to construct a design that fits the needs of regulatory agents, the sponsor, and the subjects within the trial is the essence of an adaptive design. In this section we add an additional experimental medical therapy arm to the trial. The goal is to construct a trial that learns which of the two therapies is better and then continues the trial with only the better of the two. In this scenario the sponsor prefers one of the treatments, and thus will select the preferable one if the results are similar. This could be the situation if one dose has a more difficult dosing schedule, more expensive dosing, or a less risky future safety profile. The assumptions made in Subsection 5.2.3 are retained. For example, the assumption that there is a lag-time of one month to observe the response is assumed in this discussion as well.

Algorithm 5.2 *(Adaptive design with arm dropping).* Label the therapies as Treatments A and B, respectively. The trial starts with both experimental medical therapy arms. An analysis of the data will be made when there are 50 subjects accrued in each arm, 100 total. At this first analysis one of the two treatment arms will be dropped. The following rules are used to determine which arm is dropped:

Step 1: If either treatment has a 0.05 or smaller predicted probability of success at the maximum sample size of 100, then that arm is dropped for futility.

Step 2: If there are two arms remaining in the trial then Treatment B is dropped unless Treatment B has a predictive probability of trial success (by the maximum sample size) at least 0.10 larger than Treatment A, in which case Treatment A would be dropped. This unbalanced rule is chosen because Treatment A is the regimen that is preferred unless the other has a reasonably larger probability of success.

Step 3: The single remaining treatment arm will continue to accrue until there are 75 subjects enrolled. At this analysis the trial will stop for expected success if the predictive probability of trial success with the current sample size is at least 0.90. The trial stops for futility if the probability of trial success at the maximum 100-subject look is less than 0.05.

Step 4: If the trial does not stop for futility then final data on each subject are observed and the final statistical analysis is conducted. The final statistical analysis is based on the posterior probability that the remaining treatment has a better than 0.50 posterior probability of having a success rate larger than 0.50. If this posterior probability is larger than P_{cut} then statistical success will be claimed.

∎

Example 5.5 *(Basic confirmatory trial with arm dropping).* The design above has an adaptive sample size, and the adaptive arm dropping has the potential of increasing the Type I error. The trial usually selects the better performing of the two treatments after 50 subjects are enrolled in each arm. This creates a possible "cherry-picking" effect and a possible increase to the Type I error. As in the previous examples, the value of P_{cut} is selected in order to preserve a Type I error restriction of 0.05. Table 5.7 provides the operating characteristics for various selections of P_{cut} (100,000 simulations). The probability each treatment is selected as the target treatment is reported in the "Pick" columns, and the probability

P_{cut}	Pr(Win)	Pick A	Win A	Pick B	Win B
0.95	0.0773	0.643	0.042	0.357	0.035
0.96	0.0730	0.644	0.038	0.356	0.035
0.97	0.0520	0.696	0.028	0.304	0.024
0.975	0.0463	0.699	0.025	0.301	0.021
0.98	0.0321	0.701	0.017	0.299	0.015
0.99	0.0188	0.701	0.010	0.299	0.009

Table 5.7 *Operating characteristics of the adaptive design with two experimental therapies from Section 5.3.*

p_A	p_B	Pr(Win)	Pick A	Win A	Pick B	Win B	Mean SS
0.50	0.50	0.0463	0.699	0.025	0.301	0.021	131.4
0.50	0.70	0.9099	0.091	0.011	0.909	0.899	131.8
0.70	0.50	0.9539	0.966	0.950	0.034	0.004	131.6
0.70	0.70	0.9939	0.718	0.713	0.282	0.281	128.7

Table 5.8 *Operating characteristics of the adaptive design with two experimental therapies from Section 5.3.*

each treatment is shown to have a success rate greater than 0.50 is reported in the "Win" columns.

In order to satisfy regulatory constraints, a cutoff value of 0.975 could be selected for the primary endpoint. In this design there are multiple treatment arms that start the trial and information about the two arms is used in order to select the preferred arm. Then adaptive sample size aspects are used to select the appropriate sample size. This is both a "learn" trial and a "confirm" trial. As far as the operating characteristics are concerned it is a "confirm" trial. All aspects of the trial are simulated and thus the Type I error probability is controlled.

Table 5.8 presents the operating characteristics of this design using a cutoff of $P_{cut} = 0.975$ and 100,000 simulations. Note that the decision rule around the two treatments favors Therapy A. Therefore, the second and third scenarios in Table 5.8 are not symmetric. This design allows an initial investigation of the two arms before selecting the treatment to be used in the single-arm stage of the design. This demonstrates a so-called "Type III error;" that is, the error of omitting a therapy. In the previous section we investigated a single arm in a similar adaptive design. When the true success rate is 0.70 in Table 5.5, the probability of statistical success is

0.986. It may be that there are two possible therapies and one of them is a "gold nugget," with a success rate of 0.70 and the other is ineffective, with success rate 0.50. If one of them is selected and the single-arm adaptive design is conducted then there is a 0.986 probability of a statistical success if the gold nugget therapy is selected. But, if the wrong therapy is selected then there is a 0.0454 probability of statistical success (and correctly so). In this example, where two arms are started and a decision is made after observing the results of 30 subjects, there is at least a 0.90 probability of the correct arm being selected through the empirical decision. The power is smaller than the 0.986, but the 0.986 ignores the Type III error, which is selecting the wrong therapy entirely. ∎

This was a very simple example in which there is a "learn" component to the confirmatory trial: the initial stage of the trial, where 50 subjects are enrolled in each arm before a decision is made as to which arm to continue to the confirmatory stage. All of the data on the selected arm are used in the confirmatory analysis. This is a simple example of a *seamless* phase II/III trial (see Section 5.7). The idea readily extends to additional arms and adaptive features in the learning stage of the trial.

5.4 Modeling and prediction

In Example 5.4, there was a lag in the receipt of information for subjects who had been accrued but had not yet had a final outcome reported. This is standard in clinical trials, as scenarios are rare in which immediate information about a subject's response is known. There are circumstances where the accrual is slow enough (say, 2-3 subjects accrued per month) that even a month delay in the response can be reasonably ignored.

A more common scenario is the one where a subject has earlier information observed that is informative about the final primary outcome, but is not itself the primary outcome. This information can come from early observations on an endpoint of interest, or from a different variable that is possibly informative about the primary endpoint. For example, a trial in spinal implant devices may record clinical success at 24 months after implantation. The observations of clinical success at 3, 6, and 12 months are typically highly correlated with the 24-month outcome, and thus these early observations can be critical to an efficient adaptive design. In diabetes, a primary endpoint in a confirmatory trial may be the 12-month change from baseline in HbA1c, a clinical measurement thought to be reflective of the subject's diet and medication behavior in recent weeks. Fasting blood glucose is a more immediate measure of possible drug efficacy. Regulatory agencies may not accept the 6-month outcome of a spinal implant study to be used in place of or as a surrogate for 24-month outcomes, nor do regulatory agents accept fasting blood glucose as a primary endpoint. Despite this, these variables can be utilized in an adaptive design to shape the adaptive decisions of the trial.

These early measures are referred to as *auxiliary variables*. Their role in adaptive designs is to inform the methodology and models used in the adaptive aspects of the design. The challenge in an adaptive design is to learn as much as possible about the treatments in order to make the most efficient adaptive decisions as possible. The auxiliary variables help in this learning process.

These variables are not "surrogate" markers in these trials, nor do we use the information on the auxiliary variable directly to shape the trial. Instead any correlation between the auxiliary variable and the primary outcome is harnessed. Using auxiliary variables involves creating a model for the relationship between the early endpoint and the final primary endpoint. This model is not a static model, but is informed by subjects that have early auxiliary variable observations and final primary endpoints. We create statistical models for this relationship, and these models will have parameters that are updated by the accruing information in the trial. Typically this model is selected to be flexible, yet as information on the relationship accrues, the models become critical to the adaptive decisions.

Utilizing these models allows for the predictive distribution of the final primary outcome to be calculated. Typically this predictive distribution is calculated using Bayesian multiple imputation. We demonstrate this approach by yet another extension of the setting running through this chapter.

Suppose the primary outcome is observed when a subject reaches one month. We now extend the example so that each subject observes an early reading of success or failure at the one-week visit. Let X be the primary observation at one month, and let Y be a dichotomous observation observed at one week. Here we assume that Y is an early indication of success ($Y = 1$) or failure ($Y = 0$), but it could be a different endpoint entirely, or any other dichotomous outcome observed at one week. We model the probability that a subject is a primary success, given an intermediate success (or failure) by defining

$$\gamma_0 = \Pr(X = 1 | Y = 0)$$

and

$$\gamma_1 = \Pr(X = 1 | Y = 1) \, .$$

To these parameters we assign independent beta priors,

$$\gamma_0 \sim \text{Beta}(\alpha_0, \beta_0) \quad \text{and} \quad \gamma_1 \sim \text{Beta}(\alpha_1, \beta_1) \, .$$

Therefore, at any interim analysis there will be subjects with complete information, an observed Y and X. There will also be a group of subjects with an observed Y, but no X, and a third group of subjects with no observed data (including those subjects that may be enrolled in the study in the future). As before, two interim analyses are conducted to determine if the trial stops early for expected success or for futility. The rules for the trial are identical to those of Algorithm 5.1, summarized again here:

Steps 1, 2: At the 50- and 75-subject interim analyses, if the predictive probability of success with the current sample size is at least 0.90, the trial stops for expected success (and all current subjects are followed through their final outcome). If the predictive probability of success at the maximum sample size of 100 is less than 0.05, the trial is stopped for futility.

Step 3: The final analysis is conducted when the final data on each of the subjects enrolled in the study are observed, The prior distribution for p is now fixed as a $Beta(1,1)$, and success is claimed if the posterior probability that $p > 0.50$ is at least P_{cut}.

Calculating the predictive distribution for the subjects with interim information allows us to calculate the predictive probability of eventual trial success. In this example, the predictive probability of one-month success for each subject with incomplete information depends on their interim value. In this example it is sufficient to consider three groups of subjects for predictions: those with no data, interim failures, and interim successes. Assume that the first n_X subjects have an observed X and Y, the second set of n_Y subjects have an observed Y, but not X, and n_0 have neither an X or Y, where $n = n_X + n_Y + n_0$. The predictive distribution of the number of successes for each of these subgroups is a beta-binomial and the exact probability for each outcome can be calculated. In many examples this cannot be done analytically, however, and so here we take an MCMC approach, where values of the primary endpoint are simulated for each subject. This collection of simulated final outcomes allows for the characterization of the predictive distribution. A straightforward sampling-based approach is as follows:

Algorithm 5.3 *(Using auxiliary variables).*

Step 1: An observation of γ_0 is drawn from its full conditional distribution,

$$\gamma_0 | X, Y \sim \text{Beta}\left(\alpha_0 + \sum_{i=1}^{n_X} I_{[X_i=1|Y_i=0]}, \beta_0 + \sum_{i=1}^{n_X} I_{[X_i=0|Y_i=0]}\right)$$

Step 2: An observation of γ_1 is drawn from its full conditional distribution,

$$\gamma_1 | X, Y \sim \text{Beta}\left(\alpha_1 + \sum_{i=1}^{n_X} I_{[X=1|Y=1]}, \beta_1 + \sum_{i=1}^{n_X} I_{[X=0|Y=1]}\right)$$

Step 3: For each subject with an observed Y, but no X, an imputed value of X is generated as

$$\Pr\left(X_i = 1 | Y, \gamma_0, \gamma_1\right) = \gamma_{Y_i}$$

Step 4: For each subject with no data (including those subjects yet to be accrued), an observed value is simulated as

$$\Pr\left(X_i = 1 | p\right) = p$$

Step 5: A value of p is simulated from its full conditional distribution,

$$p|X \sim \text{Beta}\left(\alpha + \sum_{i=1}^{n} I_{[X=1]}, \beta + \sum_{i=1}^{n} I_{[X=0]}\right).$$

At convergence, this MCMC process of successive simulation from the five distributions above creates an observation, $(\gamma_0, \gamma_1, X, p)$ from the joint posterior distribution.

∎

At an interim analysis, the critical aspect is the value of X for the current sample size and the full set of possible subjects. This vector of X is an observation from the predictive distribution of X. Note that this algorithm does not assume a single Bayesian model connecting all of the longitudinal values. Rather, when a subject has an interim value we create a beta-binomial model for the transitions – a separate "working model" for the transition from each interim state to the final success. This model is "restricted" to be updated only by those subjects with "transitions" from this model. We return to this issue in the context of Algorithm 5.7 below.

After each cycle through the simulation, we record whether a final set of X would result in a successful trial for both the current and final sample size. The proportion of simulated values that satisfy the final success criterion is the predictive probability of trial success. As is typical in MCMC calculations, an initial set of sampled parameter vectors are discarded (the MCMC "burn-in" period described in Algorithm 2.1). In this example, convergence is typically observed in only a handful of draws. In the calculations that follow, we discarded the first 500 iterations as MCMC burn-in.

Example 5.6 *(Confirmatory trial with auxiliary variables)*. Tables 5.9 and 5.10 provide an example set of data for an interim analysis. Table 5.9 provides the state of data at the time of the interim analysis. There are 50 subjects included at the analysis, with 20 of them reaching the 1-month endpoint, 15 as successes. There are also 20 subjects with interim information, of which 10 are successes and 10 are failures. Finally there are 10 subjects with no interim data observed. In order to calculate the predictive probabilities of success in the trial, the transition matrix reported in Table 5.10 is also needed. This table reports the transitions from 1-week results to the final outcomes at 1 month for those 20 individuals whose 1-month outcomes have been observed. Of the 15 1-month successes, 10 were

	S	F
1-Month	15	5
1-Week	10	10
No Data		10

Table 5.9 *The current status of 50 subjects for an example predictive probability calculation.*

| | 1-Month | |
	S	F
1-Week S	10	1
1-Week F	5	4
sum	15	5

Table 5.10 *The transition matrix for all subjects that have observed 1-month results.*

1-week successes and 5 were 1-week failures. Similarly, of the 5 1-month failures, 1 was a 1-week success and the other 4 were 1-week failures.

For the predictive distributions there are 10 subjects that are 1-week successes, and have a Beta(1+10,1+1) for the probability of transitioning to a 1-month success. The 1-week failures have a Beta(1+5,1+4) distribution for transitioning to 1-month success. The subjects with no interim data have a Beta(1+15,1+5) distribution for transitioning to successes.

A function for calculating the predictive probabilities at the 50- or 75-subject interim analyses is given on the book's website. The R code there provides the calculation for the example of Tables 5.9 and 5.10. The predictive probability of trial success for the current sample size of 50 subjects is 0.929. The predictive probability of success if full accrual to 100 is carried out is 0.942. According to the design of the study, accrual would stop and the full data would be collected to see if superiority is met. ∎

We carry out simulations of the described design in order to characterize the operating characteristics. We do this by embedding our R code within a larger program that simulates the accrual of subjects and the appropriate timing of the analyses, then reports the final trial results.

In order to create operating characteristics for this design, subject responses need to be simulated, including the early interim values. Therefore an assumption about the correlation between X and Y is needed. These assumptions do not affect the design in any way, but rather the operating characteristics observed. In order to simulate subjects in a straightforward manner and demonstrate the effects of the early observations we simulate subjects using the following "backward" simulation method.

First, a final observation is simulated for a subject, assuming a final probability of success, p,

$$\Pr(X = 1) = p .$$

An interim value is then simulated conditionally on the final value. With probability ρ the value of Y is assumed the same as the value of X, while with probability $1 - \rho$ the value of Y is assumed to be Bernoulli(0.5). If we assume a value of $\rho = 1$, then the early predictor, Y, is a perfect predictor of the final value, and $X = Y$. If we instead assume $\rho = 0$, then the early predictor is a Bernoulli(0.5), independent of the final value. In this case the early predictor is independent noise and will not aid the prediction. The modeling should learn that the interim value is not predictive and then account for the uncertainty. Values of ρ between 0 and 1 provide for various mixing probabilities, and thus various correlations between the interim and final values. The value of $P_{cut} = 0.965$ was selected by simulation. With the $Beta(1, 1)$ prior distribution, this results in cutoff values of 32, 46, and 60, at looks 50, 75, and 100, respectively.

As before, the probability of a Type I error, and the trial in general, is affected by the accrual rate. For example, if the accrual rate is 1 per month, then the interim analyses are done with complete information on all subjects but one. If the accrual rate is 100 per week then all interim analyses are done with no interim information. The accrual has a drastic affect on the information available at the interim analysis. This makes perfect sense since in an adaptive design, the goal is to adapt the trial to information that has been gained during the study, and in this case the study will be over before any information is learned. With the cutoff value of 0.965 the Type I error is 0.041 with an accrual rate of 1 per week, 0.037 with an accrual rate of 5 per week, and 0.030 with an accrual of 10 per week. All of these results assume $\rho = 1$, i.e., the early value is a perfect predictor; the FDA sometimes asks for results in extreme cases like this to see how well the algorithm works.

For the default scenario, we simulate 5 subjects per week and assume $\rho = 0.50$. Some example operating characteristics are presented in Table 5.11. The "bell-shape" of the sample sizes over p is a very common feature of adaptive designs with stopping for both efficacy and futility. For poor efficacy the trial is able to stop early for known futility. Likewise for strong efficacy the trial is able to stop early for known success. For moderate efficacies, however, the sample size is larger since more subjects are needed to determine the efficacy. The design is able to adjust to the data and create a more appropriate sample size (not always just a smaller one).

The probabilities of showing superiority ($p > 0.5$) for each assumed value

p	Pr(Win)	Mean SS	SD SS	Pr(50)	Pr(75)	Pr(100)
0.50	0.035	69.5	21.1	0.01	0.01	0.02
				0.48	0.23	0.25
0.55	0.187	79.4	21.8	0.04	0.04	0.11
				0.27	0.17	0.38
0.60	0.541	82.1	21.2	0.14	0.13	0.27
				0.11	0.07	0.27
0.65	0.855	74.7	21.3	0.32	0.26	0.27
				0.04	0.02	0.08
0.70	0.979	63.0	17.7	0.60	0.27	0.12
				0.01	0.00	0.01
0.75	0.997	55.0	11.3	0.82	0.16	0.02
				0.00	0.00	0.00

Table 5.11 *Operating characteristics of the adaptive design with a longitudinal model for interim results. The two numbers in each of the last three rows represent the probability of stopping for and achieving success (top) and fail (bottom).*

of p and five different weekly accrual rates, 1, 2, 5, 10, and 100, are shown in Figure 5.2. The probabilities of showing superiority are very close in each of these accrual scenarios, with a slight decrease when accrual is faster since the trial has less ability to find the correct sample size. The fastest accrual, 100/week, was selected because no data are known when 50 or 75 subjects are accrued, and thus each trial advances to 100 subjects in each simulated trial. The differences among accrual rates lie in the mean sample sizes in Figure 5.3. The faster the accrual, the more subjects are needed, yet there are essentially no differences in the probabilities of superiority. This demonstrates in adaptive designs the critical role that accrual plays in the ability of the design to be efficient. By accruing extremely fast (100/week) the sample size can be more than 50% larger, yet the conclusions are identical.

In order to evaluate the efficiency gained from modeling the early results, we vary the correlation of the early result (1 week) to the final result (1 month). We focus on the results for the scenario in which $p = 0.65$. Figure 5.4 shows the probabilities of concluding superiority (left axis; solid line) and the mean sample sizes (right axis; dashed line). The probability of concluding superiority generally increases as the predictive ability of the interim 1-week value increases. Additionally, the mean sample size generally decreases. In many adaptive designs it is the sample size that is

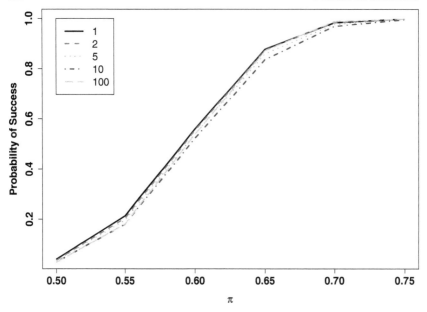

Figure 5.2 *The probability of success for five different accrual rates for the design with longitudinal modeling of an early endpoint of Section 5.4.*

affected by the ability of interim values to predict final endpoints. When information takes longer to observe in an adaptive trial, the trial needs to accrue longer before the ability to stop accrual is reached. Generally similar conclusions are drawn, but the circumstances where early predictors are available allows for these decisions to be reached more efficiently.

5.5 Prior distributions and the paradigm clash

Thus far, we have highlighted the role of the regulatory prior in confirmatory phase trials. This is the prior that is used in combination with the data to form the posterior distribution for the final analysis. Because of the nature of a confirmatory trial, it is typical that this prior represents the view of a relatively uninformed decision maker. There may be circumstances where a different analysis prior is used or desired. In these circumstances there is a clash between the role of the prior and the need to control Type I error. If a prior is used that provides favorable information for the experimental treatment, then other things being equal, the likelihood of success is increased by use of the prior. In the case where adaptive features that inflate Type I error are added to the trial the threshold for success was raised to control the Type I error. But if the threshold for success is raised to counter the effects of the prior distribution then this effectively removes

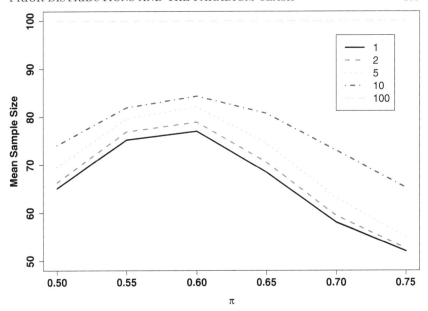

Figure 5.3 *The mean sample size for five different accrual rates for the design with longitudinal modeling of an early endpoint of Section 5.4.*

any benefit of using the prior distribution, and the two mechanisms cancel each other out.

In order to demonstrate this clash, we recall the single arm trial without adaptations from Example 5.1. Assume $n = 100$ subjects are enrolled and the final analysis must show that the posterior probability that the treatment success rate, p, is larger than 0.5 is greater than 0.95. When a Beta$(1, 1)$ prior is used, we saw in Section 5.2 that 59 or more successes resulted in a posterior probability larger than 0.95 and a Type I error of 0.0443.

Now suppose historical data that represents the entire clinical experience of the treatment in a very similar patient population resulted in 9 successes in 10 trials. Adding these data to the baseline Beta$(1, 1)$ prior results in a Beta$(10, 2)$ prior distribution. If a Beta$(10, 2)$ prior distribution is then used, then after 100 subjects a posterior probability threshold of 0.95 results in an effective cutoff of $X \geq 55$ successes. For the trial of 100 subjects, the probability that $X \geq 55$ conditional on $p = 0.5$ is 0.184. This inflation of the Type I error is due to the effects of the prior making it more likely that our posterior probability is larger than 0.95. If the approach of raising the threshold for the posterior probability to claim success is used, then this threshold must be raised to 0.9934. Of course, this threshold results in $X \geq 59$ successes again being observed out of 100 subjects. This is because

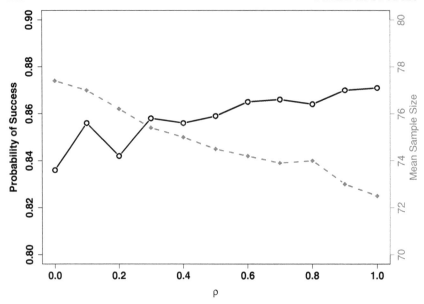

Figure 5.4 *The probability of superiority (solid line, left axis) and the mean sample size (dashed line, right axis) for the case where p = 0.65 and various values of ρ the parameter for the correlation between the early and late endpoint.*

this cutoff is determined by the frequentist Type I error, *not* a Bayesian analysis.

When the Bayesian design is required to control Type I error, it loses many of its philosophical advantages. In effect the Bayesian machinery is creating a design that is inherently frequentist. This can be the major constraint of a confirmatory trial: it must meet the conditions of the regulatory agency. There are specific rules and conditions in place, and any design must meet these rules. For this reason the role of prior distributions in confirmatory studies is rarely an issue (though see our discussion on the adaptive use of historical data in Section 6.1).

The constraint that Type I error must be controlled at a specified level creates additional conflict between the Bayesian and frequentist paradigms regarding interim data looks – for example, the adaptive design in Section 5.2.1 having interim analyses at 50 and 75 subjects. Because of these looks, the posterior probability threshold for claiming success was raised from 0.95 to 0.976. This implied that the number of successes threshold for success at the 50-, 75-, and 100-subject looks were 33, 47, and 60 respectively. In the non-adaptive design of 100 subjects, the trial is successful if 59 or more successes are observed at the 100-subject look. One trial could be run with this adaptive design, for which there could be 32, 46, and 59 successes at each of the three respective looks, and still result in an unsuccessful trial. Now suppose a second trial is run with no adaptive looks, and 59 successes are observed at 100 subjects. Suppose further that there would have been 32 and 46 successes at the interim time periods had interim analyses been conducted. In fact, assume the data for all 100 subjects are identical in each trial. The result of this second trial would be success. Therefore, we have two trials that achieve exactly the same data, yet one is successful and one is not. This result highlights a violation of the Likelihood Principle; see Subsections 2.2.3 and 2.2.7. To a Bayesian, the posterior distributions at the conclusion of each of the trials are identical. But because the rules of the trial are dictated by frequentist notions (control of Type I error), the results of the trials are different.

At some future time trials may be evaluated using fully Bayesian notions of utilities and decisions (see Section 4.6), which would enable designs to be built that do not violate the Likelihood Principle or Bayesian notions. But currently, the regulatory structure is such that confirmatory trials are usually judged and evaluated using Type I error.

5.6 Phase III cancer trials

In this section we present an example phase III cancer trial that is similar to an actual trial, but has been changed in minor ways. There is nothing cancer-specific about the design; the trial could have been constructed for a device or a drug in another therapeutic area.

The primary endpoint is time-to-failure. In an oncology setting this is typically time-to-death or time-to-disease progression. In each circumstance the "event" is a negative for the patient. Extending the time-to-failure is the desired outcome for the treatments. In this example we refer to the event as the time-to-death. Assume the historical median time of survival for subjects with this disease is 10 weeks (late stage, poor prognosis). The trial will test the standard of care (SOC) control against the standard of care plus the experimental agent (treatment). The goal is to demonstrate superiority of the treatment arm.

Assume the standard fixed design being contemplated in this circumstance is a 360-subject trial, randomized 1:1 to the treatment and SOC. Here, the primary analysis at the end of the trial, with a six-month follow-up on the last patient accrued, is a logrank test with a two-sided 0.05-level. Assuming a median survival time of 10 weeks for the SOC and 14 for the treatment arm leads to a power of 89% to demonstrate superiority. A treatment median survival time of 13 weeks provides a power of 70%. In this section we present a Bayesian adaptive alternative to this fixed design.

The structure of the trial is similar to that of the fixed trial. The randomization ratio remains 1:1 throughout, and the final analysis will remain a logrank test, though the nominal level of the test will be changed in order to control the type I error of the design.

Analyses of the data will be made for the first time when 100 subjects have been randomized. This first analysis takes place immediately upon accrual of the 100th subject, not based on the length of follow-up of the 100th subject. Therefore, if the result of the 100-subject analysis is to stop accrual, the final sample size will be 100 plus a slight overrun of subjects entering the trial. Additional analyses will be done in 20-subject increments of accrual. Thus, if the trial accrual continues, analyses will be done at 100, 120, 140, and so on to a maximum sample size of 360. The analyses are "sample size looks" only, and the conclusion of the analyses will be whether or not accrual should continue in the trial. These looks are quite different from classical O'Brien-Fleming (1979) sequential analyses. The result of these looks is not a determination of superiority, but rather a determination that the sample size is sufficient.

The rules for these sample size looks are as follows:

Algorithm 5.4 *(Phase III cancer trial design).*

Step 1: If the predictive probability of trial success with the current sample size *with 6 months additional follow-up* is larger than 0.99, then accrual will stop for *expected success*.

Step 2: If the predictive probability of trial success for the maximum sample size of 360 subjects with the full 6 months of follow-up is low less than 0.01, then accrual will be stopped for *futility*.

Step 3: If neither of the above conditions hold then accrual will continue until the next sample size analysis, or stop if the maximum of 360 subjects has been reached.

∎

If the trial stops for expected success, the last subject enrolled will be followed for the six-month minimum and the final analysis, a logrank test for superiority at the nominal level, will be performed. The sample size analyses being done shape the sample size to an appropriate value, but are different from classical sequential analyses because the analyses do not result in a determination of superiority. There is one final analysis that is conducted, after the six-months follow-up of the last subject accrued.

There are a number of aspects of the design above that have been selected without much explanation. The minimum sample size of 100 was selected to represent the smallest sample size that regulatory agencies would accept with a determination of superiority. Typically this number would be negotiated with the various scientific review bodies. The maximum sample size of 360 was selected as the sample size of the classically powered study. There is no reason that this should be the case; in fact, the strength of the trial is the ability to shape the sample size appropriately and a larger maximum would provide greater power with little impact on the mean sample size. We explore this effect on power and the mean sample size below.

The cutoff values of 0.99 and 0.01 are selected by the sponsor of the study to represent the amount of "risk" involved. The values of 0.01 and 0.99 are quite conservative. For example, in a classically powered study, a power of 80% is frequently employed to select the sample size. These stopping cutoffs represent selections with much more certainty around the final outcome. The accrual rate expected (and a range of values) and the relatively small median times of survival allow for these conservative values to be selected. If the median time of survival were larger, these "more extreme" values would be harder to reach. The minimum of 6-month follow-up is a restriction that is not always present, but in many cancer trials it is a requirement of the trial. This has some ethical aspects since this restriction assures each patient that they will contribute scientifically to the conclusions of the study.

The final analysis of the trial will be a logrank test. In order to model the interim results and the predictive distribution of the study results, a Bayesian time-to-event model is created. Due to the relatively short median times to event and historical modeling of the times of events, an exponential time-to-event model is selected with a hazard rate specific to each treatment group. Let Y_i be the time to event for subject i, for $i = 1, \ldots, n$. Let the trial arm for subject i be d_i, where $d = 1$ refers to the SOC and $d = 2$ refers to the treatment. We assume an exponential time-to-event model,

$$f(t) = \lambda_d \exp\left(-\lambda_d t\right) \text{ for } d = 1, 2 \text{ ,}$$

and independent prior distributions for the two treatment hazard rates,

$$\lambda_d \sim \text{Gamma}\left(\alpha = 1, \beta = 0.1\right) \text{ for } d = 1, 2 \text{ .}$$

These prior distributions are equivalent to assuming 1 event in 10 weeks (the unit of time in the model), and do not affect the final logrank analysis. These priors shape the sample size, but have only a small effect on the conclusions of the sample size looks. This is because at the first analysis (the 100-subject look), there will be enough follow-up and events that this "one subject worth of information" in the prior will have little weight. We refer to this model as an adaptive design *working model* because it drives the adaptive aspects of the design, but is not the final analysis, and has little impact outside of the adaptive design.

At an interim analysis, the predictive distributions are the quantities that drive the adaptive design. The calculation of the predictive probabilities of trial success via MCMC is now described. The sufficient statistics within each treatment arm d at the time of an interim analysis are the total exposure, E_d, and the number of events, X_d. The following successive steps are taken in the computation:

Algorithm 5.5 *(Phase III cancer trial MCMC sampler).*

Step 1: Simulate hazard rates for each treatment group from their full conditional distributions,

$$\lambda_d | E_d, X_d \sim \text{Gamma} \left(\alpha + X_d, \beta + E_d \right) \text{ for } d = 1, 2 \ .$$

Step 2: Simulate the final time-to-event for each subject, conditional on the hazard rate for the respective treatment group, λ_d, and the current censored time, Y_i^c, by taking advantage of the memoryless property of the exponential distribution:

$$Y_i | \lambda_d, X_d \sim Y_i^c + \text{Exponential} \left(\lambda_d \right) \ .$$

Step 3: Evaluate the logrank test for the current sample size $(Y_1, \dots, Y_n)$, and an additional 6 months of follow-up for all subjects.

Step 4: Evaluate the logrank test for the maximum sample size, $(Y_1, \dots, Y_{360})$, and an additional 6 months of follow-up for all subjects. This step involves an assumption in the calculations for the accrual rate. In an actual trial a prospective rule will need to be made for the future accrual rate, such as the average accrual over the last two months. In this example we use the true accrual rate.

Steps 1-4 are then repeated M times; note that this is a "one-off" (not iterative) Monte Carlo algorithm, so there is no need to delete any portion of the sample as burn-in. For a nominal level of the logrank test, α, we record the frequency of trials in Steps 3 and 4 that demonstrate superiority. The frequency of trials in Step 3 that demonstrate superiority is the predictive probability of superiority with the current sample size. The frequency of trials in Step 4 that demonstrate superiority is the predictive probability of superiority with the maximum sample size. ■

In order to evaluate the operating characteristics and to find an appropriate nominal α-level for the logrank test, we perform simulations of the design. Simulated trials are created, with an assumed accrual rate and assumed median survival times in each treatment group. To simulate the times-to-death we assume an exponential rate in each group with the specified median survival times. The trials are carried out exactly as described above. For each of the scenarios of interest, we simulate a mean accrual of 5 subjects per week, with an implied Poisson distribution for the number of subjects per week (due to the exponential distribution for waiting times until the next accrual).

Next we select a set of null hypotheses to evaluate the Type I error of the design. We assume the regulatory restriction is a one-sided Type I error of 0.025. Figure 5.5 shows the simulated Type I error rate for each nominal α-level used in the final superiority analysis between 0.010 and 0.025. For each nominal α level, 1000 simulated trials are conducted. The simulated Type I error is the proportion of simulated trials where the simulated data

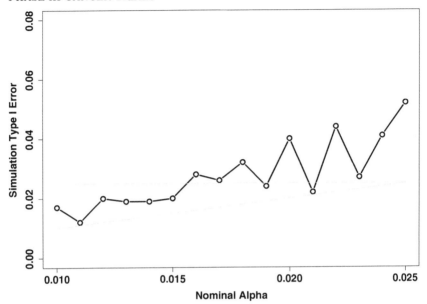

Figure 5.5 *The simulated Type I error for each nominal α-level for the cancer phase III trial.*

meets the condition of significance after 6 months of follow-up on the last subject accrued.

Due to there being just 1000 simulated trials per nominal α level, there is simulation error in the estimated Type I error rates. However, our results suggest a nominal α level of 0.015 does control the Type I error at the one-sided 0.025 level. Typically in a submission to regulatory agencies additional null scenarios as well as more simulated trials are used to justify the nominal α chosen; in this trial we use the nominal value $\alpha = 0.015$.

Simulations of the design using $\alpha = 0.015$ for the final analysis were then carried out with 1000 simulated trials per scenario. Table 5.12 presents a subset of operating characteristics for the adaptive design. In each case the median time-to-event for the control group is 10 weeks, while the median time-to-event for the treatment group is varied from 8 weeks to 16 weeks. The probability the trial concludes superiority at the final analysis is reported in the "Sup" column. The mean of the sample size is reported in the the "N" column. The probability the trial runs to the maximum sample size is reported in the "Max" column. The last six columns then report the reason for stopping accrual in the trial and the resulting conclusion at the final analysis. "Expect S" refers to stopping for expected success, "Cap" refers to stopping because of reaching the maximum sample size, and "Futility" refers to stopping for futility. If the maximum sample size of

Case	Sup	N	Max	Expect S		Cap		Futility	
				Sup	No	Sup	No	Sup	No
8	.000	128.2	.00	.00	.00	.00	.00	.00	1.0
10	.020	202.4	.07	.02	.00	.01	.03	.00	.95
11	.129	249.3	.19	.09	.00	.04	.08	.00	.79
12	.356	276.1	.34	.25	.00	.11	.14	.00	.50
13	.634	271.3	.33	.50	.00	.13	.12	.00	.24
14	.819	247.8	.23	.72	.00	.10	.07	.00	.11
15	.945	211.1	.11	.90	.00	.04	.03	.00	.03
16	.983	186.0	.04	.96	.00	.02	.01	.00	.01

Table 5.12 *Operating characteristics for the cancer phase III design. In each case the control median time-to-event is 10 weeks. The case refers to the treatment median, varied from 8 weeks to 16 weeks. The probability the trial concludes superiority is listed in the "Sup" column. The mean sample size is reported in the "N" column. The probability of the trial running to the maximum sample size of 360 is reported in the "Max" column. The last six columns report the reason the trial stopped (top row) and the conclusion of the trial, "Sup" for superiority and "No" for no superiority.*

360 is reached and the conclusion is expected success or futility, then the result is recorded as the latter rather than the former. Regardless of when it occurs, the result of the final analysis is recorded as superiority ("Sup") or non-superiority ("No").

The results demonstrate the typical bell shape to the expected sample size. For cases where there is no effect, or a negative effect, then the mean sample size is quite small. In cases where the efficacy is strong, the sample size is also small. For the more statistically challenging intermediate cases, the sample size tends to be larger. Figure 5.6 presents the mean sample size (triangles) for each of the treatment median values (circles). Figure 5.6 also presents the probability of concluding superiority for each treatment median value. This ability to understand the underlying treatment effect and shape the appropriate sample size is a positive for the sponsor, for the subjects in and out of the trial, and for the scientific community.

In cases where the treatment is detrimental or ineffective the design determines this very efficiently. In the null hypothesis case (median=10) the mean sample size is 202, only 56% of the maximum sample size. This mean sample size saves resources, prevents subjects from being randomized to ineffective treatments, and saves time. Additionally, there are limited experimental subjects and using these valuable resources on treatments that are ineffective may prevent or delay other positive treatments from being investigated. In cases where the treatment is effective, the ability to deter-

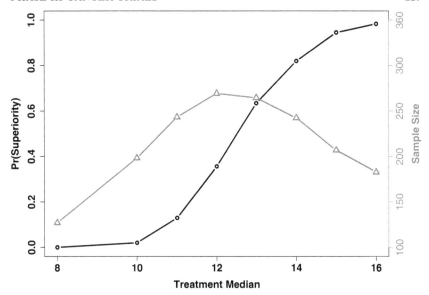

Figure 5.6 *The probability of concluding superiority (circles) and the mean sample size (triangles) for each treatment median time-to-event.*

mine this quickly and efficiently is critical. In the case where the treatment has a median time-to-event of 15 weeks, the adaptive trial has 94.5% power with a mean sample size of only 211 (59% of 360). The savings in subjects is important, but the time savings to make the conclusion is perhaps more important. The subjects outside of this trial, needing treatment, benefit greatly from the adaptive design.

The scientific community benefits as well, because the trials are more powerful per subject. Using 360 subjects unnecessarily has negative consequences to regulators and the medical community alike. As a comparison to the adaptive design, we present the results for several fixed design trials. For each of the fixed trials, the same assumptions for accrual rate and the underlying truth about the two treatment arms are made. For these fixed designs a nominal one-sided α of 0.025 is used (recall the adaptive design uses $\alpha = 0.015$). Figure 5.7 presents the probability of concluding superiority for the adaptive design (solid line). The probability of superiority for the fixed designs with 360 subjects and 100 subjects are also reported. These fixed designs are for the minimum and maximum sample sizes of the adaptive design. Note that the Bayes design does virtually as well as the full 360-patient study, but with far fewer samples on average.

There is more to the adaptive design than just understanding the treatment efficacy and then selecting the appropriate sample size. For each case we also created a fixed trial with the same sample size as the mean of the

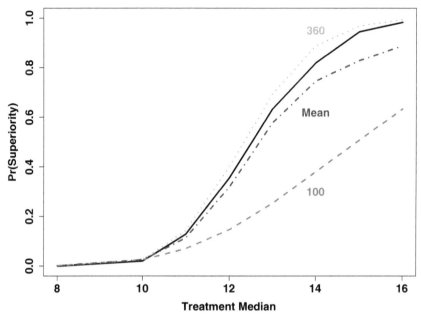

Figure 5.7 *The probability of concluding superiority for the adaptive design, a fixed design with 360 subjects, a fixed design with 100 subjects, and a fixed design where the sample size is equivalent to the mean sample size for each case.*

adaptive trial. For instance, when simulating this fixed design when the case has a treatment median of 14, a fixed sample size of 248 is used. This represents a "super smart" fixed trial, where the sample size depends on the true underlying median. The probability of superiority for this fixed design (referred to as "Mean") is also presented in Figure 5.7. Note that the adaptive design has higher power than the fixed design with exactly the same mean sample size. The strength of the adaptive design is not just getting the appropriately powered sample size, it is the ability to adjust to the results of the individual trial. Even in the case where the treatment median is 16, there are trials simulated where the results are not strong enough for superiority with 188 subjects. The power of the fixed-188 design for this case is 0.889. The adaptive design also has a mean sample size of 188, but has a power of 0.983.

5.7 Phase II/III seamless trials

Of recent interest and promise for the Bayesian approach are so-called *seamless* phase II/III designs. Typically in drug development, phase II trials, whether adaptive or not, are run for the goal of determining the next steps in the development of the drug. The data from the dose-finding phase

II trial are collected and analyzed. Decisions are then made as to whether a phase III trial should be conducted and which dose or doses will be used. Typically meetings take place with regulatory to review these decisions and to design the phase III trial. This time between the phase II trial and the phase III trial can be substantial (9 months to 2 years). Additionally, if a phase III trial is conducted, the data collected in the phase II trial is typically ignored in the evaluation of phase III.

Both of these issues have lead to the desire to develop seamless phase II/III trials. The idea of a seamless phase II/III trial is to conduct a dose-finding phase II trial, which depending on the data could spawn the start of a phase III trial, which happens "seamlessly," immediately after phase II. Randomization is taking place during the phase II aspect of the trial and a prospective decision is reached to shift to the phase III part of the trial. When this happens subjects will continue to be randomized, but typically in a different manner (perhaps a 1:1 comparison). The protocol for the trial is prospectively set up so that the trial would continue despite the shift from phase II to phase III. The seamless shift removes the time between trials, often resulting in shortened development time for the drug.

The creation of the phase III shift at the conclusion of phase II implies that phase III and the rules for shifting to phase III have to be completely prespecified before phase II starts. Thus the task of designing phase III after a typical phase II trial is done instead is undertaken before the phase II trial starts. Phase II, phase III, and the decisions to shift to phase III are all predetermined and prespecified.

There are two distinct ways in which a seamless phase II/III trial is designed. The first, referred to as an *operationally seamless* design, ignores the phase II aspect of the trial when evaluating the phase III part of the trial. In this case the phase III trial is typical in that the analysis and determination of the success of the drug is based exclusively on the data in the phase III trial. By contrast, an *inferentially seamless* trial involves analyzing all subjects from both the phase II and phase III stages of the trial for the final analysis. The benefit of an operationally seamless trial is the reduction of the time between the phase II and the phase III trial. Additionally, the sites for the design are already created and actively accruing subjects. The advantages of an inferentially seamless trial include those of the operationally seamless trial, but additionally the subjects from the phase II part of the trial are included in the final analysis of phase III. This allows for the phase II subjects to shape both the adaptive decisions of the phase II trial (the learning aspect of the trial) as well as the confirmation.

From a regulatory perspective, an inferentially seamless trial is really one large phase III trial. The first subject in the trial (at the phase II stage) is possibly included in the confirmatory analysis at the conclusion of the phase III stage. We note that some companies rely upon the results from phase II to raise capital for the phase III trial. An inferentially seamless

trial, while more efficient, usually blinds the sponsor from the results of
the data from the phase II stage of the trial and thus from using them
in raising capital. Employing an operationally seamless design allows the
sponsor to see and use the phase II trial data.

5.7.1 Example phase II/III trial

In this subsection we provide an example seamless phase II/III trial. This
is not a real trial, but is loosely based on similar trials that have been
built and conducted. The example is in spinal cord injury. In spinal cord
injury, a patient can suffer varying degrees of paralysis. The standard measure of the severity of paralysis is the American Spinal Injury Association
(ASIA) scale. The scale is categorical, with possible outcomes A (no function), B (sensory only), C (some sensory and some motor), D (useful motor
function), and E (normal). We assume that the trial enrolls subjects with
an acute injury who are initially classified as ASIA category A. A standard measure of success is the ASIA classification at 6 months. Assume
the confirmatory regulatory primary analysis is the probability a subject
progresses to ASIA C at 6 months. Each subject will have monthly measures of their ASIA score. It is possible for a subject to transition in either
direction on the ASIA score from month to month (e.g. B to A or B to C),
but positive transitions are most likely. Historically, about 10% of subjects
progress from ASIA A at entry to at least ASIA C at 6 months.

This is an ideal situation for a seamless phase II/III trial. The condition
is reasonably rare, providing a forced, slow accrual rate. The regulatory
endpoint of 6-month ASIA score is well known and well understood, and
thus there is little need for the time between trials to design the phase
III study. Finally, the phase III aspect of the trial is necessarily designed
before the phase II trial.

Four experimental doses are under consideration, and a placebo arm
is used for a control. We construct a seamless phase II/III design that
first investigates the dose-response relationship of the treatment and makes
a determination about its efficacy relative to placebo. The trial has the
possibility to shift seamlessly to a confirmatory stage. At the conclusion
of the trial the subjects in the arm selected in Stage 1 will be compared
to a placebo. The design will be inferentially seamless; all subjects from
each of the arms will be included in the final analysis, whether they were
accrued during Stage 1 or Stage 2. From a regulatory perspective this trial
is treated as a confirmatory trial. That is, from the first subject enrolled,
each is treated as though he or she is in a phase III type trial.

5.7.2 Adaptive design

Assume there are four experimental doses, $d = 1, 2, 3, 4$, and a control, $d = 0$. We label the ASIA scores as 1 (A), 2 (B), 3 (C), 4 (D), and 5 (E). Let Y_{it} be the ASIA score for subject i at monthly visit t, for $i = 1, ..., n$ and $t = 1, ..., 6$. During Stage 1 there is a possibility of a *target* experimental dose being selected to advance to Stage 2. At the conclusion of the trial, if Stage 2 is conducted, a primary analysis is conducted testing the superiority of the target dose selected in the first stage against the control.

Let p_d be the probability that a subject has an ASIA score of 3 or greater at 6 months with treatment arm d. We use T to refer to the target dose d selected in Stage 1 of the trial. We test

$$H_0 : p_T \le p_0$$

against the alternative

$$H_A : p_T > p_0 .$$

A classical frequentist test is conducted and superiority will be claimed if the test is significant at the nominal $\alpha = 0.014$ level (this value will be explained and justified to control Type I error across both stages).

We construct the following design, explaining Stage 2 first. If the decision is made to conduct Stage 2, then the trial will shift immediately from the Stage 1 design, with no delay, to Stage 2. In Stage 2 the target dose selected during Stage 1 will be randomized 1:1 to placebo, with 100 subjects accrued in each arm. Therefore, Stage 2 is a traditional-looking fixed aspect of the design.

During Stage 1 we begin with an initial allocation of 3 subjects per dose (including placebo). During this initial period a total of 15 subjects will be allocated in block fashion, 1:1:1:1:1, to the five arms. After the accrual of the 15th subject an analysis occurs and the allocation probabilities of the five arms are set. Initial analyses will be done monthly after the first analysis, and the following algorithm will be employed:

Algorithm 5.6 *(Seamless phase II-III trial design).*

Step 1: If there are at least 50 subjects in the trial and the predictive probability of the most likely effective dose 90 (ED90; defined in Subsection 5.7.4) showing superiority by the end of Stage 2 is at least 0.90, then Stage 1 ends and Stage 2 starts with the most likely ED90 as the target dose.

Step 2: If there are at least 50 subjects in the trial and the predictive probability of the most likely ED90 showing superiority by the end of Stage 2 is less than 0.10, then the trial ends for futility.

Step 3: If the maximum sample size of 150 in Stage 1 has been reached then if the predictive probability of the most likely ED90 showing superiority by the end of Stage 2 is at least 0.80 then Stage 1 ends and

Stage 2 starts with the most likely ED90 as the target dose. If the predictive probability is not at least 0.80 then the trial ends for insufficient evidence of success.

Step 4: If none of the conditions above hold then the randomization probabilities for the five arms are reset and Stage 1 continues.

The maximum sample size during Stage 1 is 150 and the maximum sample size during Stage 2 is 200. The transition between Stage 1 and Stage 2 is immediate and the decision to transition to Stage 2 happens immediately upon accrual of the 150th subject, if the transition has not been made earlier. ∎

5.7.3 Statistical modeling

For our statistical model, we use a first-order dynamic linear model (DLM; see West and Harrison, 1989) for the dose-response model for the probability of a subject having an ASIA score of 3 or better at 6 months. Let

$$p_d = \Pr\left(Y_{i6} \geq 3 | d_i = d\right).$$

We model the log-odds, $\theta_d = p_d/(1 - p_d)$, as follows. The DLM is

$$\theta_1 \sim N\left(-2, 2^2\right)$$

and

$$\theta_d \sim N\left(\theta_{d-1}, \tau^2\right) \text{ for } d = 2, 3, 4.$$

The log-odds for the placebo is modeled as

$$\theta_0 \sim N\left(-2, 2^2\right).$$

The parameter τ^2 is a variance component, referred to as the drift parameter. It dictates the amount of smoothing from dose to dose in the dose-response model. In the first-order DLM this parameter regresses the value at each dose to the neighboring doses. The second-order DLM regresses the parameter at each dose according to a linear growth model. We model the parameter τ with an inverse-gamma prior distribution,

$$\tau^2 \sim IG\left(\alpha = 2, \beta = 1\right),$$

where the pdf of the inverse-gamma distribution is taken as

$$p(\tau^2 | \alpha, \beta) = \frac{\exp\left(-\frac{1}{\beta \tau^2}\right)}{\Gamma(\alpha)\beta^\alpha \left(\tau^2\right)^{(\alpha+1)}}.$$

In order to model the early values of the ASIA scores (weeks $1, \ldots, 5$), we create an *adaptive design longitudinal model*. This model correlates the 6-month ASIA score and the earlier interim values. This model is updated by the observations of subjects at the earlier times and the 6-month value.

For each time t, we model the probability of a subject being a 6-month ASIA 3 or greater ($Y_{i6} \geq 3$) conditional on a value of $Y_{it} = 1$, $Y_{it} = 2$, and $Y_{it} = 3$,

$$\Pr\left(Y_{i6} \geq 3 | Y_{it} = k, d_i = d\right) = \frac{\exp\left(\theta_d + \gamma_{tk}\right)}{1 + \exp\left(\theta_d + \gamma_{tk}\right)} \quad \text{for } t = 1, \ldots, 5, k = 1, 2, 3 \,.$$

There are 3 parameters for each of the 5 time periods, for a total of 15 parameters. The following independent priors are selected for the γ's:

$$\gamma_{t1} \sim N\left(-2, 1\right) \text{ for } t = 1, \ldots, 5$$

$$\gamma_{t2} \sim N\left(1, 1\right) \text{ for } t = 1, \ldots, 5$$

and

$$\gamma_{t3} \sim N\left(2, 1\right) \text{ for } t = 1, \ldots, 5.$$

A value of $\gamma = 0$ implies that the likelihood of success at 6 months is equivalent to "no information," or a subject with no interim information. A value larger than 0 implies a higher likelihood of success and a value less than 0 implies a smaller likelihood of success.

5.7.4 Calculation

The joint posterior distribution is calculated using MCMC. The sequential draws are described below. The predictive probability of trial success (including the 100 additional subjects per arm in Stage 2) is calculated by simulating 6-month values for each subject in the trial and each possible prospective subject in Stage 2. The following steps are used in the MCMC routine:

Algorithm 5.7 *(MCMC for seamless phase II-III trial).*

Step 0: Set the starting value for each parameter.

Step 1: Simulate γ_{tk} for $t = 1, \ldots, 5$ and $k = 1, 2, 3$ from its full conditional distribution,

$$p\left(\gamma_{tk} | \theta, \gamma, T_{tk}^+, T_{tk}^-\right) \propto \frac{\exp\left(\theta_d + \gamma_{tK}\right)^{T_{tk}^+}}{\left[1 + \exp\left(\theta_d + \gamma_{tK}\right)\right]^{T_{tk}^+ + T_{tk}^-}} \exp\left(-\frac{\left(\gamma_{tk} - \mu_k\right)^2}{2}\right),$$

where μ_k is the prior mean for γ_{tk}, T_{tk}^+ is the number of subjects that transitioned from k at time t to a 3 or greater at time 6, and T_{tk}^- is the number of subjects that transitioned from k at time t to less than 3 at time 6. Observations are simulated using a Metropolis-Hastings step.

Step 2: Simulate Y_6 for each subject currently in Stage 1, assuming the most recent observation of $Y_t = k$:

$$\Pr\left(Y_{i6} = 3 | t, k, \gamma, \theta\right) = \begin{cases} \frac{\exp(\theta_d)}{1 + \exp(\theta_d)}, & t = 0 \\ \frac{\exp(\theta_d + \gamma_{tk})}{1 + \exp(\theta_d + \gamma_{tk})}, & t = 1, \ldots, 5 \end{cases}$$

Step 3: Simulate θ_D for $D = 0, 1, ..., 4$ from its conditional distribution,

$$p\left(\theta_D | Y_6, \theta_{D-1}, \theta_{D+1}, \tau^2\right) \propto \frac{[\exp(\theta_D)]^{\sum_{i:d_i=D} I_{[Y_{i6}=3]}}}{[1 + \exp(\theta_D)]^{n_D}} p(\theta_D),$$

where n_D is the sample size for dose D and the prior is

$$p(\theta_D) = \begin{cases} \exp\left(-\frac{(\theta_D+2)^2}{2*2^2}\right) & D = 0 \\ \exp\left(-\frac{(\theta_D+2)^2}{2*2^2} - \frac{(\theta_D - \theta_{D+1})^2}{2*\tau^2}\right) & D = 1 \\ \exp\left(-\frac{(\theta_D - \theta_{D-1})^2}{2*\tau^2} - \frac{(\theta_D - \theta_{D+1})^2}{2*\tau^2}\right) & D = 2, 3 \\ \exp\left(-\frac{(\theta_D - \theta_{D-1})^2}{2*\tau^2}\right) & D = 4 \end{cases}$$

Step 4: Simulate τ^2 from its full conditional distribution,

$$p(\tau^2 | \theta) = IG\left(\alpha + \frac{3}{2}, \left[\beta^{-1} + \frac{1}{2} \sum_{d=2}^{4} (\theta_d - \theta_{d-1})^2\right]^{-1}\right)$$

Step 5: Simulate Z_D, the number of successes in 100 subjects (Stage 2) for each arm, $D = 0, 1, 2, 3, 4$, where

$$Z_D \sim \text{Binomial}\left(100, \frac{\exp(\theta_D)}{1 + \exp(\theta_D)}\right).$$

Repeat Steps 1 through 5 $M + B$ times, where the first B are burn-in simulations and are ignored; values such as $B = 1000$ and $M = 5000$ are typically appropriate. ∎

We note that, as in Algorithm 5.3, in this algorithm we use "working models" to more easily handle the evolution of a subject's data over time. That is, if a subject has her last value at month 3 then we use the single model from month 3 to month 6; it is updated only by those subjects making that full transition from 3 to 6 months. If a subject has 4 months and we simulate the final 6-month value, we do not go back and use the subject's 3-month value *and* her imputed 6-month value.

The predictive probability of trial success at the end of the entire trial is estimated by the empirical frequency of all trial successes in both stages. That is, the final analysis includes both Stage 1 observations where $X_D = \sum_{i:d_i=d} Y_{i6}$ Stage 1 successes *and* the Stage 2 observations in Z_D in which the combination is statistically significantly superior at the one-sided nominal 0.014-level over the observations for placebo. For each of the M observations from the posterior, there is a set $(\theta_0, \ldots, \theta_4)$ that defines the probability of success in each group, $(p_0, ..., p_4)$. For each simulation, assuming the probabilities $p_0, ..., p_4$ there is an *effective dose 90*, or ED90, defined as the smallest dose that achieves at least 90% of the maximal benefit from placebo. This is the smallest d such that

$$p_d > 0.90 * (\max(p_d) - p_0) .$$

If no $p_d > p_0$ then we refer to the placebo, $d = 0$, as the ED90. The posterior probability that dose d is the ED90 is estimated by the empirical frequency of posterior simulations for which this is true. The dose with the maximum posterior probability of being the ED90 is referred to as the *most likely ED90*. At each interim analysis this dose has the possibility of being defined as the target dose and advancing to Stage 2.

Additionally, we use the posterior probability of each dose being the ED90 in order to set the randomization vector for each month, during Stage 1. When we reset the randomization probabilities each month we assign a randomization vector such that the probability of each active dose, $d = 1, \ldots, 4$, is proportional to the probability it is the ED90. The placebo's randomization probability is proportional to the maximum probability an experimental dose is the ED90. The randomization vector is then normalized to sum to 1.

5.7.5 Simulations

In order to evaluate the operating characteristics of the design and set a nominal α level, we again use simulation. In order to simulate the design as described we must simulate subjects with known probabilities of being 6-month successes, as well as each of their monthly ASIA scores, $Y_{i1}, \ldots, Y_{i6}$. We create the following mechanism for simulating subjects.

First, since states D and E are very rare, we simply group states C, D, and E into a single category ("C+"), resulting in a space with three states instead of five. We then create a Markov chain on this reduced state space, $1, 2, 3$, for the subjects and simulate transitions starting at $t = 0$ and continuing at discrete time transitions for each monthly visit for $t = 1, \ldots, 6$. We construct different transition matrices in order to create different 6-month success rates. We assume a default transition probability matrix for the categorical values, $k = 1, 2, 3$, as

$$\begin{bmatrix} 1 - \lambda_1 & \lambda_1 & 0 \\ \lambda_{-1} & 1 - \lambda_1 - \lambda_{-1} & \lambda_1 \\ 0 & \lambda_{-1} & 1 - \lambda_{-1} \end{bmatrix}$$

We assume default values of a subject improving by 1 state in a time period as $\lambda_1 = \delta_1 = 0.10$, and the default probability of a subject worsening by 1 state in one period as $\lambda_{-1} = \delta_{-1} = 0.03$. Using these default values a subject has a 0.10545 probability of being a 6-month success. In order to vary this probability we create a log-odds effect to the δ values to achieve the desired 6-month success probability. We define the "up one" and "down

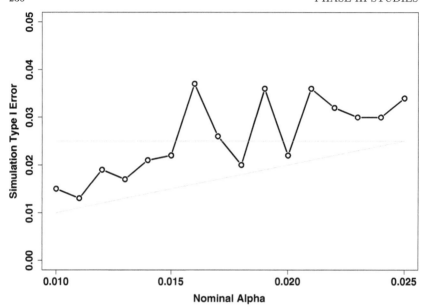

Figure 5.8 *The Type I error of the seamless design for a range of nominal α levels.*

one" transition probabilities as

$$\lambda_1 = \frac{\exp\left\{\log\left(\frac{\delta_1}{1-\delta_1}\right) + \phi\right\}}{1 + \exp\left\{\log\left(\frac{\delta_1}{1-\delta_1}\right) + \phi\right\}} \text{ and } \lambda_{-1} = \frac{\exp\left\{\log\left(\frac{\delta_{-1}}{1-\delta_{-1}}\right) - \phi\right\}}{1 + \exp\left\{\log\left(\frac{\delta_{-1}}{1-\delta_{-1}}\right) - \phi\right\}}.$$

By changing the values of ϕ, different 6-month success rate values can be created in a manner consistent with the general structure provided in the default transition matrix. For example, a value of $\phi = -0.033$ creates a 6-month rate of 0.10, which is used to simulate the results for subjects in the placebo arm. A value of $\phi = 0.725$ provides a 6-month probability of success of 0.30. Note that the methodology used to simulate patients does not affect the design itself; any approach can be used to simulate subjects.

We now provide a general structure to test the design. An accrual rate of 100 subjects per year is assumed. In each case, 10,000 simulated trials are conducted. We first simulate trials from the null hypothesis, where the true probability of success, ASIA C or better at 6 months, is 0.10 for all four experimental arms and the placebo. Figure 5.8 presents the proportion of simulated trials that select a target dose in Stage 1 and advance to Stage 2, with an outcome of superiority of the target dose at the completion of Stage 2. This would represent a Type I error for the combined trial.

We select the nominal value of 0.014 for the primary final analysis. This

Dose	p	n_I	Pr(Go)	Pr(Win)
0	.10	29.3	–	–
1	.10	21.8	.034	.005
2	.10	14.6	.012	.004
3	.10	13.9	.014	.005
4	.10	17.7	.025	.007
Total	–	97.3	.085	.021

Table 5.13 *Operating characteristics of the seamless phase II-III design under the null hypothesis.*

value controls the Type I error based on this and other simulations of null scenarios. Figure 5.8 shows that the Type I error inflation of the study is not large. Based on the general pattern of the Type I error as a function of the nominal value, there is about a 1% difference between the simulated Type I error of the adaptive design and its nominal value. Despite the design's ability to select a high-performing arm in Stage 1 of the trial, this "cherry picking" does not lead to a substantial increase in the Type I error. In part this is because a dose-response model is used for the four doses. This reduces the inflation of any arm's performance; the model uses information from neighboring doses and thus controls the multiplicities better than four paired comparisons. Additionally, the size of Stage 2, 100 per arm, is quite a bit larger than the size of Stage 1, which rarely places more than 40 subjects on a single dose.

Tables 5.13–5.17 present some operating characteristics of the seamless phase II-III design for various null and non-null scenarios. In all of these tables, the p column reports the true probability of 6-month outcomes of ASIA C or better for each dose, while the n_I column reports the mean sample size per arm in Stage 1. The "Pr(Go)" column reports the probability of each dose being selected as the target dose and advancing to Stage 2 of the design. For placebo (Dose 0), the Total Pr(Go) is the probability it is used in Stage 2, since it moves on only if the trial itself continues on. Finally, the "Pr(Win)" column is the probability that a dose is selected as the target dose *and* is shown to be superior to placebo in the final analysis.

Table 5.13 summarizes the results under the null hypothesis. The mean sample size of Stage 1 of the trial is 97.3. The probability that Stage 1 stops for futility is 0.662, with a 0.253 probability of Stage 1 going to the maximum sample size of 150 and not advancing to Stage 2. The trial advances to Stage 2 of the design with a probability of just 0.085. This represents an error of the Stage 1 aspect of the design. With this type of dose-finding design and small sample size, this is a very low Type I error

Dose	p	n_I	Pr(Go)	Pr(Win)
0	.10	32.0	–	–
1	.11	20.8	.040	.006
2	.12	15.1	.029	.014
3	.13	15.7	.039	.022
4	.15	21.4	.098	.074
Total	–	104.9	.206	.116

Table 5.14 *Operating characteristics of the seamless phase II-III design for a case where the treatment has a very minor advantage over the placebo.*

for the "phase II" aspect of this design. The probability of an arm being selected as the target dose is reported in the table. Dose 1 has the highest probability of being selected because of the desire to find the ED90; the probability for the other doses is slightly smaller. The total probability of a dose being selected as the target dose, advancing to Stage 2 and being found superior to the placebo is just 0.021. This satisfies a restriction that the entire combined phase II/III trial have a Type I error (one-sided) less than 0.025. Incidentally, Dose 0 (placebo) can never "win" (as indicated by the dash in the Pr(Win) column for this dose), but it does go on to phase III if the trial does (in this case, with probability 0.085), despite the presence of a dash in the Pr(Go) column.

We now present the results for several scenarios in which there is at least one positive experimental treatment arm. Table 5.14 presents the operating characteristics for a case in which there is a very small benefit to the experimental arms. The maximal benefit is for the largest dose, a 15% success rate at 6 months. While this represents a better treatment than the placebo, the benefit is not large enough to see a predictive power near 80%. The design does a good job of understanding the minor benefit and limiting the probability of advancing to Stage 2 to 0.206. Stage 1 stops for futility in 47% of the trials, with 32.2% advancing to the full 150 and then not advancing to Stage 2. The combined probability of finding the target arm superior to the control is 0.116. While advancing to Stage 2 is an undesired outcome for this case, about 50% of these times it chooses the largest dose, Dose 4, which is the most effective of the experimental doses.

Table 5.15 gives the simulation results for a scenario in which there is a strong treatment effect. The doses get more effective as they increase, resulting in Dose 4 being the most effective (and the ED90) with a true success rate of 30%. Doses 2 and 3 are also positive doses, but not as good as Dose 4. Dose 4 is selected as the ED90 and advances to Stage 2 in 46% of the trials (all of which ultimately lead to trial success). The second-best

Dose	p	n_I	Pr(Go)	Pr(Win)
0	.10	28.6	–	–
1	.15	14.6	.049	.017
2	.20	13.2	.080	.074
3	.25	15.5	.172	.170
4	.30	21.4	.459	.459
Total	–	93.3	.760	.720

Table 5.15 *Operating characteristics of the seamless phase II-III design for a case where the treatment has linearly increasing effectiveness with dose, to a very effective largest dose.*

Dose	p	n_I	Pr(Go)	Pr(Win)
0	.10	24.2	–	–
1	.30	16.5	.285	.282
2	.30	13.2	.191	.191
3	.30	12.6	.176	.176
4	.30	14.8	.246	.246
Total	–	81.4	.899	.896

Table 5.16 *Operating characteristics of the seamless phase II-III design for a case where each of the doses has strong efficacy.*

dose, Dose 3, is selected as the ED90 and advances to Stage 2 in 17% of the simulations. Combined, a target dose is selected to move to Stage 2 in 76% of all the trials, with another 15.6% of the trials running to the maximum sample size of 150 in Stage 1 and not advancing to Stage 2.

Table 5.16 presents the simulation results for a case in which all four of the experimental doses have a 6-month success rate of 0.30. The true ED90 is Dose 1. This dose is selected in 28.5% of the trials to advance to Stage 2. Altogether, there is an 89.9% chance of a target dose being selected and advancing seamlessly to Stage 2. When a dose is selected as the target dose to move forward, it is almost always successful in showing superiority (just 0.3% of trials went to Stage 2 and did not show superiority). While 89.9% of trials advance seamlessly to Stage 2, 7.9% run to the Stage 1 cap of 150 and do not advance to Stage 2. When a seamless shift is not made, after full follow-up of these trials, the decision could be made to conduct a phase

Dose	p	n_I	Pr(Go)	Pr(Win)
0	.10	31.3	–	–
1	.15	19.5	.077	.027
2	.30	22.2	.435	.435
3	.15	13.1	.038	.028
4	.15	15.5	.061	.043
Total	–	101.5	.612	.533

Table 5.17 *Operating characteristics of the seamless phase II-III design for a case where there is an inverted U-shaped dose-response curve.*

III trial. While the advantage of the seamless aspect is gone, this worst case scenario is quite similar to simply *not* running a seamless trial.

In the last case (Table 5.17), one quite positive dose (Dose 2) has a 30% success rate, while each of the remaining experimental arms has a less impressive 15% success rate. This is a very challenging scenario for this type of design because the best dose is an internal dose. The Bayesian dose-response model "shrinks" the results of the neighboring doses to the middle dose, thus making it harder to find that a lone internal dose is effective (this is the same strength that prevents Type I errors from occurring during Stage 1). Stage 1 is effective at placing more subjects on Dose 2, with the largest mean sample size of all experimental doses, 22.2, more than 50% larger than that of Dose 3. Dose 2 is selected as the target dose and advances to Stage 2 in 43.5% of the simulated trials. It then successfully demonstrates superiority in virtually all of these cases. All told there is a probability of 0.612 that a target dose is selected and advances to Stage 2, with Dose 2 making up 71% of these trials. The rate of trials reaching the 150 cap in Stage 1 and not advancing to Stage 2 is 21.2%, which not surprisingly is the largest of any of the cases presented here.

As a final remark, note that even after full accrual of all subjects not advancing to Stage 2, an analysis may reveal the efficacy of Dose 2, at which time an independent, traditional phase III trial can be conducted. The planning of a seamless phase II/III design enables the seamless shift to happen, but it does not in any way *prevent* a traditional phase III trial from being run. The seamless trial presented in this Section was constructed to be conservative; the hurdle for advancing to Stage 2 was reasonably high. The thought here was that if the seamless shift occurs, it was because the decision was pretty clear cut. More aggressive designs may be desirable here as well.

5.8 Case study: Ablation device to treat atrial fibrillation

In this final section we present a case study based on a confirmatory trial for the NaviStar ThermoCool^{TM} catheter. This is a medical device for the treatment of atrial fibrillation, an abnormal heart rhythm in which the heart's two upper chambers (atria) merely "quiver," instead of contracting in coordination with the lower chambers. During treatment, the source of the patient's heart arrhythmia is mapped, localized, and then destroyed (ablated) by applying radiofrequency energy through the catheter to create a small scar in the the offending area that is electrically inactive, rendering it incapable of generating arrhythmias. Additional details of the device as well as detailed trial information are available in Wilber et al. (2010). The trial was a Bayesian adaptive design with multiple looks for selecting the appropriate sample size, and with the possibility of making a claim of success before full follow-up was reached. Some of the aspects of the design must be kept confidential, but much of the detail is presented here.

Subjects with paroxysmal (recurrent but terminating in less than 7 days) atrial fibrillation were enrolled. The experimental group received treatment via the ThermoCool catheter, while the control group received antiarrhythmic drug therapy, the standard of care. Patients were randomized 7:4 in favor of the treatment group. The randomization ratio remained fixed throughout the trial. The primary endpoint for the study is a dichotomous endpoint, *chronic success*, defined as freedom from documented symptomatic atrial fibrillation and no changes in the anti-arrhythmia drug regimen during a 9-month efficacy window.

The primary outcome of the study is a dichotomous endpoint, but the endpoint is achieved by being free of "failure" during a 9-month window. Let p_T and p_C be the probability of a chronic success for a subject in the treatment group and control group, respectively. The prior distributions for each of the probabilities are taken as independent $\text{Beta}(1,1)$ distributions. The treatment will be deemed superior to the control group if the posterior probability of superiority is at least 0.98; i.e., if

$$\Pr\left(p_T > p_C | \text{Data}\right) \geq 0.98 \ .$$

The value of 0.98 was selected through simulation of the design to demonstrate the control of Type I error at the one-sided 0.025 level.

The trial design calls for a minimum accrual of 150 subjects. When the 150th subject has been accrued, an interim analysis is conducted. If reached, additional interim analyses take place at 175 and 200 subjects accrued, and if accrual continues the study stops at the maximum sample size of 230 subjects. The rules at each of the interim looks are as follows:

Algorithm 5.8 *(Atrial fibrillation (AF) trial design).*

Step 1. Expected Success: If the predictive probability of showing superiority with the current sample size is at least 0.90 for the 150-subject look or 0.80 for the 175- and 200-subject looks, then accrual stops for expected success.

Step 2. Futility: If the predictive probabilities of success for the current and maximum sample sizes (230) are each less than 0.01, then the trial stops for futility.

Step 3. Early Success: If the predictive probability of success for the current sample size is larger than 0.99, then the trial stops for expected success; immediate success is claimed, and an application is filed for immediate approval. In addition, if this early success condition is not met at the time accrual is stopped, an additional look for early success takes place 4.5 months after stopping accrual.

■

At the time of an interim analysis there will be subjects who have complete data, meaning their failure time is known or they have completed the 9-month period failure-free. There will be subjects who have interim time in the study without failing, and subjects who have no time in the study (this includes possibly future accrued subjects). We construct a model for the time until failure, which is then used for the predictive probabilities of subject and trial success. These predictive probabilities are used to guide the sample size determination, but have no effect on the primary analysis when the study is complete, except for the possible early analysis claim of success.

The dichotomous outcome of success and failure will be analyzed as described in the primary analysis section. However, analyzing the data at interim time points requires modeling the time-to-event data. The occurrence of a chronic failure is modeled as a time-to-event (failure) over the 9-month time period. For the 9-month efficacy evaluation period we model the hazard rates separately in each treatment group (the d index; 1 is control and 2 is treatment) for t in months. The time to chronic failure is assumed to be *piecewise exponential* with hazard rates

$$H_d(t) = \begin{cases} \theta_{d,1} & 0 < t \leq 0.5 \\ \theta_{d,2} & 0.5 < t \leq 2 \\ \theta_{d,3} & 2 < t \leq 9 \end{cases}.$$

A hierarchical prior distribution is used for the hazard rates within each interval, within each treatment group. The prior distributions are

$$\theta_{d,j} \sim \text{Gamma}\,(\alpha_d, \beta_d) \text{ for } d = 1, 2, \ j = 1, 2, 3\,.$$

The independent hyperpriors are

$$\alpha_d \sim \text{Exponential}\,(1)\,, \text{ for } d = 1, 2\,,$$

and

$$\beta_d \sim \text{Exponential}\,(1)\,, \text{ for } d = 1, 2\,.$$

These prior distributions were selected in discussions with regulatory agents. A typical interaction involves a proposed prior distribution and its operating characteristics. In this particular case, because this is the primary success analysis, it was desired and proposed by the sponsor that the prior distribution have little effect on the overall results. Regulatory agents agreed that such a prior distribution was appropriate. The operating characteristics of the design are calculated using this prior structure, so the ramifications of this prior are well understood.

Because accrual is slow relative to the 9-month follow-up period, we expect a reasonable number of subjects in each treatment group to have progressed through the full 9-month interval, and thus the prior distributions we explored for the hazard rates were not very important. In these circumstances, prior distributions for the parameters of the longitudinal model *can* be quite important when there is not a large number of subjects with complete data. It is not uncommon to use longitudinal models when it is expected there will be *no* subjects having complete data at the time of at least one interim analysis. In such cases, a strong prior for the longitudinal parameters is critical. Fortunately, in all the simulations of this particular trial, the accrual rate was slow enough that there were ample data to inform the longitudinal models. Therefore, in this trial, the priors for the longitudinal model also did not play an important role.

The posterior distributions of each of the parameters are updated based on each subject having greater than 0 exposure time during the primary follow-up period. Based on this modeling, the predictive distribution for each subject with no data or with partial data are defined. These predictive distributions are combined to find the predictive probability of trial success.

At an interim analysis the predictive distributions are calculated using MCMC. The approach successively simulates values from each of the model parameters as well as for each of the final observations of chronic success for each subject. Let X_i be the exposure time, F_i an indicator of whether a failure occurred, and d_i the treatment arm for subject i. If a subject reaches their full follow-up without a failure, they are labeled as $X = 9$ and $F = 0$. Letting E_{dj} and Y_{dj} be the current exposure and the number of failures, respectively, within interval j for treatment d, our MCMC algorithm is as follows:

Algorithm 5.9 *(AF trial MCMC algorithm).*

Step 0: Select initial values for each of the parameters $\theta_{1,1}, \theta_{1,2}, \theta_{1,3}, \theta_{2,1}, \theta_{2,2}, \theta_{2,3}, \alpha_1, \beta_1, \alpha_2,$ and β_2

Step 1: For each hazard rate, θ, simulate an observation from its full conditional distribution,

$$\theta_{d,j} | \mathbf{E}, \mathbf{Y}, \alpha_d, \beta_d \sim \text{Gamma}\left(\alpha_d + Y_{dj}, \beta_d + E_{dj}\right)$$

Step 2: Simulate a value of $\alpha_d, d = 1, 2$ from its full conditional distribution,

$$\alpha_d | \beta_d, \theta_{d,1}, \theta_{d,2}, \theta_{d,3} \sim \left[\frac{\beta_d^{\alpha_d}}{\Gamma(\alpha_d)} \right]^3 \left(\prod_{i=1}^{3} \theta_{d,i} \right)^{\alpha_d - 1} \exp(-\alpha_d)$$

Step 3: Simulate a value of $\beta_d, d = 1, 2$ from its full conditional distribution,

$$\beta_d | \alpha_d, \theta_{d,1}, \theta_{d,2}, \theta_{d,3} \sim \text{Gamma}\left(1 + 3\alpha_d, 1 + \sum_{i=1}^{3} \theta_{d,i} \right)$$

Step 4: For each subject with incomplete data, $X_i < 9$ and $F_i = 0$, simulate a predictive value of X_i from the piecewise exponential model with parameter $(\theta_{d_i,1}, \theta_{d_i,2}, \theta_{d_i,3})$ and conditional on no event at time X_i.

Step 5: For the complete data $X_1, ... X_n$, where n is the current sample size, evaluate whether the data constitutes a primary endpoint success. For the maximum sample size of 230, evaluate whether $X_1, \ldots, X_{230}$ constitutes a success on the primary endpoint.

The iteration of steps 1 through 5 is done $B + M$ times, where the first B observations are discarded as burn-in values. For the simulations, typical values of $B = 1000$ and $M = 5000$ are used. ∎

The proportion of times that success is achieved with the current sample size estimates the predictive probability of success with the current sample size, while the proportion of times success is achieved with the maximum sample size estimates the predictive probability of success at the maximum sample size. These predictive probabilities take in to account several sources of variability. The data for subjects with complete information remain fixed, but the data for those subjects without complete information are simulated using the Bayesian model. Therefore the predictive probability accounts for the natural variability of the future data. This model integrates over the uncertainty of the parameters of this model, namely, the hazard rates. Thus the predictive distribution accounts for the uncertainty in the longitudinal model as well.

In order to characterize the behavior of the design, we once again perform simulations. In order to simulate the design it is necessary to create "virtual subjects." The design incorporates the time-to-failure, as well as the dichotomous endpoint of 9-month failure. We simulate subject failure using the piecewise exponential longitudinal model structure (though additional simulations using different methods were also done). The default parameters assumed are $\theta_1^* = 0.65$, $\theta_2^* = 0.161$, and $\theta_3^* = 0.05$. The default probability of 9-month success is

$$\exp(-0.5\theta_1^* - 1.5\theta_2^* - 7\theta_3^*) = 0.40 \, .$$

p_T	p_C	$\Pr(S)$	$\Pr(F)$	Sample Size	Time	Sample Size 150	175	200	230
0.20	0.20	0.019	0.92	158.1	35.4	.01	.01	.00	.06
		0.004		(21.5)	(7.2)	.83	.05	.03	
0.40	0.40	0.021	0.92	158.2	35.4	.01	.01	.00	.07
		0.004		(21.4)	(7.2)	.84	.05	.03	
0.60	0.60	0.023	0.91	158.3	35.4	.01	.01	.00	.07
		0.012		(21.6)	(7.2)	.83	.05	.03	

Table 5.18 *Operating characteristics for three null hypotheses for the ThermoCool catheter trial. The first two columns report the assumed probability of chronic success in each treatment arm. The* $\Pr(S)$ *and* $\Pr(F)$ *columns report the probabilities of success for the primary endpoint and the probability of stopping for futility. The lower cell in the* $\Pr(S)$ *column is the probability of claiming success earlier than full follow-up. The fifth and sixth columns report the mean (standard deviation) of the sample and time of the trial in months. The last four columns report the probability of stopping at each sample size for expected success (upper cell) and futility (lower cell).*

In order to simulate from any arbitrary probability of chronic success, $0 < p < 1$, a value of δ is selected such that

$$\delta = \log\left(\frac{\log p}{\log 0.4}\right) .$$

The value of δ is then used to alter each individual θ as

$$\theta_j = \exp\left(\delta\right)\theta_j^* .$$

This creates a case where the probability of success for the simulated subjects is p. The default accrual rate used in the simulation is 2 per month for the first two months, 3 per month the next two months, and 5 per month starting in the fifth month. Relative to the speed of the observations of the endpoint, the accrual rate is reasonably slow.

Using the above assumptions we simulate the adaptive trial. At each planned interim analysis the steps are carried out and the results of the simulated trials are recorded. Table 5.18 presents the results of 25,000 simulated trials in which the treatment and control probability of chronic success are the same. In each case it is an error to claim superiority. These three cases represent "null" cases.

For each of these three scenarios the simulated Type I error is less than the one-sided 0.025. Numerous other null hypotheses were simulated, including different assumptions on the time-to-failure, accrual rates, and different probabilities. For each of these null scenarios the probability of con-

p_T	p_C	Pr(S)	Pr(F)	Sample Size	Time	Sample Size			
						150	175	200	230
0.30	0.20	0.316	0.46	182.3	44.7	.12	.15	.10	.30
		0.090		34.6	12.0	.34	.07	.05	
0.40	0.20	0.845	0.06	175.9	44.1	.48	.17	.09	.20
		0.429		31.6	10.6	.03	.01	.01	
0.45	0.20	0.959	0.01	164.2	39.9	.69	.14	.07	.09
		0.637		25.2	9.1	.01	.00	.00	
0.50	0.20	0.993	0.00	155.9	36.4	.85	.09	.03	.03
		0.813		16.2	6.5	.00	.00	.00	
0.50	0.40	0.260	0.53	178.9	43.2	.10	.14	.10	.26
		0.114		33.9	11.6	.41	.07	.05	
0.60	0.40	0.785	0.10	177.7	44.9	.43	.17	.11	.22
		0.644		32.2	8.7	.06	.02	.02	
0.65	0.40	0.934	0.02	166.3	42.5	.66	.15	.08	.11
		0.861		26.6	6.5	.01	.01	.00	
0.70	0.40	0.989	0.00	156.5	40.2	.84	.09	.03	.03
		0.961		17.3	4.0	.00	.00	.00	

Table 5.19 *Operating characteristics for eight cases where the device is assumed superior to the control, for the ThermoCool catheter trial. The first two columns report the assumed probability of chronic success in each treatment arm. The Pr(S) and Pr(F) columns report the probabilities of success for the primary endpoint and the probability of stopping for futility. The lower cell in the Pr(S) column is the probability of claiming success earlier than full follow-up. The fifth and sixth columns report the mean (standard deviation) of the sample and time of the trial in months. The last four columns report the probability of stopping at each sample size for expected success (upper cell) and futility (lower cell).*

cluding superiority, whether at full follow-up or an early claim of success, was less than 0.025. The final success threshold was varied in order to find the smallest value that resulted in Type I error probabilities less than 0.025 for every null case (0.98).

Table 5.19 reports the operating characteristics for cases in which the control arm has a 0.20 or 0.40 probability of success and the treatment arm varies from a 0.10 to 0.30 probability incremental improvement. The probabilities of detecting an additive improvement of 0.20 over a baseline of 0.20 or 0.40 are 0.845 and 0.785, respectively. These powers increase to 0.959 and 0.934 when the advantage enjoyed by the treatment arm increases to 0.25. In the specific case where the treatment has a 45% success rate and the control has a 20% success rate, the mean sample size is 164.2 with a standard deviation of 25.2. The probability of the trial stopping at the first look is 0.69, with only a 0.09 probability of advancing to the maximum sample size of 230. The probability of achieving an early finding of success is a robust 0.637.

The Bayesian adaptive design described here helped the device's sponsor (NaviStar) successfully navigate the approval process with the FDA. The results of the trial were announced publicly during an FDA advisory panel meeting in November 2008. The first interim analysis took place in July 2007, and the predictive probability of success for the current sample size (159 subjects) was greater than 0.999, thus resulting in a stopping of accrual and an immediate claim of superiority. The final posterior probability of superiority was greater than 0.999, which is larger than the goal cutoff of 0.98. The final Kaplan-Meier estimated success rates were 64% and 16%, for the treatment and control groups, respectively. In February 2009, the FDA approved the catheters for the treatment of atrial fibrillation.

5.9 Appendix: R Macros

The online supplement to this chapter

www.biostat.umn.edu/~brad/software/BCLM_ch5.html

provides the R code that was used to illustrate the examples in this section.

## CHAPTER 6

Special topics

In this chapter we discuss several important special topics that do not neatly fit into our earlier chapters, but are nonetheless important in the actual practice of Bayesian clinical trials. By necessity, our views reflect our own experience and interest to some extent, but the issues in this chapter do seem to come up fairly regularly, in both in-house studies as well as later-phase trials where working cooperatively with regulatory agencies comes to the fore.

6.1 Incorporating historical data

As seen earlier in this text, Bayesian clinical trial designs offer the possibility of a substantially reduced sample size, increased statistical power, and reductions in cost and ethical hazard. However when prior and current information conflict, Bayesian methods can lead to higher than expected Type I error, as well as the possibility of a costlier and lengthier trial. This motivates an investigation of the feasibility of hierarchical Bayesian methods for incorporating historical data that are *adaptively* robust to prior information that reveals itself to be inconsistent with the accumulating experimental data.

In this section, we begin with a fairly standard hierarchical model that allows sensible borrowing from historical controls, but in a way that requires the user to be fairly explicit about the degree of borrowing. We then go on to present novel modifications to the traditional power prior approach (Ibrahim and Chen, 2000) that allows the commensurability of the information in the historical and current data to determine how much historical information is used. Power priors offer a simple way to incorporate and downweight historical data, by raising the historical likelihood to a power $\alpha_0 \in [0, 1]$, and restandardizing the result to a proper distribution. These priors have been applied in a variety of contexts, including the sample size estimation problem by DeSantis (2007). We compare the frequentist performance of several methods using simulation, and close with an example from a colon cancer trial that illustrates the benefit of our proposed adaptive borrowing approach. The commensurate prior design produces more precise estimates of the model parameters, in particular conferring statistical significance to the observed reduction in tumor size for the experimental regimen as compared to the control regimen in our example.

6.1.1 Standard hierarchical models

We begin with a hierarchical model for a doubly controlled clinical trial defined as follows. Suppose that historical data exist for *both* the treatment and control groups. Let $g = 0, 1$ indicate group (historical or current), and let $i = 1, \ldots, n_g$ index the patients in each group. The full hierarchical model might look like

$$\text{Likelihood:} \quad Y_{gi} \overset{ind}{\sim} N(\theta_g + \beta_g x_{gi}, \sigma_g^2)$$

$$\text{where } x_{gi} = \begin{cases} 0 & \text{if patient } gi \text{ received control} \\ 1 & \text{if patient } gi \text{ received treatment} \end{cases}$$

$$\text{Prior:} \quad \theta_g \overset{iid}{\sim} N(\mu_\theta, \tau_\theta^2) \quad \text{and} \quad \beta_g \overset{iid}{\sim} N(\mu_\beta, \tau_\beta^2) .$$

Consider how the parameters of this model control prior shrinkage. If $\tau_\theta^2 = 0$, then $\theta_g = \mu_\theta$ for all g, and we have no borrowing among the control groups. On the other hand, if $\tau_\beta^2 = 0$, then $\beta_g = \mu_\theta$ for all g, and we have no borrowing among the treatment groups.

Next, we need a hyperprior specification to complete the model. We take flat hyperpriors on the mean parameters μ_θ and μ_β, since for most datasets these parameters will be well-estimated by the data. However, for the variances, we work (like WinBUGS) on the precision scale, and assume

$$\eta_\theta \sim G(a_\theta, b_\theta) \quad \text{and} \quad \eta_\beta \sim G(a_\beta, b_\beta) ,$$

where $\eta = 1/\tau^2$. Thus, in the treatment group, if $a_\beta = 1000$ and $b_\beta = 10$, η_β is approximately 100 and hence τ_β is approximately 0.1, a *high-shrinkage* hyperprior. If instead $a_\beta = 40$ and $b_\beta = 4$, this is a vaguer prior having $\eta_\beta \approx 10$, i.e., $\tau_\beta \approx 0.3$, a *moderate-shrinkage* hyperprior. Finally, if $a_\beta = b_\beta = \epsilon = 0.1$, the hyperprior is vague and the data must do all the work, a *low-shrinkage* hyperprior. Similar statements enabling differing levels of shrinkage assigned to the control group are possible via a_θ and b_θ.

To evaluate the quality of this hierarchical model setting, consider the simulation of its operating characteristics. Suppose we take $n_0 = n_1 = 20$, and without loss of generality take $\sigma_g^2 = 1$. We can simulate frequentist power under a variety of scenarios. For instance, we might set $\theta_0 = \theta_1 = 0$ and $\beta_0 = \beta_1 = 0$. This corresponds to complete homogeneity; there is no reason not to borrow from the historical data in both the treatment and control groups. Alternatively, we could take $\theta_0 = \theta_1 = 0$ but $\beta_0 = 0, \beta_1 = 2$. Here we specify slight heterogeneity across treatment groups, so that borrowing is somewhat suspect. Finally, if we were to take $\theta_0 = 0, \theta_1 = 30$, and $\beta_0 = 0, \beta_1 = 2$, this would correspond to enormous heterogeneity

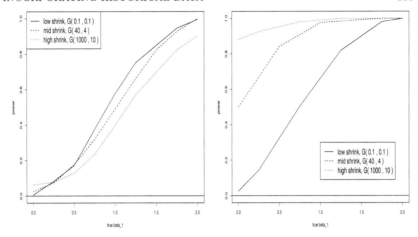

Figure 6.1 *Power curve for treatment effect in current trial (β_1): (a) true $(\theta_0, \theta_1, \beta_0) = (0, 30, 0)$; (b) true $(\theta_0, \theta_1, \beta_0) = (0, 30, 2)$.*

across control groups, and slight additional heterogeneity across treatment groups; borrowing would now be very suspect. In each case, we could lay out a grid of "true" β_1 values, choose the shrinkage level in the treatment and control group hyperpriors, and simulate frequentist power under various hypotheses.

Example 6.1 *(Test for a treatment effect in the current trial).* Consider comparing the hypotheses $H_0 : \beta_1 = 0$ and $H_a : \beta_1 \neq 0$, where we use the decision rule, "Reject H_0 if the central 95% credible interval for β_1 excludes 0." Figure 6.1 gives the power over a grid of β_1 values assuming $\theta_0 = 0$, $\theta_1 = 30$, and $\beta_0 = 0$ (left panel) vs. $\beta_0 = 2$ (right) under the high, moderate, and low shrinkage priors in the treatment group (the moderate shrinkage prior was used for the θ's in the control group). Note that the high-shrinkage hyperprior (dotted line) does well when $\beta_0 = 0$ (left panel) even though $\theta_1 \neq 0$, but has high Type I error when $\beta_0 \neq 0$ (right panel). The performance of the low shrinkage hyperprior (solid line) is almost unaffected by the true value of β_0, showing good power and Type I error behavior superior to that of the other two hyperpriors. ∎

Example 6.2 *(Test whether "to pool or not to pool").* Consider now an FDA applicant who wishes to know if she may pool her historical and experimental data in a drug or device approval study. We might now define $\Delta = \beta_1 - \beta_0$, and test the hypotheses $H_0 : \Delta \in (-c, c)$ for some $c > 0$, versus $H_a : \Delta \notin (-c, c)$. It is now convenient to use a decision rule of the form, "Reject H_0 if $P(\Delta \in (-1, 1)|\mathbf{y}) < K$," for some prespecified posterior coverage level K.

The power curves over a β_1 grid are given in Figure 6.2, which assumes

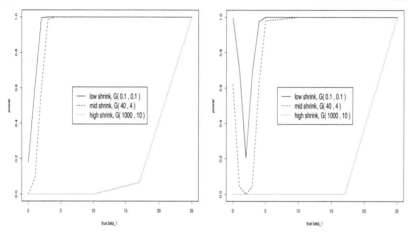

Figure 6.2 *Power curves for treatment effect difference* Δ: *(a) true* $(\theta_0, \theta_1, \beta_0) =$ $(0, 0, 0)$; *(b) true* $(\theta_0, \theta_1, \beta_0) = (0, 0, 2)$.

$c = 1$, $K = 0.80$, $\theta_0 = \theta_1 = 0$, and $\beta_0 = 0$ (left) vs. $\beta_0 = 2$ (right) for the three treatment group hyperpriors and under the low shrinkage prior for the θ's. Here the high shrinkage prior stubbornly refuses to reject H_0 unless β_1 is quite far from the null value. The low shrinkage prior has good power but perhaps slightly too much Type I error (0.18 and 0.25 in the two panels, respectively); overall the moderate shrinkage prior offers a sensible compromise. ∎

Repeating these sorts of simulations over a fine grid of $\theta_0, \theta_1, \beta_0$, and β_1 values should permit the development of guidelines for how tightly the hyperprior can be set in a given model setting, so that borrowing from historical data happens at effective yet not overly Type I error-prone levels. We could also compare these approaches head-to-head with our power prior methods below, to help attach more meaning to the hyperparameters that control the degrees of borrowing in each setting.

6.1.2 Hierarchical power prior models

A second, possibly more useful approach to incorporating historical data is through *power priors*. Adopting the notation of Ibrahim and Chen (2000), denote the historical data by $D_0 = (n_0, \mathbf{x_0})$, where n_0 denotes the sample size and $\mathbf{x_0}$ the $n_0 \times 1$ response vector, and similarly denote data from the current study by $D = (n, \mathbf{x})$. Let $L(\theta|D_0)$ denote the general likelihood function of the historical data. Then the conditional power prior for parameter θ is defined as

$$\pi(\theta|D_0, \alpha_0) \propto L(\theta|D_0)^{\alpha_0} \pi_0(\theta), \tag{6.1}$$

where $\pi_0(\theta)$ is referred to as the *initial* prior, since it represents prior knowledge about θ before D_0 is observed, and $\alpha_0 \in [0,1]$ is the *power parameter* that controls the "degree of borrowing" from the historical data. If $\alpha_0 = 0$, (6.1) reduces to the initial prior (no borrowing), whereas if $\alpha_0 = 1$, equation (6.1) returns the usual historical posterior (full borrowing).

In the case of normal historical data, $x_{0i} \overset{iid}{\sim} N(\theta, \sigma_0^2)$, σ_0^2 known, $i = 1, \ldots, n_0$, under a flat initial prior, (6.1) yields a $N\left(\bar{x}_0, \sigma_0^2/(\alpha_0 n_0)\right)$ power prior distribution for θ. Hence α_0 plays the role of a relative precision parameter for the historical data. Since $0 \le \alpha_0 \le 1$, we might also think of $\alpha_0 n_0$ as the "effective" number of historical controls being incorporated into our analysis. Ibrahim and Chen (2000) introduced power priors to the broad statistical community, and illustrated their usefulness in a variety of settings; see also Ibrahim et al. (2003) and Chen and Ibrahim (2006).

If we are willing to specify a particular value for α_0, the conditional posterior distribution for θ given D_0, D, and α_0 emerges as

$$q(\theta|D_0, D, \alpha_0) \propto \pi_0(\theta) L(\theta|D_0)^{\alpha_0} L(\theta|D) . \tag{6.2}$$

Again in the case of known-variance normal observations, $x_i \overset{iid}{\sim} N(\theta, \sigma^2)$, $i = 1, \ldots, n$, this results in another normal distribution for the posterior of θ.

We may be able to use the power parameter's interpretation as "importance of each historical patient relative to each new patient" to select a value for α_0 (say, $1/2$ or $1/3$) for approximately Gaussian likelihoods. More commonly, however, we are uncertain as to the degree to which our new data will agree with the historical data, and thus are somewhat reluctant to prespecify the degree of borrowing. In such cases, we can enable the data to help determine probable values for α_0 by adopting the usual Bayesian solution of choosing a *hyperprior* $\pi(\alpha_0)$ for α_0.

Ibrahim and Chen (2000) propose joint power priors proportional to the product of the conditional power prior in (6.1) and an independent proper prior on α_0,

$$\pi^{IC}(\theta, \alpha_0|D_0) \propto \pi_0(\theta)\pi(\alpha_0)L(\theta|D_0)^{\alpha_0}. \tag{6.3}$$

Duan et al. (2006, p. 98) and Neuenschwander et al. (2009) caution against (6.3) since it violates the Likelihood Principle (Subsection 2.2.3). To see this, note that if we use the likelihood of a sufficient statistic for θ instead of the entire random sample, we may obtain disparate joint power priors. For example, under normality, $\left[\prod_{i=1}^{n_0} Normal(x_{0i}|\theta, \sigma_0^2)\right]^{\alpha_0} \pi_0(\theta)\pi(\alpha_0)$ is not proportional to $Normal(\bar{x}_0|\theta, \frac{\sigma_0^2}{n_0})^{\alpha_0}\pi_0(\theta)\pi(\alpha_0)$ with respect to α_0, since $\left(2\pi\sigma_0^2\right)^{-\frac{\alpha_0 n_0}{2}} \ne \left(\frac{2\pi\sigma_0^2}{n_0}\right)^{-\frac{\alpha_0}{2}}$. Therefore, multiplying the historical likelihood by a constant under the α_0 exponent alters the amount of information in the power prior.

If we specify $\pi(\alpha_0)$ as a $Beta(a,b)$ distribution for fixed positive hyperparameters a and b, the joint posterior for θ and α_0 given D and D_0

becomes

$$q^{IC}(\theta, \alpha_0 | D_0, D) \propto \alpha_0^{a-1}(1 - \alpha_0)^{b-1}\pi_0(\theta)L(\theta|D_0)^{\alpha_0}L(\theta|D) . \quad (6.4)$$

In this setting, we can use the hyperparameters (a, b) to control the likely degree of borrowing; for example, $(a = 10, b = 1)$ would strongly encourage borrowing.

Duan et al. (2006) modify the joint power prior to the product of the *normalized* conditional power prior (6.1) and an independent proper prior for α_0, namely

$$\pi^D(\theta, \alpha_0 | D_0) \propto \frac{L(\theta|D_0)^{\alpha_0}\pi_0(\theta)}{\int L(\theta|D_0)^{\alpha_0}\pi_0(\theta)d\theta}\pi(\alpha_0). \quad (6.5)$$

Modified power priors obey the Likelihood Principle, and marginal posteriors for α_0 under modified power priors typically emerge as proportional to products of familiar probability distributions. Duan et al. (2006, p.98) propose modified power priors as an improvement with respect to unwarranted attenuation of historical data. Hobbs et al. (2009) present plots that offer mild support for this claim assuming small sample sizes, normal data, and $Beta(1, 1)$ hyperpriors. Furthermore, modified power priors tend to produce marginal posteriors for α_0 that are less skewed in these scenarios. This all suggests that marginal posteriors of α_0 derived from modified power priors may be less sensitive to the power parameter hyperprior than their Ibrahim-Chen counterparts. If we again specify $\pi(\alpha_0) = Beta(a, b)$ for fixed positive a and b, the joint posterior for θ and α_0 given D and D_0 replaces (6.4) in the Ibrahim-Chen approach with

$$q^D(\theta, \alpha_0 | D_0, D) \propto \alpha_0^{a-1}(1 - \alpha_0)^{b-1}\frac{L(\theta|D_0)^{\alpha_0}\pi_0(\theta)}{\int L(\theta|D_0)^{\alpha_0}\pi_0(\theta)d\theta}L(\theta|D) . \quad (6.6)$$

Commensurate power priors

A problem with the joint power priors above is that they do not directly parameterize the commensurability of the historical and new data. For example, in (6.4) or (6.6) note that the full conditional distribution for α_0 would be free of the current data D, since the current likelihood would be nothing but a multiplicative constant. Furthermore, Duan et al. (2006), Neelon et al. (2008), and Neelon and O'Malley (2010) all caution against using Ibrahim-Chen and modified power priors since they both tend to overattenuate the impact of the historical data, forcing the use of fairly large α_0 (or fairly informative hyperpriors for α_0) in order to deliver sufficient borrowing.

Suppose we assume different parameters in the historical and current group, θ_0 and θ, respectively. This bivariate parameterization allows us to extend the hierarchical model to include a parameter that directly measures the *commensurabilty* (similarity) of θ and θ_0. Suppose we pick a vague (or even flat) initial prior $\pi_0(\theta_0)$, but construct the prior for θ to be dependent upon θ_0 and τ, where τ parameterizes commensurability. We use the information in τ to guide the prior on α_0. Specifying a vague prior for τ and normalizing with respect to θ and θ_0 results in a power prior $\pi^C(\theta_0, \theta, \alpha_0, \tau|D_0)$ proportional to

$$\frac{(L(\theta_0|D_0) \times p(\theta|\theta_0, \tau))^{\alpha_0}}{\int\int (L(\theta_0|D_0) \times p(\theta|\theta_0, \tau))^{\alpha_0} d\theta_0 d\theta} \times p(\alpha_0|\tau)p(\tau) . \tag{6.7}$$

The posterior is then proportional to the product of (6.7) and the current data likelihood $L(\theta|D)$. If inference on θ_0 is not of primary interest in the current analysis, we can integrate it out to obtain the joint commensurate power prior on μ, α_0, and τ, $\pi^C(\theta, \alpha_0, \tau|D_0)$, proportional to

$$\int \frac{(L(\theta_0|D_0) \times p(\theta|\theta_0, \tau))^{\alpha_0}}{\int\int (L(\theta_0|D_0) \times p(\theta|\theta_0, \tau))^{\alpha_0} d\theta_0 d\theta} d\theta_0 \times p(\alpha_0|\tau)p(\tau) . \tag{6.8}$$

This extended power prior model requires the estimation of more parameters from the data (notably τ^2), but we can formulate the model such that the information gained is aimed directly at improving estimation of the crucial borrowing parameter α_0.

Application to Gaussian linear models

We now illustrate the application of commensurate priors in hierarchical linear models for Gaussian response data. Assume y_0 is a vector of n_0 responses from subjects in a previous investigation of an intervention that is to be used as a control in a current trial testing a newly developed intervention for which no reliable prior data exists. Let y be the vector of n responses from subjects in the current trial in both treatment and control arms. Suppose that both trials are designed to identically measure $p-1$ covariates of interest. Let X_0 be an $n_0 \times p$ design matrix and X be an $n \times p$ design matrix, both of full column rank p, such that the first columns of X_0 and X are vectors of 1s corresponding to the intercept. Now suppose $y_0 \sim N_{n_0}(X_0\beta_0, \sigma^2)$ and $y \sim N_n(X\beta + Z\lambda, \sigma^2)$ where Z is an $n \times r$ design matrix containing variables relevant only to the current trial, as well as an indicator for the new treatment. Let $D_0 = (y_0, X_0, n_0, p)$ and $D = (y, X, Z, n, p, r)$.

Suppose we assume a normal prior on β with mean β_0 and variance $\tau^2 I$, as well as a $Beta(\frac{a\sigma^2}{\tau^2}, 1)$ prior on α_0 for some $a > 0$. The variance τ^2 parameterizes commensurability, since τ^2 close to 0 corresponds to very high commensurability, while very large τ^2 implies the two datasets do not arise from similar populations. Furthermore, as τ^2 approaches 0, $\frac{a\sigma^2}{\tau^2} \to \infty$, leading to a point-mass prior at 1 on α_0. Thus, the model virtually forces borrowing from the historical data when the data are commensurate. Alternatively, as τ^2 becomes large, $\frac{a\sigma^2}{\tau^2} \to 0$, discouraging incorporation of any historical information. The hyperparameter a can be chosen to deliver acceptable Type I error and power behavior. Adding a vague prior on τ^2 completes the prior specification.

As a side comment, note that many other hyperpriors for α_0 may be appropriate. For example, we might reparameterize to

$$\alpha_0 \sim Beta(\mu\phi, (1-\mu)\phi) \,.$$

In this parameterization, μ is the hyperprior mean and ϕ is the hyperprior "precision parameter" (note the variance is decreasing in ϕ). Now we might fix ϕ, treating it like the tuning constant a above, and (setting $\sigma^2 = 1$ without loss of generality) take $\mu = 1/(1+\tau^2)$. Thus α_0 once again has prior mean 1 when $\tau^2 = 0$ and prior mean 0 when $\tau^2 = \infty$, but now with the *same precision* in both cases.

Specifying our commensurate power prior as in (6.7) leads to a full conditional prior for β_0, $\pi^C(\beta_0 \mid \beta, \lambda, \alpha_0, \tau^2, D_0)$, proportional to

$$N_p\left(\beta_0 \;\middle|\; \frac{(X_0^T X_0)^{-1}(X_0^T y_0 \tau^2 + \sigma^2 X_0^T X_0 \beta)}{\sigma^2 + \tau^2}, \; \frac{(X_0^T X_0)^{-1}\sigma^2\tau^2}{\alpha_0(\sigma^2 + \tau^2)}\right), \quad (6.9)$$

and a joint prior on β, λ, α_0, and τ^2, $\pi^C(\beta, \lambda, \alpha_0, \tau^2|D_0)$, proportional to

$$N_p\left(\beta \;\middle|\; \hat{\beta}_0, \, (X_0^T X_0)^{-1}\frac{(\sigma^2 + \tau^2)}{\alpha_0}\right) \times B\left(\alpha_0 \;\middle|\; \frac{a\sigma^2}{\tau^2}, 1\right) \times \left(\frac{1}{\tau^2}\right)^{3/2}, \quad (6.10)$$

where $\hat{\beta}_0 = (X_0^T X_0)^{-1}X_0^T y_0$. Let $V = \left(\frac{\alpha_0 X_0^T X_0}{\sigma^2 + \tau^2} + \frac{X^T(I-w)X}{\sigma^2}\right)^{-1}$ and $M = \left(\frac{\alpha_0 X_0^T y_0}{\sigma^2 + \tau^2} + \frac{X^T(I-w)y}{\sigma^2}\right)$, where $w = Z(Z^T Z)^{-1}Z^T$. Then the joint posterior $q^C(\lambda, \beta, \alpha_0, \tau^2|D_0, D)$ follows by multiplying $\pi^C(\beta, \lambda, \alpha_0, \tau^2|D_0)$ by the likelihood of y, and is proportional to

$$N\left(\lambda \;\middle|\; \hat{\lambda}, \, \sigma^2(Z^T Z)^{-1}\right) \times N_p\left(\beta \;\middle|\; VM, \, V\right) \times q^C(\alpha_0, \tau^2|D_0, D)\,, \quad (6.11)$$

where $\hat{\lambda} = (Z^T Z)^{-1}Z^T(y - X\beta)$ and, integrating β_0 out of the model, $q^C(\alpha_0, \tau^2|D_0, D) \propto \int\int q^C(\beta, \lambda, \alpha_0, \tau^2|D_0, D)d\lambda d\beta$.

Notice that the full conditional posterior mean for λ, $\hat{\lambda}$, is a function of residuals $(y - X\beta)$, whereas the conditional posterior mean of β, VM, is an average of the historical and concurrent data relative to the power and commensurate parameters, α_0 and τ^2. If we fix σ^2 to be close to the "truth", then as τ^2 becomes large and α_0 approaches 0, the marginal posterior for β converges to a normal density with mean $\left(\frac{X^T X - X^T Z(Z^T Z)^{-1}Z^T X}{\sigma^2}\right)^{-1}(X^T y$ $-X^T Z(Z^T Z)^{-1}Z^T y)$ and variance $\left(\frac{X^T X - X^T Z(Z^T Z)^{-1}Z^T X}{\sigma^2}\right)^{-1}$, recovering the result from a linear regression that ignores all of the historical data. In this case, $\hat{\lambda}$ also converges to the no borrowing estimate of the treatment difference.

Example 6.3 *(Application to Saltz/Goldberg colorectal cancer trial data).*
We consider data from two successive randomized controlled colorectal cancer clinical trials originally reported by Saltz et al. (2000) and Goldberg et
al. (2004). The initial trial randomized $N_0 = 683$ patients with previously
untreated metastatic colorectal cancer between May 1996 and May 1998
to one of three regimens: Irinotecan alone (arm A), Irinotecan and bolus
Fluorouracil plus Leucovorin (arm B; IFL), or a regimen of Fluorouracil
and Leucovorin (arm C; 5FU/LV). In an intent-to-treat analysis, arm B resulted in significantly longer progression-free survival and overall survival
than arms A and C (Saltz et al., 2000).

The subsequent trial compared three drug combinations in $N = 795$
patients with previously untreated metastatic colorectal cancer, randomized between May 1999 and April 2001. Patients in the first drug group
received the then-current "standard therapy," the IFL regimen identical
to arm B of the historical study. The second group received Oxaliplatin
and infused Fluorouracil plus Leucovorin (abbreviated FOLFOX), while
the third group received Irinotecan and Oxaliplatin (abbreviated IROX);
both of these latter two regimens were new as of the beginning of the trial.

While both trials recorded many different patient characteristics and
responses, in our analysis we concentrate on the trial's measurements of
tumor size, and how the FOLFOX regimen compared to the IFL regimen.
Therefore, the historical dataset consists of treatment arm B from the initial
study, while the current data consists of patients randomized to IFL or
FOLFOX in the subsequent trial.

Both trials recorded two measurements on each tumor for each patient at
regular cycles. The trial reported by Saltz et al. measured patients every 6
weeks for the first 24 weeks and every 12 weeks thereafter until a response
(death or disease progression), while the trial reported by Goldberg et al.
measured every 6 weeks for the first 42 weeks, or until death or disease
progression. We computed the sum of the longest diameter in cm ("ld
sum") for up to 9 tumors for each patient at each cycle. We used the
average change in ld sum from baseline to test for a significant treatment
difference in ld sum reduction among FOLFOX and control regimens. Our
analysis below also incorporates baseline ld sum as a predictor, as well as
two important covariates identically measured at baseline: age in years, and
aspartate aminotransferase (AST) in units/L.

We restricted our analysis to patients who had measurable tumors, at
least two cycles of follow-up, and a nonzero ld sum at baseline, bringing
the total sample size to 441: 171 historical and 270 current observations.
Among the current patients, there are 129 controls (IFL) and 141 patients
treated with the new regimen (FOLFOX). Suppose y_0 and y are vectors of
lengths n_0 and n for the historical and concurrent responses such that

$$y_0 \sim Normal(X_0\beta_0 \,, \sigma^2), \quad \text{and} \quad y \sim Normal(X\beta + Z\lambda \,, \sigma^2) \,, \quad (6.12)$$

	Historical data		Current data	
	estimate	95% CI	estimate	95% CI
intercept	0.880	$(-1.977, 3.738)$	-0.467	$(-2.275, 1.341)$
BL ld sum	-0.232	$(-0.310, -0.154)$	-0.397	$(-0.453, -0.340)$
age	-0.022	$(-0.067, 0.022)$	0.014	$(-0.014, 0.041)$
AST	-0.001	$(-0.017, 0.015)$	0.005	$(-0.007, 0.017)$
FOLFOX	–	–	-0.413	$(-1.017, 0.190)$

Table 6.1 *Linear regression fits to colorectal cancer data: $y_0 \sim x_0$, $DF = 167$ (left); $y \sim x + z$, $DF = 265$ (right).*

where X_0 and X are $n_0 \times 4$ and $n \times 4$ design matrices with columns corresponding to (1, ld sum at baseline, age, AST), and Z is the FOLFOX indicator function. Thus the β_0 and β parameters contain intercepts as well as regression coefficients for each of three baseline covariates, while λ represents change in average ld sum attributed to FOLFOX. Histograms of the average change in ld tumor sum from baseline (not shown) suggest that our assumption of normality here is acceptable.

Table 6.1 summarizes results from separate classical linear regression fits on the historical data (y_0, X_0) alone and the current data (y, X, Z) alone. The "current data" results thus represent the "no borrowing" analysis. Results from both datasets suggest that ld sum at baseline is highly significant while age and AST are not. Furthermore, while the estimated intercept corresponding FOLFOX in the current data is negative, -0.413, the estimate is not precise enough to conclude a significant treatment difference at the 0.05 significance level.

Information about β_0 appears to be relevant to β, so we implemented the commensurate prior linear model. We fixed the error variance, σ^2, at the historical maximum likelihood estimate of 9.32. The beta hyperparameter, a, was fixed at 0.01, which corresponds to a simulated Type I error rate (falsely rejecting the null hypothesis $\lambda = 0$) of 0.05 given $E(y)$ is set equal to $E(y_0) + \frac{3\sigma}{5}$. Other choices are certainly possible; for example, we could decrease a to deliver the same Type I error rate were mean shifts smaller than $\frac{3\sigma}{5}$ of interest.

Table 6.1 clearly shows that ld sum at baseline is a highly significant covariate. Therefore, we also generated a fake historical dataset that replaced the real baseline ld sums with values randomly generated from a $Normal(12, 9)$ distribution independent of y_0. We then fit the same commensurate power prior linear model using the real current data to see if our model could properly identify the inconsistencies and downweight the influence of the fake historical data.

| | Real x_0 | | Fake x_0 | |
	estimate	95% BCI	estimate	95% BCI
intercept	-0.058	$(-1.791, 1.684)$	-0.289	$(-2.542, 1.902)$
BL ld sum	-0.324	$(-0.375, -0.271)$	-0.380	$(-0.451, -0.310)$
age	0.003	$(-0.024, 0.030)$	0.012	$(-0.021, 0.046)$
AST	0.001	$(-0.009, 0.012)$	0.002	$(-0.012, 0.016)$
FOLFOX	-0.755	$(-1.372, -0.142)$	-0.549	$(-1.278, 0.185)$
α_0	1	$(1, 1)$	0.067	$(0.011, 0.236)$
τ^2	0	$(0,0)$	0.003	$(0.001, 0.028)$

Table 6.2 *Commensurable power prior fits to colorectal cancer data.*

Point estimates (posterior medians) and 95% equal-tail Bayesian credible intervals for both the real (left) and fake (right) data are displayed in Table 6.2. First, notice that the posterior for α_0 corresponding to the real data has converged to a point mass at 1. Therefore, our power prior linear model considers the real historical and current data to be commensurate, and thus incorporates virtually all of the historical information, increasing the precision of the parameter estimates. As a result, the 95% credible interval upper bound for λ is now less than zero, and so we can now conclude that FOLFOX resulted in a significant reduction in average ld sum when compared to the IFL regimen. This finding is consistent with those of Goldberg et al. (2004), who determined FOLFOX to have better times to progression and response rates.

On the other hand, the model properly identifies the inconsistencies in the relationship between the response and baseline covariates among the current and fake historical data. This is clear from the 95% credible interval for α_0 in this case, which is very far from 1. As a result of the decrease in precision, the posterior for λ covers 0 and the posterior summaries for β and λ mirror linear regression estimates on the right side of Table 6.1. Last, notice that the power prior credible intervals in the right side of Table 6.2 are wider than their counterparts in Table 6.1. This occurs in part because the error variance for the current data is an estimated 33% less than our fixed choice of σ^2. ∎

Hobbs et al. (2009) show that commensurate power priors also have good frequentist Type I error and power performance, but these simulations all assume Gaussian responses. Future work in this area looks toward extending to non-Gaussian settings, especially those involving categorical and time-to-event data. Another important need is the development of commensurate priors for adaptive borrowing that allows the sample size or allocation ratio in the ongoing trial to be altered if this is warranted. The idea would be to maintain the balance of samples encouraged by α_0 by defining the allocation ratio as a function of the number of effective historical controls, $n_0\alpha_0$. That is, if the model encourages greater borrowing from the historical controls, we can randomize more new subjects to the experimental treatment. Otherwise, the historical data will be suppressed, and the allocation of new subjects to treatment and placebo will remain balanced. To do this, suppose s_j and r_j denote the number of subjects randomized to treatment and control, respectively, in the current trial following the jth enrollment. Define η_j to be the effective proportion of controls after the jth enrollment,

$$\eta_j = \frac{r_j + n_0\alpha_0}{s_j + r_j + n_0\alpha_0} \ . \tag{6.13}$$

The posterior of α_0 induces a posterior for each η_j, whose median could be used as the probability that the $(j+1)^{st}$ subject is assigned to the new treatment. This imposes information balance by encouraging optimal use of new patients relative to amount of incorporated prior information. In practice this could be done in blocks, perhaps after an initial period where η_j is fixed at $1/2$.

As a final side comment, Fuquene et al. (2009) show that Cauchy priors and also a class of noninformative priors described by Berger (1985) can correctly avoid borrowing when this is unwarranted – say, due to a few large outliers in one of the two datasets. However, the commensurate prior methods are quicker to permit borrowing when this *is* warranted, the source of any "Bayesian advantage" the adaptive procedure can offer.

6.2 Equivalence studies

An increasingly common area of statistical investigation in clinical trials concerns *bioequivalence*, where we wish to know whether the rates and absorption extents of two different drugs can be thought of as equivalent. Oftentimes the two drugs are a reference product and a competing generic alternative, and we are hoping to show that the two products have similar drug concentration profiles over time, so that their therapeutic effects can be reasonably expected to be similar as well. In the United States, the FDA will not permit a generic drug to be marketed unless it can be shown to be bioequivalent to the innovator product. As such, statistical methods that are appropriate and acceptable to the FDA are crucial.

Mechanically, a typical bioequivalence study measures the concentration of drug in the blood just before and at certain set times after its administration. A sensible summary of the resulting empirical time-concentration curve, such as AUC (area under curve), C_{max} (the maximum concentration over time), or T_{max} (the time to maximum concentration), is then used as a surrogate for the drug's pharmacokinetics more generally. Since these measures are all strictly positive, it is common to take their logs as the response variable in a normal (Gaussian) statistical model. Were the goal to show a *difference* between the two drugs, an ordinary 2-sample t test might even be appropriate here.

Before getting into further statistical detail, however, we must mention that there are three distinct notions of "bioequivalence," at least as described in current FDA guidance documents (Food and Drug Administration, 1999, 2001, 2002). By far the most common is *average bioequivalence*, or ABE. This refers to equivalence between population *mean* responses in the two study groups. While this concept is easiest to understand (not to mention model statistically), note that two drugs whose drug responses are significantly different in terms of their *variability* could be declared "bioequivalent" under ABE. In *population bioequivalence*, or PBE, the variabilities of drug responses are also considered. The resulting, more stringent condition is also sometimes known as *prescribability*, since population bioequivalence implies interchangeability of the two drugs at the time of initial prescription. Finally, in *individual bioequivalence*, or IBE, we also add the notion of *switchability*, or exchangeability of the two drugs within the same patient at any time during the regimen. The thinking here is that, for a patient who had been taking the standard drug for some time, to safely switch to the new drug, one would need to show that the concentrations of the active ingredient for the two drugs are the same at any time during the regimen, not merely prior to treatment as with prescribability. Both PBE and IBE remain somewhat controversial, and virtually all practical investigations remain concerned with the demonstration of ABE. As such, in what follows we focus on ABE; however, see Erickson et al. (2006) and Ghosh and Ntzoufras (2005) for more details on these distinctions, as well as related Bayesian models and `WinBUGS` software for particular IBE and PBE settings.

In the remainder of this section, we begin with a brief description of the basic ABE problem and a few standard approaches to its solution, including fitting it into the indifference zone paradigm of Subsection 2.5.2. We then describe two specific models often used in bioequivalence studies, one for simply binary response data and the other for a more complex (though fairly standard) 2×2 crossover design.

6.2.1 Statistical issues in bioequivalence

Equivalence testing is an area of broad interest in statistics, well beyond the realm of clinical trials. But this is partly an accident of history, in the sense that it emerged as its own research area largely due to the widespread adoption of the Neyman-Pearson (N-P) statistical testing framework in the latter half of the twentieth century. As we have seen, in this framework, the usual setup for testing the significance of some treatment difference Δ,

$$H_0 : \Delta = 0 \quad \text{vs.} \quad H_A : \Delta \neq 0 , \tag{6.14}$$

presumes that the hypothesis we hope to reject is the null, H_0. Recall that in N-P testing one can never "accept" the null, only "fail to reject" it. As such, if our interest is in showing that two treatments are "equivalent," it is indeed the alternative we hope to reject. But simply switching the roles of H_0 and H_A is not sensible, since N-P testing requires the null to be a "reduction" (simplification) of the alternative, such as the one in (6.14) where Δ is set to 0. And in any event, we do not really need the treatment difference to be *exactly* 0; in the case where Δ is continuous, we would never expect any estimate $\hat{\Delta}$ to be identically equal to 0. Rather, we simply need Δ to be "close enough" to zero. One possible formulation along these lines might be

$$H_0 : \Delta \notin (-\delta, \delta) \quad \text{vs.} \quad H_A : \Delta \in (-\delta, \delta) , \tag{6.15}$$

for some prespecified $\delta > 0$. The traditional solution to this problem is the so-called *two one-sided tests (TOST)* procedure (Schuirmann, 1987). This procedure's popularity arises from its relative ease of use (it is theoretically and operationally similar to a traditional test of equality as in (6.14)) and from both regulation and encouragement by the U.S. Food and Drug Administration (1992, 1999).

We will describe the TOST approach in some detail in Subsection 6.2.2; for now, suffice to say that, while clever, it seems unattractive from a scientific point of view: surely we would prefer to avoid having to first reformulate and then swap the hypotheses, carefully crafting the "right" problem to match our available statistical technology. Moreover, since the Bayesian approach allows direct probabilistic statements about the parameter space, it would be very natural to use in assigning posterior probabilities to the two hypotheses in (6.15), and thus their relative plausibility. A traditional Bayesian solution here would compute the Bayes factor in favor of H_0 in (6.15), following the exact and approximate methods described in Subsection 2.2.3. A Bayes factor larger than 1 favors equivalence, while less than one favors inequivalence. In practice, we might insist on a larger Bayes factor threshold than 1, in order to reduce the Type I error of our procedure.

Alternatively, the indifference zone approach of Subsection 2.5.2 could be very naturally adopted here. Recall this is where we formulate the null and alternative hypotheses similar to (6.15) as

$$H_0 : \Delta \notin (\delta_L, \delta_U) \quad \text{vs.} \quad H_A : \Delta \in (\delta_L, \delta_U) , \tag{6.16}$$

for $\delta_L < \delta_U$. Referring again to Figure 2.10, which is shown again here as Figure 6.3, we recall that "equivalence" in this setting is concluded only when the 95% equal-tail posterior credible interval for $\Delta, (\Delta_L, \Delta_U)$, is entirely contained within the indifference zone (δ_L, δ_U). Again, Type I

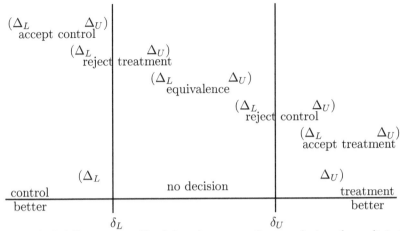

Figure 6.3 *Indifference zone* (δ_L, δ_U) *and corresponding conclusions for a clinical trial based on the location of the 95% posterior credible interval for* Δ.

error can be reduced by insisting on confidence higher than 95%, though this will of course also reduce power.

Before continuing, we mention that equivalence testing is closely related to the notion of *noninferiority testing*, where the goal is simply to show that one drug is not inferior to the other. For instance, if we want to show the treatment is not inferior to the control in Figure 6.3, we would test

$$H_0 : \Delta \leq \delta_L \quad \text{vs.} \quad H_A : \Delta > \delta_L \ ,$$

since here H_0 refers to treatment inferiority. This return to the one-sided testing makes the problem substantially easier for a frequentist; in the Bayesian paradigm, we would likely reject H_0 if $P(\Delta > \delta_L | \text{data})$ were sufficiently large, or alternatively, if the lower limit of the Bayesian credible interval Δ_L were bigger than the inferiority threshold δ_L.

6.2.2 Binomial response design

Williamson (2007) lays out the hypotheses and the standard two one-sided test (TOST) approach in the case of a simple binomial response in both treatment groups. Suppose p_1 and p_2 are the probabilities of success in the two drug groups, and let $p_\Delta = p_1 - p_2$. The hypotheses of interest are then the binomial model version of those in (6.15), which we rewrite as the *pair* of hypotheses,

$$H_{01} : p_\Delta \geq \delta \quad \text{vs.} \quad H_{A1} : p_\Delta < \delta$$
$$\text{and} \quad H_{02} : p_\Delta \leq -\delta \quad \text{vs.} \quad H_{A2} : p_\Delta > -\delta \ .$$

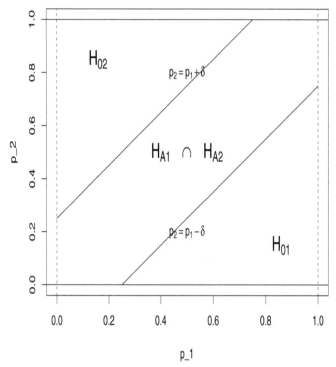

Figure 6.4 *Hypothesis of interest for the binomial response TOST.*

This setting is pictured in Figure 6.4 for $\delta = 0.25$. The basic idea behind
the TOST is that we reject H_0 if and only if H_{01} and H_{02} are *both* rejected
at a chosen level of significance, since $p_\Delta < \delta$ and $p_\Delta > -\delta$ is equivalent to
$-\delta < p_\Delta < \delta$. Note that H_{01}, H_{A1}, H_{02}, and H_{A2} correspond to inferiority,
noninferiority, superiority, and nonsuperiority of treatment 2 relative to
treatment 1.

Schuirmann (1987) showed that the TOST procedure is operationally
identical to declaring equivalence if and only if the usual $100(1 - 2\alpha)\%$
confidence interval for p_Δ is entirely contained in $(-\delta, \delta)$. Note the possibly
surprising use of 2α instead of α in this expression; see Williamson (2007,
Appendix A) for a concise and easy-to-follow proof of this fact.

Let us consider the case of two binomial responses, X_1 and X_2, giving the
number of successes in n_1 and n_2 trials, respectively, in the two treatment
groups. Here we would naturally suppose $X_i \sim Bin(n_i, p_i)$ for $i = 1, 2$, and
let $\hat{p}_i = X_i/n_i$ be the respective sample proportions. The most common
TOST interval is then the $100(1 - 2\alpha)\%$ confidence interval method applied

to the usual asymptotic interval,

$$\hat{p}_1 - \hat{p}_2 \pm z_\alpha \left(\frac{\hat{p}_1(1 - \hat{p}_1)}{n_1} + \frac{\hat{p}_2(1 - \hat{p}_2)}{n_2} \right)^{1/2},$$

which again concludes bioequivalence if this interval is contained within $(-\delta, \delta)$. Barker et al. (2001) compare this method with five other variants of it, plus two other frequentist tests, in terms of size, power, and ease of implementation. Williamson (2007) compares a subset of these tests to fully Bayesian versions based not on interval comparisons of the sort encouraged by Figure 6.3, but on Bayes factors under standard hypotheses. For instance, suppose we wish to test the hypotheses in (6.15). Williamson (2007) evaluates the Bayes factor in favor of H_0 under a flat prior for (p_1, p_2),

$$\pi(p_1, p_2) = 1, \ \ 0 < p_1 < 1, \ 0 < p_2 < 1 \,,$$

and also under a product of noninformative Jeffreys (Beta$(1/2, 1/2)$) priors,

$$\pi(p_1, p_2) = p_1^{-1/2}(1 - p_1)^{-1/2} p_2^{-1/2}(1 - p_2)^{-1/2}, \ \ 0 < p_1 < 1, \ 0 < p_2 < 1 \,.$$

In either case, the posterior probability that H_0 is true must be computed numerically, but is fairly straightforward given our conjugate prior setup.

The simulation study by Williamson (2007) compares the power and Type I error behavior of these methods with that of somewhat more informative Bayesian methods that use $Beta(2, 4)$ and $Beta(4, 4)$ priors, respectively. The noninformative Bayesian approach emerges as an attractive alternative to the TOST procedures in terms of power.

We remark that multiplicity issues like those discussed in Sections 2.2.7 and 6.3 come up again here. Suppose we wish to test $H_0 : p_i = p_j$ for all possible pairs of hypotheses (i, j), where the total number of populations is k. Lauzon and Caffo (2009) show that multiplicity is easily controlled in the TOST by simply scaling the nominal Type I error by $k - 1$ (instead of the total number of comparisons $k(k-1)/2$, the usual Bonferroni choice). This is due to the fact that the maximum error is achieved at $p_i = p_j = p$ for all adjacent p's; that is, only the $k - 1$ comparisons with the closest mean differences make any real contribution to the error. Berger and Hsu (1996) offer a critique of current TOST practice, arguing that the usual conception of size-α bioequivalence test as corresponding to a $100(1 - 2\alpha)\%$ confidence set is only true in special cases, and should be discarded in favor of more general intersection-union tests (of which the standard TOST is a special case).

6.2.3 2 × 2 crossover design

A very common framework for equivalence testing is the 2×2 *crossover design*. This setting is described in some detail by Chow and Liu (2000,

Ch. 3); here we adopt the notation of Ghosh and Rosner (2007). Suppose y_{ijk} is the log of the response in the ith sequence from the kth period for the jth subject, $i = 1, 2$, $j = 1, \ldots, n_i$, $k = 1, 2$. We model y_{ijk} as

$$y_{ijk} = m_{ik} + S_i + P_k + \delta_{ij} + \epsilon_{ijk} ,$$

where m_{ik} is the direct effect of the formulation in the ith sequence administered in the kth period, S_i is the sequence effect, P_k is the period effect, δ_{ij} is the random effect of the jth subject in the ith sequence, and ϵ_{ijk} is a within-subject random error. Without loss of generality, we may assume the first sequence is the reference formulation (R), then

$$m_{ik} = \left\{ \begin{array}{ll} m_R & \text{if } k = i \\ m_T & \text{if } k \neq i \end{array} \right. ,$$

where it is often convenient to assume $m_R + m_T = 0$. The δ_{ij} are typically assumed to be i.i.d. $N(0, \sigma^2)$ random variables, mutually independent of the ϵ_{ijk}, which are i.i.d. $N(0, \sigma_\ell^2)$, where $\ell = R$ if $i = k$ and $\ell = T$ otherwise.

Again, average bioequivalence is concluded if we reject H_0 as stated in (6.16). The FDA has suggested taking $\delta_L = \log(0.8)$ and $\delta_U = \log(1.25)$, which is sensible since the data themselves have been logged. If the posterior probability of H_A is greater than 0.5 then ABE may be concluded.

To fully specify the hierarchical model, Ghosh and Rosner (2007) actually recommend a Dirichlet process mixture prior of the form

$$
\begin{array}{rcl}
\delta_{ij} & \sim & N(\mu_j, \sigma_\delta^2) \\
\mu_j & \sim & G \\
G & \sim & DP(\alpha G_0) \\
G_0 & \sim & N(0, \sigma_G^2) \\
\text{and } \sigma_\delta^2 & \sim & IG(c, d) ,
\end{array}
$$

where DP denotes the Dirichlet process with base measure G_0 and precision parameter α, which captures our degree of confidence in our prior "best guess" G_0. Ghosh and Rosner (2007) follow Sethuraman (1994) and many other MCMC-oriented authors by regarding the infinite dimensional parameter G as an infinite mixture. A finite approximation then permits feasible WinBUGS implementation. These authors also contemplate a standard normal hierarchical model, but find the added flexibility of the DP mixture to offer worthwhile advantages, at least in the context of their real-data example.

The Bayesian hypothesis test requires estimation of the posterior probability of the null hypothesis. Using the Gibbs sampler draws $m_T^{(g)}$ and $m_R^{(g)}$ for $g = 1, \ldots, G$, we can estimate

$$P(ABE|data) \quad = \quad P(\log(0.8) < m_T - m_R < \log(1.25)|data)$$

$$\approx \; \frac{1}{G} \sum_{g=1}^{G} I(\log(0.8) < m_T^{(g)} - m_R^{(g)} < \log(1.25)) \; .$$

Again, if this estimate exceeds 0.5, we are justified in choosing the alternative hypothesis, hence concluding bioequivalence.

Up until now we have considered the analysis of just one endpoint at a time. But we may wish to evaluate bioequivalence based on a simultaneous assessment of *two* endpoints – say, the area under the blood concentration-time curve, AUC, and the maximum concentration, C_{max}. Since these endpoints are likely to be (positively) associated, this requires a multivariate response model that permits dependence among the endpoints considered. Previous approaches include work by Hauck et al. (1995), Chinchilli and Elswick (1997), and Quan et al. (2001), and have tended to achieve the desired correlations with multivariate normal models. The intersection-union tests of Berger and Hsu (1996) and Wang et al. (1999) tend to be conservative, the extent of which depends upon the between-endpoint correlation.

Ghosh and Gönen (2008) extend the semiparametric setting of Ghosh and Rosner (2007) to the case of multiple endpoints, but still using the Dirichlet process mixture (DPM) formulation. The prior is constructed to allow a positive probability of the null hypothesis for each endpoint. Prior elicitation is rather more complex here, since the model is significantly more complex and results depend crucially on the between-endpoint correlations. The authors illustrate their approach with a simultaneous analysis of AUC and C_{max} in a two-sequence, two-period crossover study of two formulations of the drug erythromycin. Interestingly, these data feature fairly strong evidence of bioinequivalence for AUC, but far more uncertainty (bordering on mild evidence of bioequivalence) for C_{max}. Ghosh and Gönen (2008) consider results over a set of assumed prior correlations ρ between the two endpoints, ranging from 0 to 0.5. The marginal probabilities of bioequivalence are modified in the expected directions as ρ increases (e.g., the probability using C_{max} starts fairly large, but drops as the impact of the less encouraging AUC data is more keenly felt).

Once again the method is fit in WinBUGS via a finite approximation to the (infinite-dimensional) DPM where a parameter L controls the number of components in the mixture. Truly joint probabilities of bioequivalence $P(ABE|data)$ are computed as

$$P(\log(0.8) < \theta_1 < \log(1.25) \cap \log(0.8) < \theta_2 < \log(1.25)|data)$$
$$\approx \tfrac{1}{G} \textstyle\sum_{g=1}^{G} I(\log(0.8) < \theta_1^{(g)} < \log(1.25) \cap \log(0.8) < \theta_2^{(g)} < \log(1.25)) \,,$$

where g indexes the Gibbs samples for the treatment differences for $AUC(\theta_1)$ and $C_{max}(\theta_2)$.

Software note: WinBUGS code to carry out this process is available from the second author's website, http://www.mskcc.org/mskcc/html/84563.cfm.

Finally, DeSouza et al. (2009) offer a fully parametric analysis of the multiple endpoint two-period crossover design of Ghosh and Gönen (2008). These authors give the relevant full conditional distributions under the usual product of minimally informative normal-inverse gamma priors, as well as an illustration using an artificial dataset taken from a bioequivalence guide published by the Brazilian government. Straightforward `WinBUGS` code is provided in Appendix A of the paper.

6.3 Multiplicity

As discussed previously in Subsection 2.2.7 and elsewhere, the problem of multiplicity is one of the most difficult for any statistician, Bayesian or frequentist. Moreover, the problem arises in virtually every data analytic context in some form or another. That is, we almost never come to a dataset intending to analyze just one particular aspect and then never touch the set again; rather, we expect to perform multiple analyses, altering our model, transforming certain variables, and so on as we go. It is sometimes difficult to say when one crosses the line between "good statistical practice" and "data dredging" that serves to inflate the perceived significance of one of many possible findings. Statistically, the problem is complicated by the fact that the frequentist and Bayesian camps can seem particularly far apart in their views as to its proper remedy. The former group typically argues for sometimes drastic corrective action, e.g., Bonferroni and other adjustments that are so conservative as to preclude significant findings in all but the very most extreme cases (where no adjustment and indeed no statistics are really necessary). On the other hand, some pure Bayesians argue that, since any marginal "slice" of a joint posterior distribution has prima facie validity in its own right, and there is no sensible way to prespecify how many of these slices one might ultimately choose to view, *no* adjustments for multiplicity are required. But this of course serves to perpetuate the problem that motivated the discussion in the first place: an overabundance of "false positives" when too many analyses are in the mix.

As usual, in clinical trials our outlook must be a practical one. Throughout this book we have advocated Bayesian methods that enjoy good frequentist properties, and it is natural to look for a similar compromise in this setting as well. Here it would mean some sort of "partial correction" that accounts for multiplicity when this is crucial (e.g., would otherwise result in an abundance of false positives), but doesn't overdo it when it is not. Hierarchical Bayesian modeling of the sort introduced in Section 2.4 is a natural tool here in cases where we can realistically expect to be able to "model our way out" of the problem to any significant extent. That is, we may be able to construct a model that (a) anticipates various structural similarities among the model parameters that could lead to problems if not acknowledged, and (b) is flexible enough to allow the accumulating data to help determine just how much correction is required.

6.3.1 Assessing drug safety

A good example of the use of hierarchical modeling to help correct for multiplicity arises in the analysis of drug safety data. Here the problem is one of determining which of several adverse events (AEs) are significantly associated with a particular experimental treatment. Typically this is in the setting of a clinical trial comparing a treatment (T) and a control (C), and we are interested in "flagging" any AE that is differentially associated between these two groups. Note that Type II errors are equally if not more important than Type I errors in such settings, since failing to flag a real drug-AE interaction is likely a greater public health risk than falsely identifying such an interaction.

A number of Bayesian methods have been proposed in drug safety assessment. In analyzing post-marketing spontaneous reports, DuMouchel (1999) proposed a gamma-Poisson shrinkage algorithm in analyzing the FDA adverse event reporting system (AERS) database, while Bate et al. (1998) used a Bayesian Confidence Propagation Neural Network (BCPNN) approach to analyze a WHO database of adverse drug reactions. In this section, we follow the model of Berry and Berry (2004), who point out two advantages the Bayesian approach offers here over the frequentist. First, the rates for those AEs *not* being considered for flagging, as well as their similarity with those that are, can be explicitly measured and fed back into the analysis. Second, a hierarchical structure may be useful in capturing the biological relationships among the various AEs. In the latter case, it's important to stress that any similarities modeled among AEs must be based on biological (or perhaps regulatory) grounds, and not merely on empirical similarity. The most obvious choice for grouping here would be based on body system: the model could assume that AEs arising from the same body system are more likely to be similar than those in different body systems.

Let us specify the problem a bit more so that appropriate statistical notation can be established. At the present time, AEs are routinely coded in *Medical Dictionary for Regulatory Activities* (MedDRA) terms with a hierarchical structure. One such coding is by system organ class (SOC), which intrinsically reflects biological relationships among various AEs in the same class. AEs in the same SOC are thus more likely to be similar, making hierarchical borrowing of strength natural. We can also allow for borrowing *across* SOCs, though our model does not impose it; instead it adapts based on the observed data. In our dataset, AEs are actually identified by their "preferred term" (PT), such as "rash, varicella-like;" MedDRA allows even further subcategorization of PTs, but in this paper we use PT as the smallest unit of analysis.

This setup essentially matches that assumed by Berry and Berry (2004), who adopt a binomial likelihood for the AE counts in the treatment (Y) and control (X) groups. That is, they let $Y_{bj} \sim Bin(N_t, t_{bj})$ and $X_{bj} \sim Bin(N_c, c_{bj})$, where t_{bj} and c_{bj} are the probabilities of adverse event for PT j and SOC b in the two groups, respectively. These authors then consider a logistic regression mean structure,

$$logit(c_{bj}) = \log(c_{bj}/(1 - c_{bj})) = \gamma_{bj} \quad \text{and} \quad logit(t_{bj}) = \gamma_{bj} + \theta_{bj} \ ,$$

so that γ_{bj} is the logit AE rate in the control group, and θ_{bj} is the relative increase in this logit rate in the treatment group. Note that this means $\theta_{bj} = \log\{[t_{bj}(1 - c_{bj})]/[c_{bj}(1 - t_{bj})]\}$ is the log-odds ratio (OR).

The hierarchical model then proceeds as follows. We begin by setting the first stage prior distributions to be

$$\gamma_{bj} \sim N(\mu_{\gamma b}, \sigma_{\gamma b}^2)$$

and

$$\theta_{bj} \sim N(\mu_{\theta b}, \sigma_{\theta b}^2) \ , \tag{6.17}$$

both for $j = 1, \ldots, J_b$ and $b = 1, \ldots, B$. These specifications encourage borrowing of strength within each SOC. Next, at the second stage we use the following prior distributions:

$$\mu_{\gamma b} \sim N(\mu_{\gamma 0}, \tau_{\gamma 0}^2), \qquad \sigma_{\gamma b}^2 \sim IG(\alpha_\gamma, \beta_\gamma)$$
$$\text{and} \quad \mu_{\theta b} \sim N(\mu_{\theta 0}, \tau_{\theta 0}^2), \qquad \sigma_{\theta b}^2 \sim IG(\alpha_\theta, \beta_\theta) \ ,$$

where again $b = 1, \ldots, B$ and IG denotes the inverse gamma distribution. This specification permits borrowing *across* SOCs where appropriate (though we do not expect such borrowing to be nearly as dramatic as that within SOC). Finally, the model specification is completed with priors for the second stage model parameters, which we take as

$$\mu_{\gamma 0} \sim N(\mu_{\gamma 00}, \tau_{\gamma 00}^2), \qquad \tau_{\gamma 0}^2 \sim IG(\alpha_{\gamma 00}, \beta_{\gamma 00}),$$
$$\mu_{\theta 0} \sim N(\mu_{\theta 00}, \tau_{\theta 00}^2), \qquad \text{and} \quad \tau_{\theta 0}^2 \sim IG(\alpha_{\theta 00}, \beta_{\theta 00}) \ .$$

We assume the hyperparameters $\mu_{\gamma 00}, \mu_{\theta 00}, \tau_{\gamma 00}^2, \tau_{\theta 00}^2, \alpha_{\gamma 00}, \beta_{\gamma 00}, \alpha_{\theta 00}, \beta_{\theta 00}, \alpha_\gamma, \beta_\gamma, \alpha_\theta,$ and β_θ are fixed constants. In our analysis, we specify minimally informative values for these as $\mu_{\gamma 00} = \mu_{\theta 00} = 0$, $\tau_{\gamma 00}^2 = \tau_{\theta 00}^2 = 10$, $\alpha_{\gamma 00} = \alpha_{\theta 00} = \alpha_\gamma = \alpha_\theta = 3$, and $\beta_{\gamma 00} = \beta_{\theta 00} = \beta_\gamma = \beta_\theta = 1$.

Berry and Berry (2004) actually recommend a slightly more sophisticated first stage model for the θ_{bj}. Specifically, they replace (6.17) with a *mixture* distribution of the form

$$\theta_{bj} \sim \pi_b \delta(0) + (1 - \pi_b) N(\mu_{\theta b}, \sigma_{\theta b}^2) \ , \tag{6.18}$$

where $0 \leq \pi_b \leq 1$ and $\delta(0)$ is the Dirac delta function (point mass) at 0. This permits a prior probability of π_b that the treatment and control rates are *exactly* the same, which is appropriate since many AEs are completely unaffected by the treatment. The remainder of the model is the same, although we now require prior distributions for the new hyperparameters π_b as follows:

$$\pi_b \sim Beta(\alpha_\pi, \beta_\pi)$$
$$\alpha_\pi \sim Exponential(\lambda_\alpha)I(\alpha_\pi > 1)$$
$$\text{and} \quad \beta_\pi \sim Exponential(\lambda_\beta)I(\beta_\pi > 1).$$

where we truncate the two exponential distributions in order to prevent too much prior mass for the π_b from accumulating near the "extreme" values of 0 and 1. We also need to add fixed values for the hyperparameters λ_α and λ_β, which we take as $\lambda_\alpha = \lambda_\beta = 0.1$.

Given the posterior distribution of our Bayesian hierarchical model, we may use the posterior *exceedance probability* to identify potential signals. For example, an AE of PT j in SOC b can be flagged if

$$P(\theta_{bj} > d \mid \mathbf{x}, \mathbf{y}) > p, \tag{6.19}$$

where d and p are prespecified constants. For safety signal detection, we might simply choose $d = 0$, indicating higher odds of AE in the treatment arm $(OR > 1)$. On the other hand, a θ_{bj} could have a high posterior probability of exceeding 0, but be clinically unimportant. As such, larger values of d (say, $\log(2)$) might be used to better capture a "clinically meaningful" effect.

The exceedance probabilities for other statistics are also easily obtainable in our Bayesian framework. For instance, we can switch from the log-OR scale to the *risk difference* (RD) scale by flagging AEs for which

$$P(t_{bj} - c_{bj} > d^* \mid \mathbf{x}, \mathbf{y}) > p, \tag{6.20}$$

where again d^* and p are appropriate constants.

Example 6.4 Xia, Ma, and Carlin (2008) apply the models above to AE data aggregated from four double-blind, placebo-controlled, phase II-III clinical trials of a particular drug. All studies were of 12 or 24 weeks in duration and were fairly similar in design and population, justifying their pooling for this analysis. The full dataset has 1245 subjects in the treatment group and 720 subjects in the control group, with reported AEs coded to 465 PTs under 24 SOCs.

Tables 6.3 and 6.4 presents various posterior exceedance probabilities from our hierarchical binomial model using the mixture prior (6.18) for the five PTs that have two-sided Fisher's exact test p-values less than 0.05 and higher observed risks on the treatment arm than on the placebo arm. The fourth column of Table 6.3 gives the posterior probability of $OR = 1$, i.e., no difference between treatment and placebo arms in our mixture setting. The last column of this table gives the posterior exceedance probabilities based on OR using the null value (1) as the cutoff. The third column of Table 6.4

SOC	PT	exact *p*-value	posterior probabilities $OR = 1$	$OR > 1$
General Disorders and Administration Site Conditions	Fatigue	0.019	0.430	0.564
Infections and Infestations	Herpes Simplex	0.025	0.459	0.532
Infections and Infestations	Sinusitis	0.012	0.302	0.697
Injury, Poisoning and Procedural Complications	Excoriation	0.030	0.680	0.296
Skin and Subcutaneous Tissue Disorders	Ecchymosis	0.005	0.457	0.535

Table 6.3 *Fisher's exact test p-values and posterior summaries under the hierarchical binomial mixture model for the four-study data.*

instead uses an OR cutoff of 2, potentially a more clinically meaningful threshold. The last two columns of Table 6.4 give the exceedance probabilities based on the risk difference scale for two potentially important differences.

The tables reveal that smaller *p*-values do not necessarily correspond to higher posterior exceedance probabilities. For example, ecchymosis has the smallest *p*-value, but does not have the largest $P(OR > 1)$. The hierarchical model assumes PTs in the same SOC to be more alike than those in different SOCs. This creates a shrinkage pattern in the log-ORs that may lead to this reordering of the AEs in terms of their departure from the null. For example, the *p*-value for ecchymosis is smaller than that for sinusitis. However, the posteriors of the AEs in the "Skin and Subcutaneous Tissue Disorders" SOC, to which ecchymosis belongs, do not show a consistent pattern of adverse effect; in fact, about half of them had *negative* treatment differences. Thus, the Bayesian model is less eager to flag ecchymosis than Fisher's exact test, which ignores the hierarchy. By contrast, in the "Infections and Infestations" SOC, to which sinusitis belongs, most AEs do show higher risk in the treatment arm. The hierarchical mixture procedure

SOC	PT	posterior probabilities		
		$OR > 2$	$RD > 2\%$	$RD > 5\%$
General Disorders and Administration Site Conditions	Fatigue	0.319	0.099	0.000
Infections and Infestations	Herpes Simplex	0.357	0.000	0.000
Infections and Infestations	Sinusitis	0.422	0.280	0.000
Injury, Poisoning and Procedural Complications	Excoriation	0.175	0.000	0.000
Skin and Subcutaneous Tissue Disorders	Ecchymosis	0.437	0.000	0.000

Table 6.4 *More posterior summaries under the hierarchical binomial mixture model for the four-study data.*

also tones down the somewhat alarming p-value of 0.03 for excoriation, obtaining a posterior probability of just 0.296 that the OR exceeds 1.

Table 6.4 also shows that the posterior probabilities of the risk difference exceeding 2% are all very low for these five AEs, further indicating that, while there may be some limited statistical significance to our findings here, their clinical significance is very much in doubt.

In the context of this example, Xia et al. (2008) also perform various simulation studies that show better power and familywise error rates for their Bayesian procedures over those based on (unadjusted) Fisher exact tests under both binomial and Poisson likelihoods. However, the authors emphasize the inevitable and now-familiar tradeoff between lower error rates and good power. ∎

Note that the models discussed above do not contemplate any sort of nonexchangeability; shrinkage both within and across groups is assumed to follow an i.i.d. normal specification, albeit with the mixture enhancement (6.18) in the case of θ_{bj}. But in some cases, there may be a "distance" metric one can use to help shrink differentially within groups. Then one could use a spatial-type model, reminiscent of those used in geostatistical data analysis (see e.g. Banerjee et al., 2004, Ch. 2). For example, the covariance between γ_{bj} and $\gamma_{bj'}$, corresponding to two AEs j and j' within SOC b, might be

$$\sigma_\gamma^2 \exp(-\rho_\gamma d_{bj,bj'}) \,,$$

where $d_{bj,bj'}$ is the "distance" between these two AEs. In the Berry and Berry (2004) setting we might set the distance between two rashes (say, measles/rubella-like and varicella-like) in Group 10 equal to 1, but use a larger distance (say, 2) between either of these rashes and eczema. Like the assignment of AEs to SOCs, the selection of these distances would be crucial, and need to be informed by biological (not empirical) mechanisms. But if one could do this, this would encourage a different (and perhaps more sensible) kind of shrinkage in the random effects that could in turn lead to better signal detection overall in the face of multiplicity. Note that the variance and range parameters above could be generalized to be SOC-specific, i.e., $\sigma_{\gamma b}^2$ and $\rho_{\gamma b}$. Alternatively, if distances between SOCs (say, b and b') can be sensibly defined, we could model spatially at this level of the hierarchy as well, e.g., using a spatial model for the correlation between $\mu_{\theta b}$ and $\mu_{\theta b'}$.

Other methodological enhancements to the basic approach are possible. The purely "nested" borrowing of strength used above (PTs within SOC, and then across SOCs) may not be the most sensible, since many SOCs are inherently different from each other. Instead, one might prefer to define a second, entirely new hierarchy that focused more on grouping PTs in similar or proximate regions of the body. This leads naturally to a model having *two* sets of random effects, say $\theta_j^{(1)}$ and $\theta_\ell^{(2)}$, with nonnested indexing systems j and ℓ that borrow strength over separate hierarchies while both contributing to log-OR. Another extension would be to the case of AE data having more than two possible outcomes. For instance, suppose each AE was coded to a severity score, such as 1=mild, 2=moderate, 3=severe, 4=life-threatening, and 5=fatal. Such data could be accommodated via a multinomial (instead of binomial) likelihood, which would in turn help decide whether two flagged AEs (say, pancreatitis and nausea) with similar posterior exceedance probabilities were really of equal concern.

In their closing paragraph, Berry and Berry (2004) mention the possibility of using their approach in other multiplicity contexts besides drug safety, and specifically mention the problem of identifying genes that are differentially expressed in cDNA microarray data. Indeed, this is an example of a setting where genetic distance offers a natural choice of $d_{bj,bj'}$ in the formula above. In the AE setting, a careful study of the MedDRA dictionary may enable a similar choice of a sensible distance metric, though the problem here is clearly less straightforward.

6.3.2 Multiplicities and false discovery rate (FDR)

The discussion in the previous subsection showed how model-based posterior inference can be used to adjust probabilities. Formally, the adjustment is implemented as hierarchical shrinkage. Inference under the hierarchical model includes posterior probabilities for each comparison, as summarized for example in Tables 6.3 and 6.4. The probabilities for each adverse event and organ class report the judgment in light of all the data, including data for other organ classes and other adverse events. In this sense the probabilities are adjusted.

However, reporting the probabilities is only part of the solution: we still need a rule of how to threshold the probabilities. In other words, we need to select adverse events to be reported for differential adverse event rates across treatment and control groups. This selection should account for the fact that we are carrying out many such comparisons simultaneously. For example, if we consider 1000 comparisons and report all comparisons with posterior probability greater than 0.9, then we could still be almost certain to include some false decisions. The use of multiple comparisons with such massive numbers of comparisons is still rare in clinical trial design. However, with the increased use of molecular markers and high-throughput data, we expect that problems related to massive multiple comparisons will become increasingly relevant in clinical trial design.

In frequentist inference, several approaches exist to address multiplicity concerns, including Bonferroni's correction as perhaps the most popular choice. Bonferroni and other adjustments control the experiment-wide error rate of reporting any false comparison. As already mentioned, for massive multiple comparisons this control becomes excessively conservative. This led to the development of alternative approaches and criteria for error control in massive multiple comparisons.

Benjamini and Hochberg (1995) proposed to control the false discovery rate (FDR). Let $\delta_i \in \{0,1\}$ denote the (unknown) truth about the ith comparison. For example, in the setting of the previous subsection, δ_i is an indicator for a non-zero true difference in rates for an adverse event. Let $d_i \in \{0,1\}$ denote the decision about the ith comparison. In the example this is an indicator for reporting differential rates across treatment and control for the i-th adverse event. Let $D = \sum d_i$ denote the number of reported comparisons. The false discovery proportion is defined as $\sum_i d_i(1-\delta_i)/D$. The FDR is the (usually frequentist) expectation

$$\text{FDR} = E\left(\frac{1}{D}\sum_i d_i(1-\delta_i)\right).$$

Benjamini and Hochberg (1995) proposed a very elegant and easily implemented algorithm that guarantees $\text{FDR} < \alpha$ for any desired error bound.

Alternatively, one could aim to control the *posterior* expectation of the false discovery proportion, leading to the posterior FDR:

$$\overline{\text{FDR}} = E\left(\frac{1}{D}\sum_i d_i(1-\delta_i) \mid y\right).$$

Here we run into some good luck: the evaluation of this posterior expectation is straightforward. Conditional on the data y, the only unknown quantities are the δ_i. The decisions d_i are functions of the data, $d_i(y)$, and are fixed conditional on y. This leaves us with $\overline{\text{FDR}} = \frac{1}{D}\sum d_i[1-E(\delta_i \mid y)]$. See, for example, Newton et al. (2004) for the use of $\overline{\text{FDR}}$ in the context of a specific model, and Müller et al. (2007) for a discussion of alternative Bayesian approaches for controlling error rates in multiple comparisons.

6.4 Subgroup analysis

6.4.1 Bayesian approach

Subgroup analysis is concerned with the question of whether an overall conclusion about the effectiveness of a treatment remains valid for subpopulations of the overall patient population. For example, in a trial for a new neuroprotective agent for stroke patients, it might be important to consider patient subpopulations defined by different stroke types (for example, ischemic vs. hemorrhagic strokes), severities, and so on. It is quite plausible that an intervention is very effective for a more homogeneous subpopulation even when investigators fail to show significant effects for the more heterogeneous patient population at large. Conversely, it is possible that a therapy that is effective for most patients may be inappropriate for important subpopulations.

Most clinical trials allow for many possible subgroups to be identified, raising concerns about data dredging when subgroup effects are investigated in an unplanned manner after a trial fails to show a significant treatment effect in the overall patient population. In particular, the large number of possible subgroups that could be considered gives rise to serious multiplicity concerns. Guidelines for good practice of subgroup analyses (Pocock et al. 2002, Rothwell 2005) include the recommendation that subgroups should be pre-specified, should be limited to a small number of clinically important subgroups, and should include appropriate adjustment for multiplicities. Dixon and Simon (1991) and Simon (2002) propose Bayesian strategies for subgroup analysis based on inference for treatment–subgroup interactions.

Simon (2002) proposes a specific approach that is suitable for generalized linear models, logistic models and proportional hazards models. For example, for the proportional hazards model he proposes to include a regression on a binary treatment indicator z, a binary covariate x, and their interaction xz. Letting $\lambda(t)$ denote the hazard, Simon uses $\lambda(t) =$

$\lambda_0(t) \exp(\alpha z + \beta x + \gamma z x)$. The discussion includes a careful consideration of the prior probability model for the interaction effect γ. The prior should be calibrated by fixing the prior probability $p(\gamma \leq \delta \mid \alpha = 0)$ of a subgroup effect beyond some minimal, clinically meaningful effect δ (for negative δ). For example, $\delta = \log(2/3)$ and $\pi = 0.025$ fixes the prior probability that the hazard reduces by more than one-third for patients in the subgroup $\{x = 1\}$ compared to $\{x = 0\}$. Posterior inference on γ formalizes the subgroup analysis.

Hodges et al. (2007) describe an approach to smoothing balanced, single-error-term ANOVA models. The method uses a hierarchical model to smooth interaction terms, which effectively remain in the model if they are important predictors, vanish from the model if they are not, and are partly smoothed away if the data are indecisive. This approach is useful for proper investigation of subgroups (whose significance depends on the significance of the interactions between the main effects), but also addresses unreplicated designs and masked contrasts in effects with many degrees of freedom.

6.4.2 Bayesian decision theoretic approach

Sivaganesan et al. (2008) and Müller et al. (2010) propose a specific implementation of inference for treatment and subgroup interactions. The proposed approach goes beyond the discussion in Simon (2002) by including formal model selection for subgroup and treatment interaction effects and a formal consideration of the decision related to subgroup reports. The approach illustrates the strength of the Bayesian perspective when inference involves a complex combination of borrowing strength across related subgroups, a trade-off between the competing goals related to the overall hypothesis versus the subgroup effects, and uncertainty about the probability model. The proposed strategy is not established standard methodology, but can be characterized as an application of familiar principles of Bayesian clinical trial design to the problem of subgroup analysis.

Subgroups are characterized by available baseline covariates. Let x_{ik}, $k = 1, \ldots, K$ denote K baseline covariates recorded for patient i. We assume that covariates are categorical, $x_{ik} \in \{1, 2, \ldots, S_k\}$. If necessary, we re-code originally non-categorical covariates. The covariate levels then define potential subgroups. When reporting subgroups with non-zero treatment effects, we include inference whether and how the non-zero treatment effect varies across the reported subgroups.

The proposed approach follows a decision theoretic motivation. For the following discussion we assume a 2-arm clinical trial, with outcome y_i for the i-th patient. Let z_i be an indicator for assignment to experimental therapy ($z_i = 1$) or control ($z_i = 0$). Let θ generically indicate a treatment effect. The treatment effect could be the difference in means for a continous outcome, or the difference in success probabilities for a binary outcome. The approach remains equally valid for any other design or outcome, with minor variations in the specific algorithm only; we will indicate necessary changes at the end of this discussion.

The proposed approach proceeds by defining a decision rule for choosing among the possible actions, namely, reporting efficacy for the overall population (H_1), for some subpopulations (A^*, see below for definition), or reporting no efficacy for any subgroups (H_0). We index a pattern of subgroup effects by a vector of indicators $\gamma_k = (\gamma_{kj};\ j = 1, \ldots, S_k)$, with $\gamma_{kj} = 0$ indicating no treatment effect for the subpopulation of patients $\{i : x_{ik} = j\}$ and $\gamma_{kj} = 1, 2, \ldots$ indicating a non-zero treatment effect for $\{x_k = j\}$, with distinct integers indicating subgroups with equal treatment effects. For example, for a covariate x_k with $S_k = 2$ levels, the possible patterns of subgroup effects are as follows. There are two possible subgroups characterized by the binary covariate x_k: $\{x_i = 1\}$ and $\{x_k = 2\}$. The possible subgroup effects distinct from H_0 and H_1 are (i) no treatment effect in the first subgroup, but non-zero effect in the second subgroup; (ii) non-zero effect in the first and zero effect in the second; (iii) non-zero and different effects in the first and second subgroup. The subgroup effects (i) through (iii) are described by $\gamma = (0, 1)$, $(1, 0)$ and $(1, 2)$. Thus let $\Gamma_k = \{(0, 1), (1, 0), (1, 2)\}$ denote the possible subgroup effects in this case. The vectors $\gamma_k = (0, 0)$ and $(1, 1)$ are not included, as they correspond to the overall null and alternative hypothesis. When reporting subgroup effects we allow reporting of subgroup patterns γ_k for multiple covariates. Let $A_K \subset \{1, \ldots, K\}$ denote the covariates for which we report subgroups. Thus a subgroup report A^* is of the form $A^* = (A_K, A_\Gamma = \{\gamma_k;\ k \in A_K\})$.

The proposed rule requires a probability model $p(M)$ over competing models. Here M could be the overall alternative H_1, the overall null H_0 or a subgroup model M_{k,γ_k}. The latter, $M_{k,\gamma}$, assumes a pattern γ_k of distinct treatment effects for subgroups defined by covariate x_k. For reference we will later describe a specific probability model. The algorithm remains valid for any alternative probability model. Let $\bar{p}(M) = p(M \mid y)$ denote the posterior probability of model M.

Decision rule: The decision rule is easy to describe, but a bit more complicated to justify. We use posterior probabilities to further restrict allowable subgroup reports. Let $\gamma_k^* = \arg\max_{\gamma_k}\{\bar{p}(M_{k,\gamma_k})\}$ denote the most likely subgroup pattern for covariate x_k. If subgroups for covariate x_k are reported, then it needs to be γ_k^*. In other words, if we decide to report non-zero treatment effects for subgroups characterized by covariate x_k, we do not allow the arbitrary selection of a possible pattern of subgroups; we only allow reporting of the most likely arrangement. The rule is to decide for $\delta^* \in \{H_1, A^*, H_0\}$ using two threshold parameters t_0 and t_1 for posterior odds in a sequence of pairwise comparisons

$$\delta^* = \begin{cases} H_1 & \text{if } \frac{\bar{p}(H_1)}{\bar{p}(H_0)} > t_0 \text{ and } \frac{\bar{p}(\gamma_k^*)}{\bar{p}(H_1)} < t_1 \text{ for all } k \\ A^* & \text{if for some } k : \frac{\bar{p}(\gamma_k^*)}{\bar{p}(H_0)} > t_0 t_1 \text{ and } \frac{\bar{p}(\gamma_k^*)}{\bar{p}(H_1)} > t_1 \\ H_0 & \text{if neither } H_1 \text{ nor } A^* \text{ are chosen} \end{cases} \quad (6.21)$$

In the implementation we use thresholds $t_0 = t_1 = 1.0$ as default choices.

Model probabilities: We use model probabilities $p(M)$ indexed by two hyperparameters, p and α:

$$p(M) = \begin{cases} p^2 & \text{for } M = H_0 \\ (1-p)^2/(1+\alpha) & \text{for } M = H_1 \\ cp^{n_{k0}}\alpha^{G_k-1}\frac{\prod_{g=1}^{G_k}(n_{kg}-1)!}{\prod_{j=2}^{S_k}(\alpha+j-1)} & \text{for } M = \text{ all other } M_{k,\gamma_k} \end{cases} , (6.22)$$

with $G_k = \max_j \gamma_{kj}$ and $n_{kg} = \sum_j I(\gamma_{kj} = g)$. The specification of these prior probabilities involves two more hyperparameters, p and α, and can be described as a zero-enriched Polya urn. As default choices we suggest $p = 0.6$ and $\alpha = 1.0$. The model is completed with any sampling model $p(y \mid M)$.

Utility function: The rule (6.21) can be justified as an approximate Bayes rule under the probability model (6.22) and an assumed utility function. The utility function assigns a value $u(\delta, M, y)$ for any decision δ under assumed future data and a hypothetical truth M. Specifically,

$$u(\delta, M, y) = \begin{cases} u_0 I(M = H_0) & \text{if } \delta = H_0 \\ u_1 I(M = H_1) & \text{if } \delta = H_1 \\ u_2 I(M = M_{k\gamma_k}) & \text{if } \delta = A^* \text{ and } k \in A_K \text{ and } \gamma_k = \gamma_k^* \\ 0 & \text{otherwise} \end{cases}$$

The utilities u_0, u_1, u_2 determine the thresholds $t_0 = u_0/u_1$ and $t_1 = u_1/u_2$; see Müller et al. (2010) for details.

The approach is summarized in the following algorithm.

Algorithm 6.1 *(Decision-theoretic subgroup analysis).*

Step 0. Initialization: Fix thresholds t_0, t_1 and hyperparameters p and α. Use defaults $t_0 = t_1 = 1$, $p = 0.6$ and $\alpha = 1.0$.
Determine all the possible subgroup patterns for each covariate, Γ_k.

Step 1. Marginal posterior probabilities: Evaluate marginal posterior probabilities $\bar{p}(M) \equiv p(M \mid y)$ for $M = H_0$, H_1 and M_{k,γ_k}, $\gamma_k \in \Gamma_k$.

Step 2. MAP subgroup patterns: Record the maximum *a posteriori* (MAP) pattern of subgroup effects for each covariate, computed as $\gamma_k^* = \arg\max_{\gamma_k} \bar{p}(M_{k,\gamma_k})$. Let $A_K = \{k : \frac{\bar{p}(\gamma_k^*)}{\bar{p}(H_0)} > t_0 t_1 \text{ and } \frac{\bar{p}(\gamma_k^*)}{\bar{p}(H_1)} > t_1\}$. Note the set A_k could be empty.

Step 3. Report (approximate) Bayes rule δ^*: Evaluate rule (6.21).

- If $\overline{p}(H_1)/\overline{p}(H_0) > t_0$ and $\overline{p}(\gamma_k^* \mid y)/\overline{p}(H_1) < t_1$ for all k, then report H_1, an overall non-zero treatment effect.
- If $A_K \neq \emptyset$, then report $A^* = (A_K, A_\Gamma = \{\gamma_k^*, \ k \in A_K\})$.
- Report H_0 if neither H_1 nor A^* are chosen.

■

6.5 Appendix: R Macros

The online supplement to this chapter

$$\texttt{www.biostat.umn.edu/\~{}brad/software/BCLM\_ch6.html}$$

provides the R and BRugs code that was used to illustrate the examples in this chapter.

References

Abbruzzese, J.L., Grunewald, R., Weeks, E.A., Gravel, D., Adams, T., Nowak, B., Mineishi, S., Tarassoff, P., Satterlee, W., and Raber, M.N. (1991). A phase I clinical, plasma, and cellular pharmacology study of gemcitabine. *J. Clin. Oncology*, **9**, 491-498.

Albert, J.H. (1996). *Bayesian Computation Using Minitab*. Belmont, CA: Wadsworth.

Albert, J.H. (2007). *Bayesian Computation with R*. New York: Springer.

Albert, J.H. and Chib, S. (1993). Bayesian analysis of binary and polychotomous response data. *J. Amer. Statist. Assoc.*, **88**, 669–679.

Aranda-Ordaz, F.J. (1983). On two families of transformations to additivity for binary response data. *Biometrika*, **68**, 357–363.

Babb, J. and Rogatko, A. (2001). Patient specific dosing in a cancer phase I clinical trial. *Statistics in Medicine*, **20**, 2079-2090.

Babb, J. and Rogatko, A. (2004). Bayesian methods for cancer phase I clinical trials. In *Contemporary Biostatistical Methods in Clinical Trials*, ed. N. Geller, New York: Marcel Dekker, pp. 1–40.

Babb, J., Rogatko, A., and Zacks, S. (1998). Cancer phase I clinical trials: efficient dose escalation with overdose control. *Statistics in Medicine*, **17**, 1103–1120.

Banerjee, S., Carlin, B.P., and Gelfand, A.E. (2004). *Hierarchical Modeling and Analysis for Spatial Data*. Boca Raton, FL: Chapman and Hall/CRC Press.

Barker, A.D., Sigman, C.C., Kelloff, G.J., Hylton, N.M., Berry, D.A., and Esserman, L.J. (2009). I-SPY 2: An adaptive breast cancer trial design in the setting of neoadjuvant chemotherapy. *Clinical Pharmacology and Therapeutics*, **86**, 97–100.

Barker, L., Rolka, H., Rolka, D., and Brown, C. (2001). Equivalence testing for binomial random variables: which test to use? *The American Statistician*, **55**, 279–287.

Bate, A., Lindquist, M., Edwards, I.R., Olsson, S., Orre, R., Lansner, A., and De Freitas, R.M. (1998). A Bayesian neural network method for adverse drug reaction signal generation. *Eur. J. Clin. Pharmacol.*, **54**, 315–321.

Bayes, T. (1763). An essay towards solving a problem in the doctrine of chances. *Philos. Trans. Roy. Soc. London*, **53**, 370–418. Reprinted, with an introduction by George Barnard, in 1958 in *Biometrika*, **45**, 293–315.

Bekele, B., Ji, Y., Shen, Y., and Thall, P. (2008). Monitoring late-onset toxicities in phase I trials using predicted risks. *Biostatistics*, **9**, 442–57.

Bekele, B. and Shen, Y. (2005). A Bayesian approach to jointly modeling toxicity and biomarker expression in a phase I/II dose-finding trial. *Biometrics*, **61**, 343–354.

Benjamini, Y. and Hochberg, Y. (1995). Controlling the false discovery rate: A practical and powerful approach to multiple testing. *J. Roy. Statist. Soc., Ser. B*, **57**, 289–300.

Berger, J.O. (1985). *Statistical Decision Theory and Bayesian Analysis*, 2nd ed. New York: Springer-Verlag.

Berger, J.O. and Berry, D.A. (1988). Statistical analysis and the illusion of objectivity. *American Scientist*, **76**, 159–165.

Berger, J.O. and Pericchi, L.R. (1996). The intrinsic Bayes factor for linear models. In *Bayesian Statistics 5*, eds. J.M. Bernardo, J.O. Berger, A.P. Dawid, and A.F.M. Smith, Oxford: Oxford University Press, pp. 25–44.

Berger, J.O. and Wolpert, R. (1984). *The Likelihood Principle*. Hayward, CA: Institute of Mathematical Statistics Monograph Series.

Berger, R.L. and Hsu, J.C. (1996). Bioequivalence trials, intersection-union tests and equivalence confidence sets. *Statistical Science*, **11**, 283–319.

Bernardo, J.M. and Smith, A.F.M. (1994). *Bayesian Theory*. New York: John Wiley & Sons.

Berry, D.A. (1989). Monitoring accumulating data in a clinical trial. *Biometrics*, **45**, 1197–1211.

Berry, D.A. (1991). Bayesian methods in phase III trials. *Drug Information Journal*, **25**, 345–368.

Berry, D.A. (1993). A case for Bayesianism in clinical trials (with discussion). *Statistics in Medicine*, **12**, 1377–1404.

Berry, D.A. (1996). *Statistics: A Bayesian Perspective*. Belmont, CA: Duxbury.

Berry, D.A. (2005). Introduction to Bayesian methods III: use and interpretation of Bayesian tools in design and analysis (with discussion). *Clinical Trials*, **2**, 295–300; discussion 301–304, 364–378.

Berry, D.A. (2006). Bayesian clinical trials. *Nature Reviews Drug Discovery*, **5**, 27–36.

Berry, D.A. and Eick, S. (1995). Adaptive assignment versus balanced randomization in clinical trials: a decision analysis. *Statistics in Medicine*, **14**, 231–246.

Berry, D.A. and Ho, C.-H. (1988). One-sided sequential stopping boundaries for clinical trials: A decision-theoretic approach. *Biometrics*, **44**, 219–227.

Berry, D.A. and Hochberg, Y. (1999). Bayesian perspectives on multiple comparisons. *J. Statist. Plann. Inf.*, **82**, 215-227.

Berry, D.A., Müller, P., Grieve, A.P., Smith, M., Parke, T., Blazek, R., Mitchard, N., and Krams, M. (2001). Adaptive Bayesian designs for dose-ranging drug trials (with discussion and rejoinder). In *Case Studies in Bayesian Statistics, Volume V*, eds. C. Gatsonis, R.E. Kass, B.P. Carlin, A. Carriquiry, A. Gelman, I. Verdinelli, and M. West, Lecture Notes in Statistics, New York: Springer-Verlag, pp. 99–181.

Berry, D.A. and Stangl, D.K., eds. (1996). *Bayesian Biostatistics*. New York: Marcel Dekker.

Berry, D.A. and Stangl, D.K., eds. (2000). *Meta-Analysis in Medicine and Health Policy*. Boca Raton, FL: Chapman and Hall/CRC Press.

Berry, S.M. and Berry, D.A. (2004). Accounting for multiplicities in assessing drug safety: a three-level hierarchical mixture model. *Biometrics*, **60**, 418–426.

Birnbaum, A. (1962). On the foundations of statistical inference (with discussion). *J. Amer. Statist. Assoc.*, **57**, 269–326.

Biswas, S., Liu, D.D., Lee, J.J., and Berry, D.A. (2009). Bayesian clinical trials at the University of Texas M.D. Anderson Cancer Center. *Clinical Trials*, **6**, 205–216.

Box, G.E.P. and Tiao, G. (1973). *Bayesian Inference in Statistical Analysis*. London: Addison-Wesley.

Braun, T.M. (2002). The bivariate continual reassessment method: extending the CRM to phase I trials of two competing outcomes. *Controlled Clinical Trials*, **23**, 240–255.

Braun, T.M., Yuan, Z., and Thall, P.F. (2005). Determining a maximum-tolerated schedule of a cytotoxic agent. *Biometrics*, **61**, 335–343.

Brockwell, A.E. and Kadane, J.B. (2003). A gridding method for Bayesian sequential decision problems. *Journal of Computational and Graphical Statistics*, **12**, 566–584.

Brook, R.H., Chassin, M.R., Fink, A., Solomon, D.H., Kosecoff, J., and Park, R.E. (1986). A method for the detailed assessment of the appropriateness of medical technologies. *International Journal of Technology Assessment and Health Care*, **2**, 53–63.

Brooks, S.P. and Gelman, A. (1998). General methods for monitoring convergence of iterative simulations. *J. Comp. Graph. Statist.*, **7**, 434–455.

Bryant, J. and Day, R. (1995). Incorporating toxicity considerations into the design of two-stage phase II clinical trials. *Biometrics*, **51**, 1372–1383.

Buzdar, A.U., Ibrahim, N.K., Francis, D., Booser, D.J., Thomas, E.S., Rivera, E., Theriault, R.L., Murray, J.L., Pusztai, L., Rosales, M.F., Green, M.J., Walters, R., Arun, B.K., Giordano, S.H., Cristofanilli, M., Frye, D.K., Smith, T.L., Hunt, K.K., Singletary, S.E., Sahin, A.A., Ewer, M.S., Buchholz, T.A., Berry, D.A., and Hortobagyi, G.N. (2005). Significantly higher pathological complete remission rate following neoadjuvant therapy with trastuzumab, paclitaxel and epirubicin-containing chemotherapy: results of a randomized trial in HER-2-positive operable breast cancer. *Journal of Clinical Oncology*, **23**, 3676–3685.

Carlin, B.P., Kadane, J.B., and Gelfand, A.E. (1998). Approaches for optimal sequential decision analysis in clinical trials. *Biometrics*, **54**, 964–975.

Carlin, B.P. and Louis, T.A. (2009). *Bayesian Methods for Data Analysis*, 3rd ed. Boca Raton, FL: Chapman and Hall/CRC Press.

Carmer, S.G. and Walker, W.M. (1982). Baby bear's dilemma: a statistical tale. *Agronomy Journal*, **74**, 122–124.

Chen, M.-H. and Ibrahim, J.G. (2006). The relationship between the power prior and hierarchical models. *Bayesian Analysis*, **1**, 554–571.

Chen, M.-H., Shao, Q.-M., and Ibrahim, J.G. (2000). *Monte Carlo Methods in Bayesian Computation*. New York: Springer-Verlag.

Chen, T.T. (1997). Optimal three-stage designs for phase II cancer clinical trials. *Statist. Med.*, **16**, 2701–2711.

Chen, T.T. and Ng, T.H. (1998). Optimal flexible designs in phase II clinical trials. *Statist. Med.*, **17**, 2301-2312.

Cheung, Y.K. and Chappell, R. (2000). Sequential designs for phase I clinical trials with late-onset toxicities. *Biometrics*, **56**, 1177–1182.

Cheung, Y.K., Inoue, L.Y.T., Wathen, J.K., and Thall, P.F. (2006). Continuous Bayesian adaptive randomization based on event times with covariates. *Statistics in Medicine*, **25**, 55–70.

Chib, S. and Jacobi, L. (2008). Analysis of treatment response data from eligibility designs. *J. of Econometrics*, **144**, 465–478.

Chinchilli, V.M. and Elswick, R.K. (1997). The multivariate assessment of bioequivalence. *J. Biopharmaceutical Statistics*, **7**, 113-123.

Chow, S.-C. and Liu, J.-P. (2000). *Design and Analysis of Bioavailability and Bioequivalence Studies*, 2nd ed. New York: Marcel Dekker.

Chu, P.-L., Lin, Y., and Shih, W.J. (2009). Unifying CRM and EWOC designs for phase I cancer clinical trials. *J. Statist. Plann. Inf.*, **139**, 1146–1163.

Collins, J.M., Grieshaber, C.K., and Chabner, B.A. (1990). Pharmacologically guided phase I clinical trials based upon preclinical drug development. *J. Natl. Cancer Inst.*, **82**, 1321–1326.

Collins, J.M., Zaharko, D.S., Dedrick, R.L., and Chabner, B.A. (1986). Potential roles for preclinical pharmacology in Phase I clinical trials. *Cancer Treat. Rep.*, **70**, 73-80.

Cook, T.D. and Demets, D.L., eds. (2008). *Introduction to Statistical Methods for Clinical Trials*. Boca Raton, FL: Chapman & Hall/CRC Press.

Cornfield, J. (1966a). Sequential trials, sequential analysis and the likelihood principle. *The American Statistician*, **20**, 18–23.

Cornfield, J. (1966b). A Bayesian test of some classical hypotheses – with applications to sequential clinical trials. *J. Amer. Statist. Assoc.*, **61**, 577–594.

Cornfield, J. (1969). The Bayesian outlook and its applications. *Biometrics*, **25**, 617–657.

Cowles, M.K. and Carlin, B.P. (1996). Markov chain Monte Carlo convergence diagnostics: A comparative review. *J. Amer. Statist. Assoc.*, **91**, 883–904.

DeGroot, M.H. (1970). *Optimal Statistical Decisions*. New York: McGraw-Hill.

DeFinetti, B. (1992). *Theory of Probability: A Critical Introductory Treatment, Volumes 1 & 2*. New York: John Wiley (Classics Library).

DeSantis, F. (2007). Using historical data for Bayesian sample size determination. *J. Roy. Statist. Soc., Ser. A*, **170**, 95–113.

DeSouza, R.M., Achcar, J.A., and Martinez, E.Z. (2009). Use of Bayesian methods for multivariate bioequivalence measures. *J. Biopharmaceutical Statistics*, **19**, 42–66.

Dixon, D.O. and Simon, R. (1991). Bayesian subset analysis. *Biometrics*, **47**, 871–882.

Dixon, W.J. and Mood, A.M. (1948). A method for obtaining and analyzing sensitivity data. *J. Amer. Statist. Assoc.*, **43**, 109–126.

Duan, Y., Ye, K., and Smith, E.P. (2006). Evaluating water quality using power priors to incorporate historical information. *Environmetrics*, **17**, 95–106.

DuMouchel, W. (1990). Bayesian meta-analysis. In *Statistical Methods for Pharmacology*, ed. D. Berry, New York: Marcel Dekker, pp. 509–529.

DuMouchel, W. (1999). Bayesian data mining in large frequency tables, with an application to the FDA Spontaneous Reporting System (with discussion). *The American Statistician*, **53**, 177–202.

Edwards, W., Lindman, H., and Savage, L.J. (1963). Bayesian statistical inference for psychological research. *Psych. Rev.*, **70**, 193–242.

Efron, B. and Feldman, D. (1991). Compliance as an explanatory variable in clinical trials. *J. Amer. Statist. Assoc.*, **86**, 9–17.

Eisenhauer, E.A., Therasse, P., Bogaerts, J., Schwartz, L.H., Sargent, D., Ford, R., Dancey, J., Arbuck, S., Gwyther, S., Mooney, M., Rubinstein, L., Shankar, L., Dodd, L., Kaplan, R., Lacombe, D., and Verweij, J. (2009). New response evaluation criteria in solid tumours: Revised RECIST guideline (version 1.1). *Eur. J. Cancer*, **45(2)**, 228–247.

Ensign, L.G., Gehan, E.A., Kamen, D.S., and Thall, P.F. (1994). An optimal three-stage design for phase II clinical trials. *Statistics in Medicine*, **13**, 1727–1736.

Erickson, J.S., Stamey, J.D., and Seaman, J.W. (2006). Bayesian methods for bioequivalence studies. *Advances and Applications in Statistics*, **6**, 71–85.

Fan, S.K. and Chaloner, K. (2004). Optimal designs and limiting optimal designs for a trinomial response. *J. Statist. Plann. Inf.*, **126**, 347–360.

Faries, D. (1994). Practical modifications of the continual reassessment method for phase I cancer clinical trials. *J. Biopharmaceutical Statistics*, **4**, 147–164.

Fleming, T.R. (1982). One-sample multiple testing procedure for phase II clinical trials. *Biometrics*, **38**, 143–151.

Food and Drug Administration (1992). Bioavailability and bioequivalence requirements. *U.S. Code of Federal Regulations*, Vol. 21, Chap. 320. Washington, DC: U.S. Government Printing Office.

Food and Drug Administration (1999). *Statistical Approaches to Establishing Bioequivalence*. U.S. Department of Health and Human Services, FDA, Center for Drug Evaluation and Research (CDER), Rockville, MD (`www.fda.gov/cder/guidance`).

Food and Drug Administration (2001). *Average, Population, and Individual Approaches to Establishing Bioequivalence*. U.S. Department of Health and Human Services, FDA, Center for Drug Evaluation and Research (CDER), Rockville, MD (`www.fda.gov/cder/guidance`).

Food and Drug Administration (2002). *Bioavailability and Bioequivalence Studies for Orally Administered Drug Products – General Considerations*. U.S. Department of Health and Human Services, FDA, Center for Drug Evaluation and Research (CDER), Rockville, MD (`www.fda.gov/cder/guidance`).

Freedman, L.S., Lowe, D., and Macaskill, P. (1984). Stopping rules for clinical trials incorporating clinical opinion. *Biometrics*, **40**, 575–586.

Freedman, L.S. and Spiegelhalter, D.J. (1983). The assessment of subjective opinion and its use in relation to stopping rules for clinical trials. *The Statistician*, **32**, 153–160.

Freedman, L.S. and Spiegelhalter, D.J. (1989). Comparison of Bayesian with group sequential methods for monitoring clinical trials. *Controlled Clinical Trials*, **10**, 357–367.

Freedman, L.S. and Spiegelhalter, D.J. (1992). Application of Bayesian statistics to decision making during a clinical trial. *Statistics in Medicine*, **11**, 23–35.

Freireich, E.J., Gehan, E., Frei, E., Schroeder, L.R., Wolman, I.J., Anbari, R., Burgert, E.O., Mills, S.D., Pinkel, D., Selanry, O.S., Moon, J.H., Gendel, B.R.,

Spurr, C.L., Storrs, R., Haurani, F., Hoogstraten, B., and Lee, S. (1963). The effect of 6-mercaptopurine on the duration of steroid-induced remissions in acute leukemia: a model for evaluation of other potentially useful therapy. *Blood*, **21**, 699–716.

Frühwirth-Schnatter, S. (1994). Data augmentation and dynamic linear models. *Journal of Time Series Analysis*, **15**, 183–202.

Fuquene, J.P., Cook, J.D., and Pericchi, L.R. (2009). A case for robust Bayesian priors with applications to clinical trials. *Bayesian Analysis*, **4**, 817–846.

Gamerman, D. and Lopes, H.F. (2006). *Markov Chain Monte Carlo: Stochastic Simulation for Bayesian Inference*, 2nd ed. Boca Raton, FL: Chapman and Hall/CRC Press.

Gehan, E.A. (1961). The determination of the number of patients required in a preliminary and a follow-up trial of a new chemotherapeutic agent. *Journal of Chronic Diseases*, **13**, 346–353.

Gelfand, A.E. and Ghosh, S.K. (1998). Model choice: A minimum posterior predictive loss approach. *Biometrika*, **85**, 1–11.

Gelfand, A.E. and Smith, A.F.M. (1990). Sampling-based approaches to calculating marginal densities. *J. Amer. Statist. Assoc.*, **85**, 398–409.

Gelman, A. (2006). Prior distributions for variance parameters in hierarchical models. *Bayesian Analysis*, **1**, 515–534.

Gelman, A., Carlin, J., Stern, H., and Rubin, D.B. (2004). *Bayesian Data Analysis*, 2nd ed. Boca Raton, FL: Chapman and Hall/CRC Press.

Gelman, A., Roberts, G.O., and Gilks, W.R. (1996). Efficient Metropolis jumping rules. In *Bayesian Statistics 5*, eds. J.M. Bernardo, J.O. Berger, A.P. Dawid, and A.F.M. Smith, Oxford: Oxford University Press, pp. 599–607.

Gelman, A. and Rubin, D.B. (1992). Inference from iterative simulation using multiple sequences (with discussion). *Statistical Science*, **7**, 457–511.

Geman, S. and Geman, D. (1984). Stochastic relaxation, Gibbs distributions and the Bayesian restoration of images. *IEEE Transactions on Pattern Analysis and Machine Intelligence*, **6**, 721-741.

Geyer, C.J. (1992). Practical Markov Chain Monte Carlo (with discussion). *Statistical Science*, **7**, 473–511.

Ghosh, P. and Gönen, M. (2008). Bayesian modeling of multivariate average bioequivalence. *Statistics in Medicine*, **27**, 2402–2419.

Ghosh, P. and Khattree, R. (2003). Bayesian approach to average bioequivalence using Bayes' factor. *J. Biopharmaceutical Statistics*, **13**, 719–734.

Ghosh, P. and Ntzoufras, I. (2005). Testing population and individual bioequivalence: a hierarchical Bayesian approach. Technical report, Department of Statistics, Athens University of Economics and Business.

Ghosh, P. and Rosner, G.L. (2007). A semi-parametric Bayesian approach to average bioequivalence. *Statistics in Medicine*, **26**, 1224–1236.

Giles, F.J., Kantarjian, H.M., Cortes, J.E., Garcia-Manero, G., Verstovsek, S., Faderl, S., Thomas, D.A., Ferrajoli, A., O'Brien, S., Wathen, J.K., Xiao, L.-C., Berry, D.A., and Estey, E.H. (2003). Adaptive randomized study of idarubicin and cytarabine versus troxacitabine and cytarabine versus troxacitabine and idarubicin in untreated patients 50 years or older with adverse karyotype acute myeloid leukemia. *Journal of Clinical Oncology*, **21**, 1722–1727.

Gilks, W.R., Richardson, S., and Spiegelhalter, D.J., eds. (1996). *Markov Chain Monte Carlo in Practice*. London: Chapman and Hall.

Gilks, W.R. and Wild, P. (1992). Adaptive rejection sampling for Gibbs sampling. *J. Roy. Statist. Soc., Ser. C (Applied Statistics)*, **41**, 337–348.

Goldberg, R.M., Sargent, D.J., Morton, R.F., Fuchs, C.S., Ramanathan, R.K., Williamson, S.K., Findlay, B.P., Pitot, H.C., and Alberts, S.R. (2004). A randomized controlled trial of Fluorouracil Plus Leucovorin, Irinotecan, and Oxaliplatin combinations in patients with previously untreated metastatic colorectal cancer. *J. Clin. Oncol.*, **22**, 23–30.

Goodman, S.N., Zahurak, M.L., and Piantadosi, S. (1995). Some practical improvements in the continual reassessment method for phase I studies. *Statistics in Medicine*, **14**, 1149–1161.

Gopalan, R. and Berry, D.A. (1998). Bayesian multiple comparisons using Dirichlet process priors. *J. Amer. Statist. Assoc.*, **93**, 1130-1139.

Gray, R., Manola, J., Saxman, S., Wright, J., Dutcher, J., Atkins, M., Carducci, M., See, W., Sweeney, C., Liu, G., Stein, M., Dreicer, R., Wilding, G., and DiPaola, R.S. (2006). Phase II clinical trial design: methods in translational research from the genitourinary committee at the Eastern Cooperative Oncology Group. *Clinical Cancer Research*, **12**, 1966–1969.

Green, S.J. and Dahlberg, S. (1992). Planned versus attained design in phase II clinical trials. *Statist. Med.*, **11**, 853-862.

Greenland, S., Lanes, S., and Jara, M. (2008). Estimating effects from randomized trials with discontinuations: The need for intent-to-treat design and G-estimation. *Clinical Trials*, **5**, 5–13.

Grieve, A.P. (1985). A Bayesian analysis of two-period crossover design for clinical trials. *Biometrics*, **41**, 979–990.

Haario, H., Saksman, E., and Tamminen, J. (2001). An adaptive Metropolis algorithm. *Bernoulli*, **7**, 223–242.

Hadjicostas, P. (1998). Improper and proper posteriors with improper priors in a hierarchical model with a beta-binomial likelihood. *Communications in Statistics – Theory and Methods*, **27**, 1905–1914.

Hastings, W.K. (1970). Monte Carlo sampling methods using Markov chains and their applications. *Biometrika*, **57**, 97–109.

Hauck, W.W., Hyslop, T., Anderson, S., Bois, F.Y., and Tozer, T.N. (1995). Statistical and regulatory considerations for multiple measures in bioequivalence testing. *Clinical Research and Regulatory Affairs*, **12**, 249-265.

Hernán, M.A. and Robins, J.M. (to appear). *Causal Inference*. Boca Raton, FL: Chapman and Hall/CRC Press.

Herndon II, J.E. (1998). A design alternative for two-stage, phase II, multicenter cancer clinical trials. *Controlled Clinical Trials*, **19**, 440-450.

Heyd, J.M. and Carlin, B.P. (1999). Adaptive design improvements in the continual reassessment method for phase I studies. *Statistics in Medicine*, **18**, 1307–1321.

Hirano, K., Imbens, G.W., Rubin, D.B., and Zhou, X.-H. (2000). Assessing the effect of an influenza vaccine in an encouragement design. *Biostatistics*, **1**, 69–88.

Hobbs, B.P. and Carlin, B.P. (2008). Practical Bayesian design and analysis for drug and device clinical trials. *J. Biopharmaceutical Statistics*, **18**, 54–80.

Hobbs, B.P., Carlin, B.P., Mandrekar, S., and Sargent, D.J. (2009). Hierarchical power prior models for adaptive incorporation of historical information in clinical trials. Research Report 2009–017, Division of Biostatistics, University of Minnesota.

Hodges, J.S., Cui, Y., Sargent, D.J., and Carlin, B.P. (2007). Smoothing balanced single-error-term analysis of variance. *Technometrics*, **49**, 12–25.

Holland, P. (1986). Statistics and causal inference. *J. Amer. Statist. Assoc.*, **81**, 945–970.

Houede, N., Thall, P.F., Nguyen, H., Paoletti, X., and Kramar, A. (2010). Utility-based optimization of combination therapy using ordinal toxicity and efficacy in Phase I/II trials. To appear *Biometrics*.

Huang, X., Biswas, S., Oki, Y., Issa, J.-P., and Berry, D.A. (2007). A parallel Phase I/II clinical trial design for combination therapies. *Biometrics*, **63**, 429–436.

Huang, X., Ning, J., Li, Y., Estey, E., Issa, J.-P., and Berry, D.A. (2009). Using short-term response information to facilitate adaptive randomization for survival clinical trials. *Statistics in Medicine*, **28**, 1680–1689.

Ibrahim, J.G. and Chen, M.-H. (2000). Power prior distributions for regression models. *Statistical Science*, **15**, 46–60.

Ibrahim, J.G., Chen, M.-H., and Sinha, D. (2003). On optimality properties of the power prior. *J. Amer. Statist. Assoc.*, **98**, 204–213.

Imbens, G.W. and Rubin, D.B. (1997). Bayesian inference for causal effects in randomized experiments with noncompliance. *Ann. Statist.*, **25**, 305–327.

Inoue, L.Y.T., Thall, P., and Berry, D.A.. (2002) Seamlessly expanding a randomized phase II trial to phase III. *Biometrics*, **58**, 823–831.

Janicak, P.G., Pandey, G.N., Davis, J.M, Boshes, R., Bresnahan, D., and Sharma, R. (1988). Response of psychotic and nonpsychotic depression to phenelzine. *Amer. J. Psychiatry*, **145**, 93–95.

Jennison, C. and Turnbull, B.W. (2000). *Group Sequential Methods with Applications to Clinical Trials*. Boca Raton, FL: Chapman and Hall/CRC Press.

Ji, Y., Li, Y., and Bekele, B.N. (2007) Dose-finding in oncology clinical trials based on toxicity probability intervals. *Clinical Trials*, **4**, 235–244.

Ji, Y., Li, Y., and Yin, G. (2007). Bayesian dose-finding designs for phase I clinical trials. *Statistica Sinica*, **17**, 531–547.

Jin, H. and Rubin, D.B. (2008). Principal stratification for causal inference with extended partial compliance. *J. Amer. Statist. Assoc.*, **103**, 101–111.

Johnson, V.E. and Albert, J.H. (2000). *Ordinal Data Modeling*. New York: Springer-Verlag.

Johnson, V.E. and Cook, J.D. (2009). Bayesian design of single-arm phase II clinical trials with continuous monitoring. *Clinical Trials*, **6**, 217–226.

Johnson, V.E. and Rossell, D. (2010). On the use of non-local prior densities for default Bayesian hypothesis tests. *J. Roy. Statist. Soc., Ser. B*, **72**, 143–170.

Kadane, J.B., ed. (1996). *Bayesian Methods and Ethics in a Clinical Trial Design*. New York: John Wiley & Sons.

Kadane, J.B., Dickey, J.M., Winkler, R.L., Smith, W.S., and Peters, S.C. (1980). Interactive elicitation of opinion for a normal linear model. *J. Amer. Statist.*

Assoc., **75**, 845–854.

Kass, R.E., Carlin, B.P., Gelman, A., and Neal, R. (1998). Markov chain Monte Carlo in practice: A roundtable discussion. *The American Statistician*, **52**, 93–100.

Kass, R.E. and Greenhouse, J.B. (1989). A Bayesian perspective. Invited comment on "Investigating therapies of potentially great benefit: ECMO," by J.H. Ware. *Statistical Science*, **4**, 310–317.

Kass, R.E. and Raftery, A.E. (1995). Bayes factors. *J. Amer. Statist. Assoc.*, **90**, 773–795.

Kola, I. and Landis, J. (2004). Can the pharmaceutical industry reduce attrition rates? *Nature Reviews Drug Discovery*, **3**, 711–715.

Korn, E.L., Midthune, D., Chen, T.T., Rubinstein, L.V., Christian, M.C., and Simon, R.M. (1994). A comparison of two phase I trial designs. *Statistics in Medicine*, **13**, 1799–1806.

Krams, M., Lees, K.R., and Berry, D.A. (2005). The past is the future: innovative designs in acute stroke therapy trials. *Stroke*, **36**, 1341–1347.

Lan, K.K.G. and DeMets, D.L. (1983). Discrete sequential boundaries for clinical trials. *Biometrika*, **70**, 659–663.

Lauzon, C. and Caffo, B. (2009). Easy multiplicity control in equivalence testing using two one-sided tests. *The American Statistician*, **63**, 147–154.

Le Tourneau, C., Lee, J.J., and Siu, L.L. (2009). Dose escalation methods in phase I cancer clinical trials. *J. Natl. Cancer Inst.*, **101**, 708–720.

Lee, J.J. and Feng, L. (2005). Randomized phase II designs in cancer clinical trials: current status and future directions. *Journal of Clinical Oncology*, **23**, 4450–4457.

Lee, J.J. and Liu, D.D. (2008). A predictive probability design for phase II cancer clinical trials. *Clinical Trials*, **5**, 93–106.

Lee, P.M. (1997). *Bayesian Statistics: An Introduction*, 2nd ed. London: Arnold.

Lin, Y. and Shih, W.J. (2001). Statistical properties of the traditional algorithm-based designs for phase I cancer clinical trials. *Biostatistics*, **2**, 203–215.

Lindley, D.V. (1972). *Bayesian statistics: A review*. Philadelphia: SIAM.

Lindley, D.V. (1998). Decision analysis and bioequivalence trials. *Statistical Science*, **13**, 136–141.

Liu, P.Y., LeBlanc, M., and Desai, M. (1999). False positive rates of randomized phase II designs. *Controlled Clinical Trials*, **20**, 343–352.

Liu, J.S. (2008). *Monte Carlo Strategies in Scientific Computing*. New York: Springer.

Louis, T.A. (1975). Optimal allocation in sequential tests comparing the means of two Gaussian populations. *Biometrika*, **62**, 359–370 (correction: **63**, 218).

Louis, T.A. (1977). Sequential allocation in clinical trials comparing two exponential survival curves. *Biometrics*, **33**, 627–634.

Lumley, T. and Maechler, M. (2007). R package `adapt` – multidimensional numerical integration. Available online at `http://cran.r-project.org/src/contrib/Archive/adapt/`.

MacEachern, S.N. and Berliner, L.M. (1994). Subsampling the Gibbs sampler. *The American Statistician*, **48**, 188–190.

Mandrekar, S.J., Cui, Y., and Sargent, D.J. (2007). An adaptive phase I design for identifying a biologically optimal dose for dual agent drug combinations. *Statistics in Medicine*, **26**, 2317–2330.

Mariani, L. and Marubini, E. (1996). Design and analysis of phase II cancer trials: a review of statistical methods and guidelines for medical researchers. *International Statistical Review*, **64**, 61–88.

Marin, J.-M. and Robert, C.P. (2007) *Bayesian Core: A Practical Approach to Computational Bayesian Statistics*. New York: Springer.

McCarthy, A. (2009). Is it time to change the design of clinical trials? *Cure*, September 12, 2009; available online at www.curetoday.com/index.cfm/fuseaction/article.PrintArticle/article_id/371.

Mealli, F. and Rubin, D.B. (2002). Assumptions when analyzing randomized experiments with noncompliance and missing outcomes. *Health Services and Outcomes Research Methodology*, **3**, 225–232.

Mengersen, K.L., Robert, C.P., and Guihenneuc-Jouyaux, C. (1999). MCMC convergence diagnostics: A reviewww (with discussion). In *Bayesian Statistics 6*, eds. J.M. Bernardo, J.O. Berger, A.P. Dawid, and A.F.M. Smith. Oxford: Oxford University Press, pp. 415–440.

Metropolis, N., Rosenbluth, A.W., Rosenbluth, M.N., Teller, A.H., and Teller, E. (1953). Equations of state calculations by fast computing machines. *J. Chemical Physics*, **21**, 1087–1091.

Mook, S., Van't Veer, L.J., Rutgers, E.J., Piccart-Gebhart, M.J. and Cardoso, F. (2007). Individualization of therapy using MammaPrint: from development to the MINDACT trial. *Cancer Genomics Proteomics*, **4**, 147–155.

Müller, P., Berry, D., Grieve, A., and Krams, M. (2006). A Bayesian decision-theoretic dose finding trial. *Decision Analysis*, **3**, 197–207.

Müller, P., Parmigiani, G., and Rice, K. (2007). FDR and Bayesian multiple comparisons rules. In *Bayesian Statistics 8*, eds. J.M. Bernardo, M.J. Bayarri, J.O. Berger, A.P. Dawid, D. Heckerman, A.F.M. Smith, and M. West, Oxford: Oxford University Press, pp. 349–370.

Müller, P., Sivaganesan, S., and Laud, P.W. (2010). A Bayes rule for subgroup reporting. To appear in *Frontiers of Statistical Decision Making and Bayesian Analysis*, eds. M.-H. Chen, D.K. Dey, P. Müller, D. Sun, and K. Ye, New York: Springer-Verlag.

Natarajan, R. and McCulloch, C.E. (1995). A note on the existence of the posterior distribution for a class of mixed models for binomial responses. *Biometrika*, **82**, 639–643.

Neal, R.M. (2003). Slice sampling (with discussion). *Annals of Statistics*, **31**, 705–767.

Neaton, J.D., Normand, S.-L., Gelijns, A., Starling, R.C., Mann, D.L., and Konstam, M.A., for the HFSA Working Group (2007). Designs for mechanical circulatory support device studies. *J. Cardiac Failure*, **13**, 63–74.

Neelon, B. and O'Malley, A.J. (2010). The use of power prior distributions for incorporating historical data into a Bayesian analysis. CEHI Working Paper 2010-01, Nicholas School of Business, Duke University.

Neelon, B., O'Malley, A.J., and Margolis, P.A. (2008). Bayesian analysis using historical data with aplication to pediatric quality of care. *ASA Proceedings of the Bayesian Statistical Sciences Section*, **2008**, 2960–2967.

Nelsen, R.B. (1999). *An Introduction to Copulas*. New York: Springer-Verlag.

Neuenschwander, B., Branson, M., and Gsponer, T. (2008). Critical aspects of the Bayesian approach to phase I cancer trials. *Statistics in Medicine*, **27**, 2420–2439.

Neuenschwander, B., Branson, M., and Spiegelhalter, D.J. (2009). A note on the power prior. *Statistics in Medicine*, **28**, 3562-3566,

Neuenschwander, B., Capkun-Niggli, G., Branson, M., and Spiegelhalter, D.J. (2010). Summarizing historical information on controls in clinical trials. *Clinical Trials*, **7**, 5-18.

Newton, M., Noueriry, A., Sarkar, D. and Ahlquist, P. (2004). Detecting differential gene expression with a semiparametric heirarchical mixture model. *Biostatistics*, **5**, 155–176.

O'Brien, P.C. (1983). The appropriateness of analysis of variance and multiple-comparison procedures. *Biometrics*, **39**, 787–788.

O'Brien, P.C. and Fleming, T.R., (1979). A multiple testing procedure for clinical trials. *Biometrics*, **35**, 549–556.

O'Hagan, A. (1995). Fractional Bayes factors for model comparison (with discussion). *J. Roy. Statist. Soc., Ser. B*, **57**, 99–138.

O'Hagan, A., Buck, C.E., Daneshkhah, A., Eiser, J.R., Garthwaite, P.H., Jenkinson, D.J., Oakley, J.E., and Rakow, T. (2006). *Uncertain Judgements: Eliciting Experts' Probabilities*. Chichester, UK: John Wiley & Sons.

O'Hagan, A. and Forster, J. (2004). *Bayesian Inference: Kendall's Advanced Theory of Statistics Volume 2B*, 2nd ed. London: Edward Arnold.

O'Hagan, A. and Stevens, J.W. (2001). Bayesian assessment of sample size for clinical trials of cost-effectiveness. *Medical Decision Making*, **21**, 219–230.

O'Hagan, A., Stevens, J.W., and Montmartin, J. (2000). Inference for the C/E acceptability curve and C/E ratio. *PharmacoEconomics*, **17**, 339–349.

O'Hagan, A., Stevens, J.W., and Montmartin, J. (2001). Bayesian cost effectiveness analysis from clinical trial data. *Statistics in Medicine*, **20**, 733–753.

O'Quigley, J., Pepe, M., and Fisher, L. (1990). Continual reassessment method: a practical design for phase I clinical trials in cancer. *Biometrics*, **46**, 33–48.

Pazdur, R., Newman, R.A., Newman, B.M., Fuentes, A., Benvenuto, J., Bready, B., Moore, Jr., D., Jaiyesimi, I., Vreeland, F, Bayssas, M.M.G., and Raber, M.N. (1992). Phase I trial of taxotere: five-day schedule. *J. Natl. Cancer Inst.*, **84**, 1781–1788.

Pearl, J. (2000). *Causality: Models, Reasoning, and Inference*. Cambridge, UK: Cambridge University Press.

Piantadosi, S. (2005). *Clinical Trials : A Methodologic Perspective*. Hoboken, NJ: Wiley-Interscience.

Piantadosi, S., Fisher, J.D., and Grossman, S. (1998). Practical implementation of a modified continual reassessment method for dose-finding trials. *Cancer Chemother. Pharmacol.*, **41**, 429–436.

Pocock, S.J. (1976). The combination of randomized and historical controls in clinical trials. *J. Chronic Disease*, **29**, 175–188.

Pocock, S.J. (1977). Group sequential methods in the design and analysis of clinical trials. *Biometrika*, **64**, 191–199.

Pocock, S.J. (1983). *Clinical Trials: A Practical Approach*. Chichester, UK: Wiley.

Pocock, S.J., Assmann, S.E., Enos, L.E., and Kasten, L.E. (2002). Subgroup analysis, covariate adjustment and baseline comparisons in clinical trial reporting: Current practice and problems. *Statistics in Medicine*, **21**, 2917–2930.

Prentice, R.L., Langer, R.D., Stefanick, M.L., Howard, B.V., Pettinger, M., Anderson, G.L., Barad, D., Curb, J.D., Kotchen, J., Kuller, L., Limacher, M., and Wactawski-Wende, J., for the Women's Health Initiative Investigators (2006). Combined analysis of Women's Health Initiative observational and clinical trial data on postmenopausal hormone treatment and cardiovascular disease. *Amer. J. Epid.*, **163**, 589–599.

Quan, H., Bolognese, J., and Yuan, W. (2001). Assessment of equivalence on multiple endpoints. *Statistics in Medicine*, **20**, 3159-3173.

Racine-Poon, A., Grieve, A.P., Fluhler, H., and Smith, A.F.M. (1987). A two stage procedure for bioequivalence studies. *Biometrics*, **43**, 847–856.

Robert, C.P. (2001). *The Bayesian Choice*, 2nd ed. New York: Springer-Verlag.

Robert, C.P. and Casella, G. (2005). *Monte Carlo Statistical Methods*, 2nd ed. New York: Springer-Verlag.

Roberts, G.O. and Rosenthal, J.S. (2007). Coupling and ergodicity of adaptive Markov chain Monte Carlo algorithms. *J. Applied Probability*, **44**, 458–475.

Roberts, G.O. and Smith, A.F.M. (1993). Simple conditions for the convergence of the Gibbs sampler and Metropolis-Hastings algorithms. *Stochastic Processes and their Applications*, **49**, 207–216.

Robertson, T., Wright, F.T., and Dykstra, R.L. (1988). *Order Restricted Statistical Inference*. Chichester, UK: John Wiley and Sons.

Robins, J.M. (1998). Correction for non-compliance in equivalence trials. *Statistics in Medicine*, **17**, 269–302.

Robins, J.M. and Tsiatis, A.A. (1991). Correcting for non-compliance in randomized trials using rank preserving structural failure time models. *Communications in Statistics, Ser. A*, **20**, 2609–2631.

Robins, J.M. and Greenland, S. (1994). Adjusting for differential rates of PCP prophylaxis in high- versus low-dose AZT treatment arms in an AIDS randomized trial. *J. Amer. Statist. Assoc.*, **89**, 737–749.

Rogatko, A., Tighiouart, M., and Xu, R. (2008). *EWOC User's Guide, Version 2.1*. Winship Cancer Institute, Emory University, Atlanta, GA. http://sisyphus.emory.edu/software_ewoc.php

Rossell, D., Müller, P., and Rosner, G. (2007). Screening designs for drug development. *Biostatistics*, **8**, 595–608.

Rossi, P.E., Allenby, G., and McCulloch, R. (2005). *Bayesian Statistics and Marketing*. New York: John Wiley and Sons.

Rothman, K.J. (1990). No adjustments are needed for multiple comparisons. *Epidemiology*, **1**, 43-46.

Rothwell, P.M. (2005). Subgroup analysis in randomised controlled trials: importance, indications, and interpretation. *Lancet*, **365** 176–186.

Rubin, D.B. (1984). Bayesianly justifiable and relevant frequency calculations for the applied statistician. *Ann. Statist.*, **12**, 1151–1172.

Rubin, D.B. (2005). Causal inference using potential outcomes: design, modeling, decisions. *J. Amer. Statist. Assoc.*, **100**, 322–331.

Saltz, L.B., Cox, J.V., Blanke, C., Rosen, L.S., Fehrenbacher, L., Moore, M.J.,

Maroun, J.A., Ackland, S.P., Locker, P.K., Pirotta, N., Elfring, G.L., and Miller, L.L., for the Irinotecan Study Group (2000). Irinotecan plus fluorouracil and leucovorin for metastatic colorectal cancer. *New Engl. J. Med.*, **343**, 905–914.

Savage, L.J. (1972). *The Foundations of Statistics*, revised edition. New York: Dover Publications.

Scher, H.I. and Heller, G. (2002). Picking the winners in a sea of plenty. *Clinical Cancer Research*, **8**, 400–404.

Schuirmann, D. (1987). A comparison of the two one-sided tests procedure and the power approach for assessing the equivalence of average bioavailability. *J. Pharmacokinetics and Pharmacodynamics*, **15**, 657–680.

Schultz, J.R., Nichol, F.R., Elfring, G.L., and Weed, S.D. (1973). Multiple-stage procedures for drug screening. *Biometrics*, **29**, 293–300.

Schwarz, G. (1978). Estimating the dimension of a model. *Ann. Statist.*, **6**, 461–464.

Sethuraman, J. (1994). A constructive definition of Dirichlet priors. *Statistica Sinica*, **4**, 639-650.

Seymour, L., Ivy, P., Sargent, D., Spriggs, D., Baker, L., Rubinstein, L., Ratain, M., Le Blanc, M., Stewart, D., Crowley, J., Groshen, S., Humphrey, J., West, P., and Berry, D. (2010). The design of Phase II clinical trials testing cancer therapeutics: Consensus recommendations from the clinical trial design task force of the National Cancer Institute Investigational Drug Steering Committee. *Clinical Cancer Research*, **16**, 1764–1769.

Shih, J.H. and Louis, T.A. (1995). Inferences on the association parameter in copula models for bivariate survival data. *Biometrics*, **51**, 1384–1399.

Simon, R. (1989). Optimal two-stage designs for phase II clinical trials. *Controlled Clinical Trials*, **10**, 1–10.

Simon, R. (2002). Bayesian subset analysis: application to studying treatment-by-gender interactions. *Statistics in Medicine*, **21**, 2909–2916.

Simon, R., Freidlin, B., Rubinstein, L., Arbuck, S.G., Collins, J., and Christian, M.C. (1997). Accelerated titration designs for phase I clinical trials in oncology. *J. Natl. Cancer Inst.*, **89**, 1138–1147.

Simon, R., Wittes, R.E., and Ellenberg, S.S. (1985). Randomized phase II clinical trials. *Cancer Treatment Reports*, **69**, 1375–1381.

Sivaganesan, S., Laud, P., and Müller, P. (2008). A Bayesian subgroup analysis with a zero-enriched Polya urn scheme. Technical report, Department of Mathematical Sciences, University of Cincinnati.

Smith, M., Jones, I., Morris, M., Grieve, A., and Tan, K. (2006). Implementation of a Bayesian adaptive design in a proof of concept study. *Pharmaceutical Statistics*, **5**, 39–50.

Smith, M.K. and Richardson, H. (2007). WinBUGSio: A SAS macro for the remote execution of WinBUGS. *J. Statistical Software*, **23**(9).

Smith, T.C., Spiegelhalter, D.J., and Parmar, M.K.B. (1996). Bayesian meta-analysis of randomized trials using graphical models and BUGS. In *Bayesian Biostatistics*, eds. D.A. Berry and D.K. Stangl, New York: Marcel Dekker, pp. 411-427.

Smith, T.L., Lee, J.J., Kantarjian, H.M., Legha, S.S., and Raber, M.N. (1996).

Design and results of phase I cancer clinical trials: three-year experience at M.D. Anderson Cancer Center. *J. Clin. Oncology*, **14**, 287–295.

Spiegelhalter, D.J., Abrams, K.R., and Myles, J.P. (2004). *Bayesian Approaches to Clinical Trials and Health-Care Evaluation*. Chichester, UK: John Wiley & Sons.

Spiegelhalter, D.J., Best, N., Carlin, B.P., and van der Linde, A. (2002). Bayesian measures of model complexity and fit (with discussion). *J. Roy. Statist. Soc., Ser. B*, **64**, 583–639.

Spiegelhalter, D.J., Freedman, L.S., and Parmar, M.K.B. (1994). Bayesian approaches to randomised trials (with discussion). *J. Roy. Statist. Soc., Ser. A*, **157**, 357–416.

Storer, B.E. (1989). Design and analysis of phase I clinical trials. *Biometrics*, **45**, 925–937.

Storer, B.E. (2001). An evaluation of phase I clinical trial designs in the continuous dose-response setting. *Statistics in Medicine*, **20**, 2399–2408.

Tanner, M.A. (1998). *Tools for Statistical Inference: Methods for the Exploration of Posterior Distributions and Likelihood Functions*, 3rd ed. New York: Springer-Verlag.

Thall, P.F. and Cook, J.D. (2004). Dose-finding based on efficacy-toxicity trade-offs. *Biometrics*, **60**, 684–693.

Thall, P.F., Cook, J.D., and Estey, E.H. (2006). Adaptive dose selection using efficacy-toxicity trade-offs: illustrations and practical considerations. *J. Biopharmaceutical Statistics*, **16**, 623–638.

Thall, P.F., Millikan, R.E., Müller, P., and Lee, S.-J. (2003). Dose-finding with two agents in phase I oncology trials. *Biometrics*, **59**, 487–496.

Thall, P.F. and Simon, R.M. (1994). Practical Bayesian guidelines for phase IIB clinical trials. *Biometrics*, **50**, 337–349.

Thall, P.F., Simon, R.M., and Estey, E.H. (1995). Bayesian sequential monitoring designs for single-arm clinical trials with multiple outcomes. *Statistics in Medicine*, **14**, 357–379.

Thall, P. and Wathen, J. (2005). Covariate-adjusted adaptive randomization in a sarcoma trial with multi-stage treatments. *Statistics in Medicine*, **24**, 1947–1964.

Thall, P. and Wathen, J. (2007). Practical Bayesian adaptive randomisation in clinical trials. *European Journal of Cancer*, **43**, 859–866.

Thall, P.F., Wathen, J.K., Bekele, B.N., Champlin, R.E., Baker, L.H., and Benjamin, R.S. (2003). Hierarchical Bayesian approaches to phase II trials in diseases with multiple subtypes. *Statistics in Medicine*, **22**, 763–780.

Thall, P., Wooten, L., and Tannir, N. (2005). Monitoring event times in early phase clinical trials: some practical issues. *Clinical Trials*, **2**, 467–478.

Therasse, P., Arbruck, S.G., Eisenhauer, E.A., Wanders, J., Kaplan, R.S., Rubinstein, L., Verweij, J., Van Glabbeke, M., van Oosterom, A.T., Christian, M.C., and Gwyther, S.G. (2000). New guidelines to evaluate the response to treatment in solid tumors. *Journal of the National Cancer Institute*, **92**, 205–216.

Therasse, P., Eisenhauer E.A., and Verweij, J. (2006). RECIST revisited: A review of validation studies on tumour assessment. *European Journal of Cancer*,

42, 1031–1039.

Thompson, W. (1933). On the likelihood that one unknown probability exceeds another in view of the evidence of two samples. *Biometrika*, **25**, 285–294.

Tierney, L. (1994). Markov chains for exploring posterior distributions (with discussion). *Ann. Statist.*, **22**, 1701–1762.

Wang, W., Hwang, J.T.G., and Dasgupta, A. (1999). Statistical tests for multivariate bioequivalence. *Biometrika*, **86**, 395-402.

Ware, J.H. (1989). Investigating therapies of potentially great benefit: ECMO (with discussion). *Statistical Science*, **4**, 298–340.

Wathen, J. and Cook, J. (2006). Power and bias in adaptively randomized clinical trials. Technical report, Department of Biostatistics, M.D. Anderson Cancer Center, http://www.mdanderson.org/pdf/biostats_utmdabtr_002_06.pdf.

West, M. and Harrison, P.J. (1989). *Bayesian Forecasting and Dynamic Models*. New York: Springer-Verlag.

Wilber, D., Pappone, C., Neuzil, P., De Paola, A., Marchlinski, F., Natale, A., Macle, L., Daoud, E.G., Calkins, H., Hall, B., Reddy, V., Augello, G., Reynolds, M.R., Vinekar, C., Liu, C.Y., Berry, S.M., and Berry, D.A. for the ThermoCool AF Trial Investigators (2010). Comparison of antiarrhythmic drug therapy and radiofrequency catheter ablation in patients with paroxysmal atrial fibrillation: a randomized controlled trial. *J. Amer. Med. Assoc.*, **303**, 333–340.

Williamson, P.P. (2007). Bayesian equivalence testing for binomial random variables. *J. Statist. Computation and Simulation*, **77**, 739–755.

Xia, H.A., Ma, H., and Carlin, B.P. (2008). Bayesian hierarchical modeling for detecting safety signals in clinical trials. Research Report 2008-017, Division of Biostatistics, University of Minnesota.

Yin, G., Li, Y., and Ji, Y. (2006). Bayesian dose-finding in Phase I/II clinical trials using toxicity and efficacy odds ratios. *Biometrics*, **62**, 777–787.

Yin, G. and Yuan, Y. (2009a). A latent contingency table approach to dose finding for combinations of two agents. *Biometrics*, **65**, 866–875.

Yin, G. and Yuan, Y. (2009b). Bayesian dose finding in oncology for drug combinations by copula regression. *J. Roy. Statist. Soc., Ser. C (Applied Statistics)*, **58**, 211-224.

Zacks, S., Rogatko, A., and Babb, J. (1998). Optimal Bayesian feasible dose escalation for cancer phase I trials. *Statistics and Probability Letters*, **38**, 215–220.

Zhang, W., Sargent, D.J., and Mandrekar, S. (2006). An adaptive dose-finding design incorporating both toxicity and efficacy. *Statistics in Medicine*, **25**, 2365–2383.

Zhou, X., Liu, S., Kim, E.S., Herbst, R.S., and Lee, J.J. (2008). Bayesian adaptive design for targeted therapy development in lung cancer – a step toward personalized medicine. *Clinical Trials*, **5**, 181–193.

Zohar, S. and Chevret, S. (2007). Recent developments in adaptive designs for phase I/II dose-finding studies. *J. Biopharmaceutical Statistics*, **17**, 1071–1083.

Author index

Index

For Product Safety Concerns and Information please contact our EU
representative GPSR@taylorandfrancis.com
Taylor & Francis Verlag GmbH, Kaufingerstraße 24, 80331 München, Germany

www.ingramcontent.com/pod-product-compliance
Ingram Content Group UK Ltd.
Pitfield, Milton Keynes, MK11 3LW, UK
UKHW021117180425
457613UK00005B/118